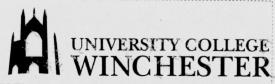

Martial Rose Library
Tel: 01962 827306

	- 3 OCT 2007	
2 3 JAN 2006	- 7 DEC 2007	
	1 6 DEC 2008	
1 8 OCT 2006	- 2 MAR 2010	
3/0 OCT 2006		
NO RENEWAL	- 4 NOV 2011	
- 6 FEB 2007		
2 2 JAN 2007		

SEVEN DAY LOAN ITEM

To be returned on or before the day marked above subject to recall.

A

B O O K

The Philip E. Lilienthal imprint
honors special books
in commemoration of a man whose work
at the University of California Press from 1954 to 1979
was marked by dedication to young authors
and to high standards in the field of Asian Studies.
Friends, family, authors, and foundations have together
endowed the Lilienthal Fund, which enables the Press
to publish under this imprint selected books
in a way that reflects the taste and judgment
of a great and beloved editor.

The publisher gratefully acknowledges the generous contribution to this book provided by the Philip E. Lilienthal Asian Studies Endowment Fund of the University of California Press Associates, which is supported by a major gift from Sally Lilienthal.

Hygienic Modernity

ASIA: LOCAL STUDIES/GLOBAL THEMES

Jeffrey N. Wasserstrom, Kären Wigen, and Hue-Tam Ho Tai, Editors

Hygienic Modernity

Meanings of Health and Disease in Treaty-Port China

RUTH ROGASKI

University of California Press

BERKELEY   LOS ANGELES   LONDON

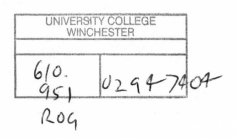

University of California Press
Berkeley and Los Angeles, California

University of California Press, Ltd.
London, England

© 2004 by
The Regents of the University of California

Library of Congress Cataloging-in-Publication Data

Rogaski, Ruth.
    Hygienic modernity : meanings of health and disease in treaty-port
China / Ruth Rogaski.
        p.   cm. — (Asia: Local studies/global themes ; 9)
    Includes bibliographical references and index.
    ISBN 0-520-24001-4 (cloth : alk. paper).
    1. Health behavior—China.   2. Public health—China.
I. Title. II. Series.

    RA776.5.R59   2004
    362.1'0951'09034—dc22   2003019001

Manufactured in the United States of America

13   12   11   10   09   08   07   06   05   04
10   9   8   7   6   5   4   3   2   1

The paper used in this publication is both acid-free and totally chlorine-free
(TCF). It meets the minimum requirements of ANSI/NISO Z39.48-1992
(R 1997) (Permanence of Paper).♾

Contents

Illustrations

Acknowledgments

Thinking back on it now, it is quite obvious that influences from my upstate New York childhood inspired this study of health and hygiene in China. My mother's old medical technician's textbooks from the 1940s introduced me to a laboratory world that held the conquest of bacteria as its greatest achievement. Growing up in a rural area gave me an appreciation of the engineering feats and large public investments that lie behind the invisible miracles of modern sanitation. We had relatives who still used outhouses. A plan for the costly construction of a local sewer system became the greatest political debate of the 1970s in my home town. And it's not too far-fetched to think that the years I spent pushing wheelbarrows full of horse manure from our stable to the back of our property somehow imbued me with a kind of transhistorical empathy for the night-soil carriers of Tianjin. The first expression of gratitude, then, should go to my parents, who raised me in a small town but encouraged me to explore the world beyond it.

The remarkable faculty and facilities at the University of Pennsylvania allowed me as an undergraduate to explore my interests in Chinese culture and in the natural sciences. I hope that the appearance of this book on medical history might assure my instructors in the sciences that their efforts were not all for naught. It was a particular privilege to study under the University of Pennsylvania's faculty in Oriental Studies in the early 1980s: Robert Hartwell, Hongjun Liu, Victor Mair, Susan Naquin, W. Allyn Rickett, and Nathan Sivin. Their tireless efforts in undergraduate education provided me with the strong basis in Chinese language, history, and literature that I still rely on today.

At Yale I was most fortunate to study under Jonathan Spence, who nurtured my love of narrative history and at the same time encouraged me to discover meanings behind the narrative. Emily Honig imparted her wisdom on doing urban history in mainland China. Beatrice Bartlett, Deborah Davis, Valerie Hansen, Helen Siu, and John Harley Warner all contributed to my broader understanding of the points where Chinese history and medical history might intersect. I owe the shape and scope of this project to their collective expertise.

A number of unique individuals in Tianjin opened doors, smoothed out crises, and provided support for me during my long sojourn there. Professor Feng Chengbo of Nankai University gave me my first memorable tour of Tianjin and served as the anchor of the intellectual community I grew to know there. Chen Zhenjiang introduced me to the resources of Nankai's history department. Fang Zhaolin at the Tianjin People's Political Consultative Committee local history institute, and Chen Ke, formerly of the Tianjin Historical Museum, provided access to invaluable local history materials and arranged interviews with local elders. Gao Wangling worked wonders in Tianjin at a distance from his residence in Beijing, as did Kwan Man-bun from his residence in Cincinnati. The late Lou Xiangzhe worked tirelessly on my behalf. The city of Tianjin is a diminished place without him. Finally, Liu Haiyan of the Historical Research Institute at the Tianjin Academy of Social Sciences, with tremendous generosity and good humor, took me under his wing in the early 1990s and continues to guide me through the very rocky shoals of PRC research.

The staff at the Tianjin Municipal Archives was patient and exceedingly helpful, as was the staff at the Tianjin Municipal Library. In the United States, I benefited greatly from living next door to some of the best East Asian collections in the world, Yale University's Sterling Library and Princeton's Gest Library. Special appreciation is due to Gest's Chinese and Western bibliographer, Martin Heijdra, for knowing both the Gest Library and my own research topics inside and out.

The faculty of Princeton University's Department of History and the Program in the History of Science challenged me to think as an historian first and as a scholar of China second, while colleagues in the Department of East Asian Studies made sure I remained deeply engaged in the languages and cultures of China and Japan. Teaching with and learning from the late Gerry Geison shaped my understanding of European and American medical history. Michael Mahoney's constant query upon encountering flagrant deconstructors of science—"I wonder if they have their children vaccinated?"—has served as a reminder for me to always look at the benefits of technology as I unravel its structures of power. Angela Creager, Dirk Hartog, and Christine Stansell were steady sources of encouragement and advice. I profited immensely from teaching and talking with my colleagues in Japanese history, Sheldon Garon and David Howell. Susan Naquin provided constant intellectual stimulation, unflagging support, and an example of integrity in scholarship and teaching. Finally, new colleagues at Vanderbilt University provided a congenial environment in which the manuscript's final preparations were completed.

Over the years this project received generous funding from many sources: the Committee for Scholarly Communication with the People's Republic of China, the Fulbright-Hays Doctoral Dissertation Research Abroad Fellowship, a Yale University Prize Fellowship in East Asian Studies, the Princeton University Committee on Research in the Humanities and Social Sciences, and the Princeton University Department of History. This support also made it possible for me to employ four talented women who helped me with research matters over the years: Nancy Lin, Kathleen Liu, Gu Haiyan, and Aminda Smith.

Carol Benedict and Angela Leung read the manuscript in full for the University of California Press and offered invaluable critiques; Tak Fujitani also read the manuscript in full for the Press editorial committee and provided encouragement and insight. Sheila Levine patiently supported the project from its earliest inception. Reed Malcolm and Suzanne Knott took over to shepherd the manuscript through production with tremendous skill. Bridie Andrews, Peter Carroll, Benjamin Elman, Joseph Esherick, Marta Hanson, James Hevia, Gail Hershatter, Yoshikuni Igarashi, and Ka-che Yip have either commented on papers that made up the study, read parts of the draft, or listened patiently as I thought things through out loud. Their feedback has been greatly appreciated. Flaws that remain in my work are entirely of my own doing.

The experiences of the past few years have demonstrated to me that writing a book is a profoundly selfish undertaking. I have also discovered that few activities are as diametrically opposed as writing a book on Chinese history and raising a small child. Neither the book writing nor the child raising would have succeeded without the help of my husband, Gerald Figal, who often set aside his own scholarship on Japanese history in order to shore up our domestic life. I owe a tremendous debt to his intellectual and emotional fortitude. I would also like to recognize the efforts of the staff at Lawrence Day School who helped care for my daughter while my husband and I worked. Finally, an apology and a thank you are due to my daughter Safa: an apology for being absent at times when you may have needed me, and a thank you for already understanding, at the tender age of three, that in addition to being a mother, I also teach and write books.

Prologue

SUN THE PERFECTED ONE'S SONG OF GUARDING LIFE
(*SUN ZHENREN WEISHENG GE*)

Between Heaven and Earth, Man is most precious,
His head resembles Heaven, his feet resemble Earth.
The best way to cherish the body your father and mother gave you,
Is to diligently study this "Five Happiness Longevity" technique.

To guard life *(wei sheng)* one must know the three things to avoid:
Great anger, great desire, and great drunkenness.
If of the three, one still lurks,
You must be on guard against the harm it may do to your True
    Original Qi.

If you desire long life, first abstain from sex.
If the Fire does not appear, then the Spirit is naturally calm.
Just as Wood that avoids Fire does not become ash,
He who can abstain from sex can extend his life.
To harbor unchecked desire exhausts Seminal Essence;
Take care that you do not lose your Original Spirit,
If you exhaust the Form and scatter your Qi,

How then can you preserve your Body?
If the Heart is greatly exerted, it becomes exhausted,
If the Form is greatly exhausted, it becomes weak,
If the Spirit is greatly injured, it becomes depleted,
If the Qi is greatly harmed, it will be extinguished.

For generations men have desired to know the Way of Guarding Life
    [*wei sheng zhi dao*]:
Be happy often, rarely be angry,
A sincere heart and righteous intentions will naturally make concerns
    disappear.

Act according to Principle *[li]*, cultivate yourself *[xiushen]* and worries
   will depart.

"Xu" in the spring will make your eyes bright, in the summer "ah"
   your Heart,
In the autumn, "pi," in the winter "cui," and your Lung and Kidney
   will be tranquil,
"Hu" throughout the four seasons so your Spleen will transform food,
"Xi" your Triple Burner and its heat will be impossible to stop.

As hair should be combed frequently, so should Qi be exercised,
Knock your teeth several times, and swallow your saliva.
If you wish for a long life, cultivate Kunlun,
Frequently rub your face with your two hands.

In the Spring months it is best to avoid Sour and eat more Sweet,
In the Winter months it is best to eat Bitter and avoid Salty,
In the Summer increase Pungent and reduce Bitter,
In the Autumn you can reduce Pungent but increase Sour.
If according to season you reduce Salty and avoid Sweet,
The Five Viscera will naturally remain trouble-free.
If you are able to reduce all the Flavors then you will be healthy
If the Flavors tend to excess, then it is difficult to not have illness. . . .

We can not control the tangled obligations of love and benevolence,
In the midst of striving for fame and profit, make part of your time for
   rest.
Be generous with your children and your home will naturally be happy,
and you can avoid turning prematurely gray in middle age.
It is not easy to exist with our heads touching Heaven, our feet firmly
   planted on Earth:
Even if we have enough to eat and warm clothes to wear,
we are unable to keep a peaceful conscience.
Don't worry about repaying the vast benevolence you have received,
Don't burn incense morning and night out of feelings of guilt.

What is the way to achieve health, longevity, and happiness?
Pacify your heart, accumulate good works,
Cherish life, cherish the body, cherish Qi,
And learn by heart this Song of Guarding Life.[1]

Introduction

The goal of this book is to place meanings of health and disease at the center of Chinese experiences of modernity. It does so by focusing on the multiple manifestations across time of a single Chinese word: *weisheng*. Today this term is variously rendered into English as "hygiene," "sanitary," "health," or "public health." Before the nineteenth century, *weisheng* was associated with a variety of regimens of diet, meditation, and self-medication that were practiced by the individual in order to guard fragile internal vitalities. With the arrival of armed imperialism, some of the most fundamental debates about how China and the Chinese could achieve a modern existence began to coalesce strongly around this word. Its meaning shifted away from Chinese cosmology and moved to encompass state power, scientific standards of progress, the cleanliness of bodies, and the fitness of races. The persistent association of *weisheng* with questions of China's place in the modern world has inspired me to translate it as "hygienic modernity." This study illuminates how *weisheng* transformed a city, and how it became a central term through which Chinese elites "named the conditions of their existence" under foreign imperialism in the nineteenth and twentieth centuries.[1]

In today's People's Republic of China (PRC) it is impossible not to notice *weisheng*. The word is a pervasive adjective/noun that fails to be contained by any one-to-one correspondence with the word *hygiene*. One may encounter *weisheng* chopsticks (made of cheap wood, wrapped in paper, and designed for one use only), *weisheng* paper (toilet paper), and *weisheng* spheres, or mothballs. One can "do *weisheng*" (*daosao weisheng* or *gao weisheng*), which means to accomplish a thorough cleaning at home or in the workplace. The bathrooms in private homes and toilets in public spaces are referred to as *weisheng* rooms (*weisheng jian*). The national government bureau that oversees the medical profession, hospitals, epidemic control, and pharmaceutical standards is called the Ministry of *Weisheng*. Municipalities and counties have their own Bureau of *Weisheng* responsible for the public health in each locale. Although in many occurrences *weisheng* can (and should) be translated simply as "hygiene/hygienic" or "sanitation/sanitary," its pervasive presence in Chinese society indicates a significance beyond the mere concern for cleanliness that is conveyed by these terms in contemporary American English.

It is perhaps its frequent use in conjunction with "the people," cities, and even the nation that *weisheng* reveals itself as a central part of contemporary China's struggle to achieve what seems to be an ever-elusive state of modernity. Frequent municipal campaigns urge the public to "pay attention to *weisheng*" *(jiang weisheng)*, reminding people that in a modern society, people wash their hands, keep their dwellings clean, and most important, refrain from spitting in public. Slogans painted on walls and buildings urge residents to create "civilized and hygienic cities" *(wenming weisheng chengshi)* as part of the policy of reforming the country and opening up to the outside world *(gaige kaifang)*. In conversations with Chinese of a certain educational background, one might encounter an admiration for Singapore because it is *weisheng* and a general sense of dissatisfaction with China because it is not. And although most mass mobilization campaigns have dissipated in the post-Deng era, the government still regularly coordinates nationwide Patriotic Hygiene Campaigns (Aiguo weisheng yundong) as a method of improving China's health, appearance, and national status. In these manifestations, *weisheng* is a central element in the definition of modernity, not only for the individual but also for the built environment of cities and even for the imagined totality of the nation. The meanings of this "hygiene" go far beyond anything ever associated with the word before the late nineteenth century.

This study seeks to understand the process through which these novel meanings became associated with the term *weisheng*. Understanding this process may shed new light on the underlying nature of social and intellectual change in urban China in the nineteenth and twentieth centuries. John Fitzgerald has described how national elites in the twentieth century undertook a project of "awakening" China from a condition of national subjugation, a condition that elites perceived as stemming from weaknesses inherent in the Chinese themselves.[2] This study suggests that much of this awakening project was centered on the term *weisheng*. In the first decades of the twentieth century, Chinese elites accepted a medicalized view of their country's problems and embraced a medicalized solution for the deficiencies of both the Chinese state and the Chinese body. Focusing on medical developments in one treaty-port city, this study considers the century-long process of how health and disease emerged as a discursive center of Chinese deficiency under conditions of imperialism and traces specific projects of "awakening" the Chinese nation, race, and body to a state of corporal modernity.[3]

One of my main goals is to locate changing meanings of health within the urban environments that helped generate those meanings. The early twentieth century saw an outpouring of writings on health and hygiene, but these works were produced by people who lived in environments that encompassed epidemics, graveyards, floods, marketplaces, streets, temples, brothels, and foreigners. In order to capture this context, I focus on one locale: the northern treaty-port city of Tianjin, which was (and still is) a bustling city, one of China's largest. From 1860 to 1943, the city was also a remarkable example of a treaty port, divided into a Chinese-administered zone and as many as nine different foreign concessions. The resulting multiplicity of boundaries, architectures, government policies, and interactions among Chinese and foreigners embodied China's unique experience under imperialism—at once not a colony, yet still the site of multiple colonialisms. Tianjin provides the perfect setting for the study of the condition that has been called "semicolonialism."[4]

Setting this study in one locale also facilitates the creation of a narrative of change over time. Tianjin experienced highly significant moments of encounter and influence in the course of its long history as a treaty port: the arrival of "Western medicine" with the British navy in 1858, the occupation by foreign forces in 1900 and the Qing recovery of the city in 1902, the Japanese occupation of the city in the 1930s and 1940s. This study narrates the intersections between these political events and the transformation of practices related to health—taking medicine, drinking water, arranging space, managing excreta. Within this narrative, I remain sensitive to how elites imbued these changes with a significance that went well beyond their quotidian effects. Overall, a local history approach facilitates the simultaneous consideration of both the mundane (if not the profane) and the sublime: it investigates where people went to the bathroom as well as how people envisioned the nation. This study tries to find the meaningful connections between the two.

The task of connecting the privy to the nation through the thread of hygienic modernity involves several stages and touches upon several different scholarships. The first challenge is to place the shift to hygienic modernity within the context of the history of medicine in general and the history of colonial medicine in particular. The shift away from old meanings of health and hygiene was a global phenomenon, but one with specific meanings for societies under colonialism. The second task is to consider how hygienic modernity altered urban landscapes—both material and human—as it became a marker of civilization and sovereignty. Finally translations of texts helped produce new meanings of *health* and *hygiene* not by bringing together two monolithic cultures or transferring an absolute science from one language to another but by negotiating meanings between two languages at highly specific moments in the histories of local sciences and local societies. This tale of health and disease in a Chinese treaty port rests at the intersection of three scholarships: the history of medicine, urban history, and translation studies.

THE (GLOBAL) TRANSFORMATION OF HYGIENE AND THE RISE OF (CHINESE) DEFICIENCY

In 1220, Genghis Khan sent his personal minister, Liu Wen, accompanied by twenty warriors and bearing a golden tablet in the shape of a tiger's head, to summon a Daoist master named Qiu Changchun from his home temple in Shandong province. After an exceedingly dangerous and expensive journey covering thousands of miles, the Daoist master finally found himself face to face with the Mongol conqueror in the imperial tents at Samarkand. According to one of Changchun's disciples, their initial conversation went something like this:

THE EMPEROR ASKED: "Perfected One, what Medicine of Immortality (*chang sheng zhi yao*) have you brought me from afar?"

THE MASTER REPLIED: "I possess the Way of Guarding Life (*wei sheng zhi dao*), but no medicine that will prolong life (*chang sheng zhi yao*)."[5]

It is not surprising that Genghis's first question to Changchun is about an elixir of immortality, or *chang sheng zhi yao*. By the thirteenth century there already existed a millennium's worth of history and folktales about emperors who sought the secrets of physical transcendence from Daoist advisors. In his project of building a great Eurasian empire, it was only natural that Genghis Khan would try to bring China's most valuable strategic resources under his command—including the knowledge that might enable him to live, if not forever, then certainly for a very long time. In response to this query, Changchun the Perfected One boldly puns on the emperor's words, replying that although there is no drug *(yao)* that can *chang sheng* (literally, lengthen life), there is, however, a Way *(Dao)* that can *wei sheng* (literally, guard life). The Daoist master offers a regimen that could strengthen the body's resistance to illness, reduce the effects of aging, and help the Khan live out the number of years allotted him by Heaven. Changchun warns Genghis Khan about the dangers of sex ("Try sleeping alone for one month; you will be surprised what an improvement there will be in your spirits and energy"), outlines the benefits of a simple diet harmonized with the seasons, and extols the virtues of quiet meditation.[6] This, in essence, was a summary of a Chinese path to hygiene, the Dao of *weisheng.*

As illustrated in the classic tale of Changchun the Perfected One, *weisheng* was once a confident Chinese "Way of Guarding Life," a set of advanced hygiene techniques closely associated with Chinese culture and coveted by foreign powers. By the twentieth century, however, *weisheng* was deployed as a discourse of Chinese deficiency: a gauge that measured the distance that lay between China and a foreign-defined modernity. In the twentieth century, meanings of *weisheng* changed to encompass modern biomedicine, public health, and personal decorum. In the writings about *weisheng* by Chinese elites in the twentieth century there was an explicit understanding that Chinese were not as clean, not as organized, not as disciplined, and not as healthy as an imagined West. The present study traces the irony and historical significance embodied in this linguistic shift.

Certainly China was not the only place where the content of "hygiene" changed in the modern era. Andrew Wear has pointed out that the meaning of the word *hygiene* in Europe also underwent a radical change during the nineteenth century. From antiquity to the early modern era, hygiene encompassed a wide variety of health-giving practices such as exercise, diet, and rest. Today, Wear observes, "Hygiene means cleanliness, and its scope is narrower."[7] Shifts in the meaning of hygiene in the West and China were similar, but they had profoundly different social and political implications in the two places.

Changchun's *weisheng* advice to Genghis Khan bore distinct similarities to a classical Western view of hygiene. The Daoist master warned the Mongol to moderate his diet, to act according to the seasons, and to limit his sexual activities. Hippocratic treatises such as *Regimen in Health* (fifth century B.C.E.) called upon individuals to alter their patterns of eating, drinking, sleeping, and activity according to the seasons and according to their own bodily constitutions. These writings outlined the different natures of food and medicines, prescribed general times for baths, and recommended parameters for frequency of sexual intercourse, much as the Daoist adept advised Genghis Khan. The second-century Roman physician Galen advised moderation in exercise, diet, and drink in his treatise *De sanitate tuenda* (Hygiene). In *Ars medica* (Art of medicine), Galen identified the six categories of air, food and drink, sleep and waking, movement and rest, retention and evacuations, and the passions of the soul as the major external factors that influenced health, elements that later became the cornerstones of hygiene known as the "six nonnaturals." Moderation and seasonality were the watchwords of this hygiene philosophy. Consistent adherence to wisdom laid out by the Greeks and Romans typified writings on the maintenance of health from the Middle Ages and the Renaissance. The early modern period saw a flourishing of hygiene advice books, some of which offered variations in time-honored regimens, but scholars have argued that into the eighteenth century there was very little departure from the holistic approaches to hygiene set out by Galen.[8]

Radical departures in approaches to health emerged in the eighteenth century with the development of a "public hygiene" in France, England, and Prussia. In the minds of some administrators, intellectuals, and revolutionaries, the most important health was the health of the nation. It was the job of the government to prevent diseases of the national body through sanitary policing, public works, and state-sponsored medical institutions.[9] At the same time, hygiene became more associated with cleanliness, manners, and class status. A concern about cleanliness was later augmented by a fear of germs.[10] By the mid–twentieth century, the fractured nature of health was symbolized in English through use of different words that constituted two worlds: an expansive realm of public health and a narrow realm of personal hygiene. The conceptual basis for holistic approaches to health—a concern with humors and seasons—had essentially disappeared, and there was no longer any single word that could convey a path to health through diet, exercise, rest, and moderation.

These transitions have garnered relatively little attention from historians of Western medical traditions. In his many studies of popular perceptions of health and healing, Roy Porter highlighted the perpetuation of beliefs about humors and balance among patients in the eighteenth century, even as physicians began to shift away from Galenic views of the body.[11] Charles Rosenberg and others have noted how American physicians were reluctant to jettison humors and holistic approaches to therapy in the nineteenth century, in spite of the influence of Paris medicine and the rise of the germ theory of disease in Germany.[12] But for the most part these phenomena were thought of as transitional moments, as lag times between a tradi-

tional past and an inevitable achievement of medical modernity. Medical anthropologists have questioned the thoroughness of this transition among
the lay populace, while historians of the "medical fringe" have highlighted
nineteenth-century movements that resisted the growing hegemony of
"medical orthodoxy."[13] But overall, the historian's focus on "the rise of modern medicine" (particularly modern therapeutics) has resulted in an overall disregard of the history of preventive medicine and changes in general
conceptualizations of health. Through routine exposure of the masses to
modern biomedicine and the public health apparatus of the state, older approaches to hygiene in the West seem to have faded away with little
difficulty, little complaint, and with few consequences to the society as a
whole.

Scholarship on the history of health and medicine in non-European societies is not as sanguine. Many scholars of "colonial medicine" have dwelt
on the shock and displacement that European approaches to health and healing brought to indigenous societies.[14] The classical study in this vein is David
Arnold's 1993 work, *Colonizing the Body*. Arnold highlights the "corporal" aspects of British colonialism as British administrators counted, quar-
antined, vaccinated, and inspected Indian bodies. Particularly during outbreaks of epidemic disease such as bubonic plague, Western medicine and
Western methods of disease prevention appear as an "assault on the body,"
a violent and coercive corporal colonization carried out in the name of modern health and hygiene. Other scholars, most notably Megan Vaughan and
Warwick Anderson, have similarly emphasized colonial medicine's violent
interventions in Africa and Southeast Asia, as British missionaries or
American troops scrutinized the blood and fecal matter of indigenous populations. Here the focus has been on the development of Western discourses
that turned indigenous peoples into diseased and chaotic medical objects,
and the coercive techniques used to act upon native bodies as objects.[15]
Arnold also sees the Indian body as a site of "contestation and not just colonial appropriation," as indigenous people protested and resisted the interventions of colonial medicine. He suggests, however, that Western medicine
became "part of a new cultural hegemony and incipient political order" as
it "infiltrated the lives of an influential section of the Indian population,"
although in this work he is more interested in charting the intent of the colonizers and the reactions of the "masses" than exploring the adoption of
Western medicine by Indian elites.[16]

Other scholars have acknowledged the violence and interventions of colonial public health but chose to emphasize instead the ability of indigenous
populations to appropriate and refashion the concepts of health and disease

brought by colonizers. Indigenous elites "contested colonial hegemony" and turned colonial medicine into "contested knowledge" by producing hybrid forms of medicine, or by finding within their own traditions the basis to launch critiques of Western medical systems.[17] These contestations and combinations often took place through the process of translation. In an insightful study, Bridie Andrews has demonstrated that Chinese physicians translated information about bacteria and the germ theory of disease within a Chinese framework, linguistically conceptualizing germs as akin to other discrete, animal-like pathogens already prevalent in popular concepts of disease etiology.[18] Gyan Prakash has highlighted how Indian elites, through the process of translation, questioned whether Western science had a monopoly on the truth, particularly truths about the functioning of the body.[19] Ashis Nandy has highlighted how Gandhi and others accomplished a deep critique of Western medicine by turning to Indian philosophies of health.[20] In all these cases, indigenous actors shaped and questioned Western knowledge from a position firmly grounded in strong indigenous practices of health, healing, and hygiene.

Both of these general trends of "colonizing the body" and "contesting colonial hegemony" are present in the Chinese experience of Western approaches to health and the body in the nineteenth and twentieth centuries. There were numerous moments when colonizers "touched the body" and enforced coercive regimes of medical control on an unwilling populace. Chinese medical thinkers also creatively used Chinese health concepts to challenge and reformulate Western concepts. However, certain general trends become more apparent when one looks at a specific setting across long periods of time. Many studies focus on isolated moments of "encounter" between European medicine and indigenous medicine: a specific set of translations, a particular epidemic, or the thought of one individual at the height of his influence. In part as a result of their limited time frame, they emphasize significant moments of resistance and agency. The present study attempts a more holistic approach to the history of health and hygiene by considering multiple actors, a complex urban setting, and a period of approximately one hundred years. This approach deconstructs the monolith of "Western medicine" and captures its transformations and multiple manifestations in both the metropole and abroad. It reveals moments when indigenous elites challenged and reformulated what they perceived as the errors in Western concepts of health and disease. Most important, it conveys the fluctuations in imperialism's character across time and space, highlights moments of cooperation as well as coercion, and looks at the sometimes intimate collaborations between multiple "colonizers" and various members of "the colonized."

In spite of these fluctuations and moments of resistance, however, the resulting overall picture reveals a growing hegemony of biomedical approaches to health in the public discourse of Chinese elites, and a concurrent acceptance of a picture of the Chinese people as inherently lacking when compared with Western-defined standards of health. *Weisheng* as hygienic modernity becomes a definitive example of a "derivative discourse" of nationalism, one based on an argument of native deficiency originally devised by colonial powers.[21] In China, few if any alternative voices emerged from the treaty-port elite to challenge its underlying power.

The historical development of biomedical discourses of deficiency has begun to concern scholars of colonial medicine. Ann Laura Stoler has traced how the project of creating a bourgeois society in Europe relied upon marking distinctions and establishing boundaries between colonizer and colonized outside of Europe.[22] Mark Harrison has suggested that a rise in a European mentality that thought of many Indians as inherently diseased and deficient accompanied the erosion of an "optimism about acclimatization and the colonization of India" after 1800. The belief that whites could not adjust to a pathogenic Indian environment "was closely related to the emergence of ideas of race and the consolidation of colonial rule."[23] What survived into the twentieth century, even after the environment was no longer seen as a major cause of disease, was the notion that '"natives'" themselves produced disease through inherent deficiencies of body and behavior. The rise in the germ theory of disease accentuated this tendency to locate disease within the inherent "racial" habits of indigenous populations.[24]

Although scholars have been working on connecting the shifts in concepts of health, race, and class that occurred within the West to the same changing formulations that occurred in the colonies, to date no truly synthetic work has emerged.[25] Warwick Anderson has suggested that scholars of medical history undertake a truly postcolonial history of medicine by exploring the ways in which modern biomedicine has acted as a colonizing force on the body in the West, not only in the colonies.[26] A global history of changing concepts of hygiene would provide fruitful terrain for such an endeavor.[27] The present study, however, is unabashedly about meanings of health and daily life in a Chinese treaty port: I will leave any exposé of the colonizing nature of modern biomedicine in the West to scholars who specialize in that particular region of the globe. This study does, however, strive to place the global within the local. It is highly aware of how Chinese, through interaction with representatives of multiple colonialisms/medicines (French, British, German, Japanese, and American), changed the meaning of health in a city that was one of the major crossroads of imperialism.

TIANJIN, HYPERCOLONY, AND SEMICOLONIALISM

Situating this investigation in one of China's largest and most complex treaty ports helps to illuminate how foreign and indigenous actors reshaped approaches to health under the conditions of China's '"semicolonialism.'" I have chosen the former treaty-port city of Tianjin, in northern China, as the anchor for my study. This local narrative approach has many advantages. It allows us to imagine how people might have perceived the benefits and dangers of their specific environment: the mists rising from marshes, the intense heat of the summer sun, the taste of brackish water from a well dug in salty soil. It allows us to ask certain concrete questions about the relationship between disease and society: When did epidemics run through the city, and how did people make sense of them? How did different groups— administrators, physicians, lay people—respond to these specific challenges? How did class differences, regional differences, and migration affect approaches to health? By grounding a study of health in one place, we can better visualize the texture of life experienced by both physicians and sufferers. A local history may seem constrained and narrow, but within a single locale the rich details of everyday life appear more vibrant and more meaningful.

As a single locale, Tianjin is by no means insignificant. Tianjin is China's third largest city, and its population of close to six million people makes it one of the largest cities in the world. I initially chose Tianjin as the site for my study because it is the home to some of China's most important medical "firsts." Tianjin was the first Chinese city to have a native-administered municipal department of health (1902), founded during the New Reforms period under Yuan Shikai. Tianjin was also home to the first government hospital of Western medicine in China: the Beiyang Medical Academy, founded by British missionaries in 1880 and taken over by the Qing government in 1888. But what makes these medical "firsts" even more interesting is the unique setting of foreign and Chinese interaction in which they took place.

From 1860 to 1945, Tianjin was home to as many as eight different foreign concessions, the most of any Chinese treaty port. Shanghai, China's most famous treaty port, had two foreign zones, the French Concession and the

International Settlement (primarily British). Tianjin, however, contained a Japanese, French, British, German, Belgian, Russian, Austro-Hungarian, and Italian Concession. Eventually only the Japanese, French, British, and Italian Concessions lasted beyond World War I, but in the first decades of the twentieth century, Tianjin could be viewed as a "hypercolony," a chaotic crossroads of Chinese and foreigners and a booming showcase of imperialism.[28]

I have coined the term *hypercolony* from Sun Yat-sen's famous formulation of China as a "hypo-colony." Sun claimed that *semicolonial,* the term that many used to describe China's condition of not being a total colony, simply meant that China was partially colonized by a large assortment of foreign powers. Borrowing the term *ci* (hypo-) from chemistry, Sun described China's status as that of a *ci zhimindi,* a "hypo-colony," a weak nation that had more difficulty developing identity and a sense of unity than "true" colonies such as Korea or Vietnam.[29] The ironic implication of Sun's statement is that China would have been better off colonized by only one foreign nation, a conclusion at odds with my appreciation of the complexities of Tianjin's political and cultural circumstances at the turn of the century.

By suggesting that Tianjin could be described as a "hypercolony," I am not seeking to generate a new theoretical model: I am simply drawing attention to the potential implications that arise when one urban space is divided among multiple imperialisms. Tianjin's status as a hypercolony placed Chinese urban dwellers under the gaze—and sometimes the control—of several different imperial powers. At the same time, this condition offered Chinese a perspective on several variant models of urban modernity and colonial ideology. The presence of multiple imperialisms influenced the imperialists as well. The close juxtaposition of so many settlements within one urban space affected the practices and self-representations of the foreign powers at the local level. This became particularly important for the large Japanese Concession that was literally and figuratively positioned between the Chinese city and the European concessions. Each concession had to represent and negotiate its identity on the ground vis-à-vis other imperial powers. They did so through the deployment of architecture, the creation of specific forms of local administration, and by creating different policies governing the Chinese who made up the vast majority of residents in each concession. This study explores how health and hygiene became an important strategy in these imperial representations.

The search for a term that adequately captures the complexity of China's experience with colonialism has captivated many scholars of modern Chinese history. Recent work has taken up the previously disfavored Marxist term *semicolonial,* seeking to outline its contours and contrast it with the purely *colonial,* represented primarily by scholarship on India. As semicolonialism has been put back to work, much has been required of it. The term must suggest at the same time the incompleteness of a colonizing process in China as well as the effects of having multiple colonizers within China's borders. Shu-mei Shih, in her sophisticated study of the relationship of Chinese writers to imperialism and modernity, has employed *semicolonial* to mean "the multiple, layered, intensified, as well as incomplete and fragmentary nature of China's colonial structure."[30] The term is supposed to suggest that the foreign presence in China was scant but also potentially oppressive: China's cup of imperialism was at times less than half full, but at other times it overflowed.

In spite of a recognition of this paradox, scholars have tended to use the term *semicolonialism* to emphasize the "half-full" nature of the foreign presence in China. To explain why so many Chinese intellectuals seemed to embrace modernity without ambivalence (in contrast with India), Shu-mei Shih finds that the incomplete nature of foreign administration "afforded Chinese intellectuals more varied ideological, political, and cultural positions than in formal colonies." Foreign powers in China not only "lack[ed] systematic institutional infrastructure," they also did not "impose a colonial epistemology by force."[31] Bryna Goodman has suggested a spectrum of approaches to the question of power and imperialism in China's modern history.[32] At one end Goodman places scholarship, such as recent Chinese studies of treaty ports, that emphasizes reciprocity between Chinese and foreigners and "tends to downplay the prejudices and power differentials of semicolonialism." At another end she places studies by Tani Barlow and other scholars affiliated with the journal *positions* who, according to Goodman, overemphasize the extreme violence and dominance of the foreign presence in China and do not distinguish between colonialism and semicolonialism. Following Jürgen Osterhammel, Goodman calls for a scholarship on semicolonialism that avoids the extremes of mutual benefit and total domination by mapping "when, where, how, and to what effect did which extraneous forces impinge on Chinese life."[33] However, Goodman, like Shih, is suspicious of approaches that emphasize foreign violence or characterize the foreign presence as a powerful threat to China's sovereignty. For her study of late nineteenth century Shanghai, she finds Chinese in confident positions vis-à-vis foreigners, able to conduct negotiations and appropriations in a relatively unconstrained political environment. Foreign violence may have opened the treaty ports, but this violence is a vague memory that does not affect the everyday interactions between foreigners and Chinese in Shanghai.

By narrating the changing concepts of health within the specific setting of Tianjin, this study attempts to pinpoint "when, where, how, and to what effect" foreign forces "impinged on Chinese life." The result suggests that no one treaty-port history can stand in for all the others, and that *semicolonialism* is not an adequate term to capture the complexity of the one-hundred-year history of imperialism in China. There are distinct differences in the intensity, power, and violence of the foreign presence over time and from place to place. This variation is not only present in the social and economic realms, but is tremendously evident in a "cultural" realm like conceptions of health and disease. The violent battles of imperialism, perhaps nothing more than a vague memory for Shanghai, had visited the northern city of Tianjin several times in the nineteenth and twentieth centuries. Perhaps in other locales, foreigners "lack[ed] systematic institutional infrastructure" and did not "impose a colonial epistemology by force." The Chinese city of Tianjin, however, had been ruled for two years by an international army that enforced new ways of behavior at gunpoint. This occupying force also determined the conditions under which the indigenous government could regain its sovereignty over Tianjin, and thus radically shaped the native government of the city after reversion.

Scholars have also suggested that the lack of foreign dominance and violence in Chinese treaty ports is what allowed Chinese intellectuals to turn a blind eye to the imperialist constructs of modernity. In contrast, what is most striking about Tianjin is how Chinese elites were quite willing to embrace a foreign-defined modernity—particularly its aspects related to public health and hygiene—at the very height of imperialist violence and coercion and to extend that embrace once the violence ended. To use a formulation proposed by Shih, Tianjin's elites seemed to accomplish the bifurcations (separating modernity from imperialism) and suppressions (suppressing the racist hierarchies implicit in modernity) required to embrace modernity, but they did so under surprisingly contradictory conditions of both "colonial" coercion and " semicolonial" sovereignty.

A focus on Tianjin helps to shed light on this complex process by foregrounding the crucial mediating role played by Japan. In the scramble for concessions unleashed by the suppression of the Boxer Uprising in 1900, Japan appeared simultaneously as an invading foreign power and as a brother. For most of the period of this study, Japan served as a model of a successful "Asian modernity" that could serve as a bridge to modernity for China. From the perspective of many Tianjin elites, Japan was a force that could bring order, rationality, and health to a subaltern society that had become unmanageable. If the history of hygienic modernity is essentially the story of the adoption by Chinese elites of a technology of imperialism, that adoption was facilitated by the presence of Japan.

Japan's role becomes particularly apparent when one looks at efforts and ideas surrounding *weisheng*. The word *weisheng* as "hygienic modernity" was itself the creation of Japanese physicians who used an ancient Chinese term to translate European concepts of national health. After the suppression of the Boxer Uprising, Japanese advisors helped create Tianjin's sanitary police force, military medical school, and its first department of health. Tianjin was home to the most important formal Japanese Concession in China proper—Mark Peattie has called it "the jewel of Japan's privileged territories in China"—and as a result, tens of thousands of Chinese lived daily life under Japanese hygienic administration.[34] Finally, the Japanese occupation of the city (1937–45) brought a type of hygienic modernity to Tianjin that was to have a profound influence on the city long after the Japanese empire had disappeared. Grounding a study of changing meanings of health in the city of Tianjin highlights the important role of Japan in the formation of Chinese modernity.

Setting this study in Tianjin also provides an opportunity to recreate the past of a Chinese city, with its smells, foods, street life, and sufferings. In some ways this study adopts a Foucault-inspired approach to history: It generates a genealogy of a discourse and shows how that discourse acquired a powerful ability to define the conditions of existence in the modern world. However, I am not of the belief that discourses speak for themselves. What a person sees out his window, what temples he frequents, how he gets his drinking water, what epidemics he fears, and how many times he is vaccinated by soldiers are all important details that contribute to our understanding of how health and disease were interpreted in the past. Through recourse to narrative, this study seeks to highlight the way daily life contributes to the authorship of historical meaning.[35] Ultimately, I take the creation of historicity to be one of the more important and pleasurable tasks of the historian. Perhaps it also allows me to indulge in a certain kind of nostalgia for a lost Tianjin, one filled with active temples, its streets alive with multiple manifestations of social and economic life.[36]

Finally, delving into the lives and settings of local actors helps to rectify a particularly obvious gap in studies of colonial medicine by offering a more nuanced picture of indigenous society. Previous works have emphasized the intent of the colonizer, while the thoughts and intentions of the colonized have remained obscure. Some recent studies on health and medicine in Asia and Africa under colonialism have focused on meanings generated by indigenous actors.[37] The Chinese case is greatly aided by the presence of voluminous writings by indigenous elites and by the existence of a massive (though not always accessible) archive generated by indigenous governments. By understanding foreign views of health and healing as a form of "contested knowledge" that is evaluated by multiple actors from a variety of subject positions, we can better understand processes of appropriation without attributing all outcomes either to the inherent superiority of Western knowledge or the quaint resistances of cultural conservatives. At the same time, however, it is essential to remain sensitive to the ways that imperialism has inexorably altered both the terms and the conditions of life in modern China.

LANGUAGE, TRANSLATION, AND VISIONS OF HEALTH

Readers unfamiliar with Chinese or Japanese may find it strange that I use the Chinese word *weisheng* (Japanese, *eisei*) throughout this study. This is not because *weisheng*, like some mystical Chinese concept, is impossible to translate into English. From the mid-nineteenth to the mid-twentieth centuries, *weisheng* is, in fact, eminently translatable into many different words and phrases—health, hygienic, physiology, nutrition, clean, medicine, protecting internal vitalities, sanitary science, promoting fertility, public health, and conquering death, to name a few—and therein lies the problem. Ultimately the word refers to the actions that humans can take to ensure health. This may be loosely conveyed with the English word *hygiene.* Yet the meaning of the English word *hygiene* has certainly changed over time in Europe and United States over the past two centuries. To settle on a one-to-one correspondence between *weisheng* and *hygiene* would run the risk of both freezing its meaning across time and denying the possibility that the word could have multiple meanings at the same time. I take care to suggest what I think *weisheng* means to different people at different junctures, but I often leave the term untranslated in order to suggest that it is a vessel into which numerous meanings are poured. This book seeks to understand how Chinese in various circles brought their own understanding of health and disease to the construction of "hygienic modernity," a process that Lydia Liu has called "translingual practice."[38]

Weisheng provides an ideal case study of translingual practice for a variety of reasons. First, because we have an account of the "birth" of the term in its modern guise from a Japanese physician/bureaucrat, Nagayo Sensai, who claimed to have taken a term from an ancient Daoist text and used it to translate a matrix of European words that suggested both the government management of the people's health and the creation of hygienically disciplined citizens.[39] This moment of translation in Japan is crucial to understanding the nature of *weisheng* in China in the twentieth century. Nagayo Sensai's translation demonstrates how Meiji medical elites realized that technologies of medicine, surveillance, and policing were central to the European blueprint for modernity. In an uncanny way, Nagayo Sensai (and East Asian modernizers after him) used the single term *weisheng* (Japanese, *eisei*) to encompass what Foucault termed "bio-power," a series of techniques through which the state undertakes the administration of life, and "governmentality," the idea that individuals internalize disciplinary regimes and thus harmonize their own behaviors with the goals of the state.[40] I am not suggesting that Nagayo Sensai was anticipating Foucault. However, Japanese elites, engaged in their own quest to order society, quickly grasped some of the core elements that made Europe appear modern and sought to employ them as "full kits" to transform their own societies. Japanese elites then transferred this impulse to China. Therefore, although this study is focused on Tianjin, it dedicates a separate chapter to a consideration of the context of *weisheng*'s significant transformation in Meiji Japan.

That moment of translation was only the beginning of the term's contentious circulation. What would the term *weisheng* mean to a Chinese man in the late Qing who was well versed in the classics but who had never been to London or Berlin? How was the meaning of the word shaped through acts of translation, acts of administration, or acts of consumption? Did it behave like an oddly familiar "returned graphic loan" or a startling neologism, and at what point did it assert a natural presence within the lexicon?[41] And what were the implications for a society that felt at home with a word that was both native and alien at the same time? This study seeks to embed language and translation within the social struggles and intellectual accidents that gave rise to both a new language and a new way of being in twentieth-century China.

The advantages of pursuing translation studies have become evident to many scholars of China in the past several years, but the approach contains several pitfalls.[42] Preeminent among them is that texts might be mistaken for civilizations, and variations in meaning generated through the process of translation might be mistaken for an incommensurability between civilizations.[43] There is a danger, particularly in exploration of science translations, of assuming that a single text represents "Western medicine," or that the translator represents a monolithic "Chinese tradition." Perhaps the most important strategy for avoiding false "East/West" dichotomies is to pay attention to change over time not only in China, but also in the various imperial powers under consideration. We must not assume that the West (and Japan) provided an unchanging standard of scientific modernity for China. This study has not one, but as many as four "moving targets." Immense changes in medicine, hygiene, and public health not only occurred in China, but in Europe, the United States, and Japan as well during the nineteenth and twentieth centuries. These ideas were not imported sui generis into China, but were introduced into specific locales by specific agents, some of whom had their own eccentric beliefs and agendas. Tracing specific aspects of Western medicine as they were encountered by Chinese not only helps to debunk the idea that Western concepts of health and disease were inherently superior, it also reveals the surprising similarities between certain Chinese and Western approaches to health at different historical junctures.

There is a danger that the single-minded pursuit of one word might narrow the field of inquiry and even produce historical inaccuracies. For example, in the present study, I observe that before the twentieth century concepts such as "the public" and "impurity" were rarely if ever associated with the term *weisheng*. However, this does not mean that concepts such as the government responsibility for health, environmental sanitation, or personal cleanliness did not exist in China before the arrival of European imperialism. The scholarship of several historians of premodern China has demonstrated that these things most surely did exist. Ancient dynasties appointed imperial health officers to treat the diseases of the people. Medical education was supported and regulated by the court at various points in China's history. Concepts of miasma and impurities associated with environments were widespread. The Chinese bathed—probably more often than Europeans before the early modern period—and they even used soap.[44]

The difference between premodern and modern Chinese concepts of health is that before the arrival of European (and Japanese) imperialism, these various practices were dispersed through the cultural terrain and had little if any relation to one single term. There was no clear sense that practices as disparate as brushing teeth and regulating medical education should somehow be grouped together, nor was there a sense that these practices, as an aggregate object, could be used as a symbol of civilization or difference. It was the arrival of foreign imperialism and European-Japanese conceptualizations of health that resulted in the creation of a discourse of *weisheng,* bringing together public and private meanings of health into a powerful model of modernity. A focus on the word *weisheng*, rather than conveying continuities with the ancient Chinese past, reveals ruptures and reconfigurations of conceptions of health and disease, worked out along stress lines that were created by the presence of violent foreign imperialism. This study does not hold that diverse "modern" hygienic practices did not exist in the Chinese past. Instead it contends that a radically new *weisheng* emerged in the twentieth century, one that did things it never did before: set standards for individual behavior, determined the structure of urban space, defined the autonomy of countries, and measured the quality of a people.

The making of a modern *weisheng* also does not mean that earlier associations of the term were entirely eliminated from a Chinese understanding of health. If anything, one of the most noteworthy aspects of Chinese modernity is the survival (and the popularity) of indigenous health practices such as Chinese medicine, "tai-ch'i," and qigong. However, those elements associated with earlier meanings of *weisheng*—including practices of meditation and yoga, the ingestion of specific foods, and the adherence to lifestyle regimes based on cosmological schema—were divorced from the realm of science in which *weisheng* now dwells, and were shifted on to other words that belonged to the realm of "tradition." By the first decades of the twentieth century, *weisheng* encompassed a wide variety of meanings that derived their validity from their association with science, not their association with Chinese cosmology. *Weisheng* today speaks in the language of science and bureaucracy. It is no longer available to conversations about *qi*, Warming or Cooling foods, or seasonal rhythms. Words that do encompass these '"traditional'" concepts, particularly *yangsheng*, are outside of the secure realm of the scientific, or dwell uneasily on its edges. Prasenjit Duara, in his influential work *Rescuing History from the Nation*, has called upon historians of China to be more aware of the way that hegemonic constructions of China's national history have suppressed alternative visions of China's past and China's future.[45] Such visions are never entirely suppressed, but persist and threaten to overflow the neat confines of present constructions of modernity. This study is dedicated to tracing the emergence of a hegemonic vision of health as defined by modernizing elites and the state. Ultimately we must admit that the modernizing state, in its embrace of science and rationality, may never be able to eliminate alternative constructions of modernity entirely. But the present study suggests that the state, through a redeployment of intensely meaningful language, can make some of those alternative constructions far more problematic to use than others.

The chapters of this book interweave the writings of physicians and health administrators with narratives of events in and around Tianjin. Chapters 1 and 2 can be read together as an exploration of premodern meanings of *weisheng*. Chapter 1, "Conquering the Hundred Diseases," examines occurrences of *weisheng* in Chinese texts published before the twentieth century in order to sketch out an earlier matrix of meaning and practice associated with the word. Rather than translate premodern *weisheng* as "health" or "hygiene," I have chosen to render it literally as "guarding life." This chapter will explain the logic behind that choice. Chapter 2, "Health and Disease in Heaven's Ford," reads practices of *weisheng* in the daily life of Tianjin before the city was open to foreign settlement. Using Tianjin's herbs, foods, and popular meditation manuals, the city's residents strengthened their bodies against the vagaries of the environment and the exigencies of Tianjin's social crises. These crises included the arrival of foreign armies in the middle of the nineteenth century and the opening of the city as a treaty port in 1860.

Chapter 3, "Medical Encounters and Divergences," explores just what exactly constituted the "Western medicine" that first arrived in Tianjin aboard British warships in the 1860s and compares it with midcentury Chinese approaches to health and healing. Basic debates of medical theory and therapeutics raged in England in the mid–nineteenth century, but the nation's great sanitary revolution had already begun. Chinese and British medical practitioners may have shared certain outlooks on disease and therapeutics, but changes in European politics had given rise to a unique formulation of public health that was to constitute an important divergence between the Great Qing and Great Britain.

Chapters 4 and 5 take a detour away from Tianjin to consider the translation processes, conducted in Shanghai and Tokyo, through which *weisheng* became "hygienic modernity." Chapter 4, "Reshaping *Weisheng* in Treaty-Port China," provides a close reading of China's first translations that presented Western ways of hygiene under the rubric *weisheng*. Centered on late nineteenth-century Euro-American debates over temperance, this translated *weisheng* appeared highly selective, eccentric, and contradictory. Nevertheless, these translations began *weisheng*'s significant shift toward the laboratory and away from correlative cosmology. Chapter 5 considers the "birth" of hygienic modernity as Meiji physician-bureaucrats used the term *weisheng* to convey a philosophy that linked the health of the individual to the health of the nation. The regime of *eisei* (Chinese, *weisheng*) that these physician-bureaucrats created would become extremely important in China after 1900.

Chapter 6 considers the sudden changes that engulfed Tianjin during the Boxer Uprising of 1900, when an international force comprised of the troops of eight different imperial powers invaded and occupied the city. A careful examination of the city's two-year occupation reveals the centrality of health and hygiene to the new government's control of the city, and simultaneously reveals the centrality of the Japanese presence in the occupation government. After 1900, *weisheng* acquired a politically significant definition as "hygienic modernity": even national sovereignty was predicated on a mastery of health technologies that were judged to be adequately modern in the eyes of foreign imperial powers. In order to regain sovereignty over Tianjin, the Qing government was forced to establish a department of health *(weisheng ju)* analogous to the one created by the foreign occupiers. Ironically, at the same time that *weisheng* became a cornerstone of Chinese sovereignty, it began to form an essential core in a Sino-foreign discourse of Chinese deficiency.

Chapters 7 and 8 suggest how *weisheng* changed the physical and cultural terrain of Tianjin in the first three decades of the twentieth century. Chapter 7, "Seen and Unseen," examines modernity's impulse to hide and separate functions of life in order to create a hygienic urban environment. Visions of an ordered and odorless Tianjin, however, were thwarted by poverty and by the tenacious presence of the thousands of men who transported water and waste through the city's streets. Chapter 8, "*Weisheng* and the Desire for Modernity," surveys multiple representations of *weisheng* in Tianjin during the 1920s and 1930s. Although many Chinese subscribed to the idea of *weisheng* as central to Chinese deficiency, the responses to this lack ranged widely, from a longing for the consumer trappings of a hygienically modern life to an embrace of new theories of racial hygiene, or *minzu weisheng.* By the end of this period, it had become increasingly difficult, if not impossible, to formulate alternate visions of a hygienic modernity that incorporated traditional forms of "guarding life."

The final chapters examine the impact of midcentury imperialism on the experience of health and disease in Tianjin. Japanese science during the war sought both to cause epidemics and to prevent them. The result was a paradox of extreme hygienic efficiency coexisting with the use of germ warfare. China's war-time legacy of germs as enemies set the stage for the Communist manipulation of *weisheng* to incorporate meanings of enemies as germs during the Korean War Patriotic Hygiene Campaign of 1952. As millions of Chinese were organized in this massive battle against germs, *weisheng* completed its transformation from a set of individual-based techniques for preserving health to a war against nature that involved the entire Chinese nation. With the rise of *weisheng* as hygienic modernity, individual practices of health based on Chinese cosmologies still continued to thrive in China, but for the most part they existed separately from the scientifically sanctioned realm of *weisheng*. Linguistic divisions, engendered by a century-long experience with imperialism, created fault lines that held (and continue to hold) categories of tradition and modernity in uneasy separation.

1 "Conquering the One Hundred Diseases"

Weisheng *before the Twentieth Century*

What associations would the term *weisheng* create in the mind of a Chinese scholar living in a nineteenth-century city? To understand how *weisheng* as "hygienic modernity" emerged in the twentieth century requires an understanding of *weisheng*'s textual antecedents. By the end of the Qing period (1644–1911), the term *weisheng* appeared within a print matrix that encompassed well-known medical texts, household health manuals, and the Chinese classics. In the mind of a literate gentleman, *weisheng* might invoke a loose web of quotations and aphorisms about health and the body. Such an individual might know that the locus classicus for *weisheng* was in a Daoist text written in the third century before the common era. His library might hold *weisheng* titles originally penned during the thirteenth century. With servants, space, and leisure time, the well-off urbanite might even pursue the sometimes esoteric health and meditation techniques laid out in manuals of "guarding life." These textual references resonated in the minds of treaty-port Chinese as they encountered new configurations of *weisheng* at the end of the nineteenth century.

The goal of this chapter is not to generate a stable and precise definition of "premodern" *weisheng*. Instead, it seeks to demonstrate that few, if any, of the multiple meanings associated with the term *weisheng* during the late imperial period overlapped with concepts conveyed by the word in the twentieth century. Before the twentieth century, *weisheng* did not constitute an instrumental form of knowledge. It was instead a loose, luminous orb of a word that invoked multiple associations, all of which were related to techniques that the individual could employ in order to improve individual health. It was not associated with cleanliness, smells, or dirt. Nor was it associated with the state, the nation, race, or the public. By the early twentieth century, a powerful new set of meanings coalesced strongly around the word *weisheng,* causing it to split from its previous associations. The term became one of the most significant ways of naming the modern condition: a hierarchical principle that determined who would be included or excluded from the realm of civilization, a discourse that defined the difference between a sovereign nation and a subjected tribe. To distinguish this pre-twentieth-century *weisheng* from its modern meanings, I frequently render it literally as "guarding life," after the two characters that comprise it. I also translate it variously as "hygiene" or even as generally as "health," but *weisheng* as "guarding life" is significantly different from its modern parameters.

By 1900, translators in China and Japan were using the term *weisheng* to convey an approach to health that was dictated by the laboratory and the state. But at the same time, *weisheng* also invoked other understandings about health and disease, understandings that were woven into the very basis of lived Chinese culture. For a short time in the early twentieth century, the "Way of Guarding Life" *(weisheng zhi dao)* was still strengthened by associations with the ancients and still revered for its efficacious ability to "conquer the one hundred diseases." There was a window of time when Chinese elites used the cultural resonances of *weisheng* to contest and interpret the meaning of modernity.

TEXTUAL ORIGINS: QUOTATIONS FROM THE MASTERS

An elite nineteenth-century reader would quite likely know that the locus classicus for *weisheng* is in the Daoist classic *Zhuangzi* ([The book of] Master Zhuang, third century B.C.E.). For the late Qing man with aspirations for cultural advancement, the works of some "masters" were more important than others. During the Qing dynasty, the official examinations that led to degrees and government posts emphasized the memorization and analysis of works attributed to Master Kong (Confucius, sixth century B.C.E.) and his follower, Master Meng (Mencius, fourth century B.C.E.), as annotated by a twelfth-century master, Zhu Xi. But cultural literacy of a more eloquent and expansive degree would require a familiarity with other masters from other philosophical traditions, including the masters of Daoism, Laozi and Zhuangzi.

The *Zhuangzi,* together with the *Dao de jing* (The canon of the way and virtue, late fourth–early third century B.C.E.) attributed to the "Old Master" (Master Lao, Laozi), constitute the two foundational texts of Daoism. Late Qing scholars would likely know that the locus classicus for the word *weisheng* was in the "Gengsang Chu," the twenty-third chapter of *Zhuangzi*. This chapter of *Zhuangzi* features Gengsang Chu, an eccentric old man who is a direct disciple of Laozi. A certain aged gentleman named Nanrong Chu (rendered by Victor Mair as "Rufus Southglory") has tried to study the Way under Gengsang Chu, but his obtuse teachings have only confused the hapless pupil. Hoping for clarification, Nanrong Chu packs up his belongings and seeks out Laozi himself. In desperation, Nanrong Chu begs the Old Master to dispense with profound dissertations on the Way. All he wishes to hear about are "the basic rules for guarding life [*weisheng zhi jing*], that's all." A man of advanced years, it appears that Nanrong Chu is more concerned with curing the infirmities of his body than improving the well-being of his spirit. He complains that listening to Gengsang Chu's advice on the Dao was like taking a medicine that only made him sicker. Nanrong Chu is probably not prepared for the Old Master's remarkable reply:

> The basic rules for guarding life are:
> Can you embrace Unity?
> Can you keep from losing it?
> . . . Can you stop when it's time to stop?
> Can you cease when it's time to cease?
> Can you give up looking for it in others and seek for it in yourself?[1]

The Old Master tells Nanrong Chu that he should become as naive and as spontaneous as a child. A child has tremendous strength, energy, and concentration: It is able to cry all day without wearing out its throat, stare all day without blinking.[2] The child "walks but knows not where, remains stationary but knows not why. It is intertwined with things and ripples along together with them." That, summarizes the Old Master, is the basic rule for guarding life. The implication is immediately clear: for Laozi, "the basic rule for guarding life" is to live entirely in harmony with the way of nature.

The aged Nanrong Chu's practical request for "the standard method for guarding life" and Laozi's mystical reply highlight some of the murky links between early Daoism, the origins of Chinese health practices, and the quest for immortality. Donald Harper has observed that the "scholarly convention" holds that Chinese health practices and the pursuit of immortality all originated in the "belief system loosely called Daoist."[3] However, recent work on Chinese societies before the first unification under the Qin (c. 221–206 B.C.E.) demonstrates that the conceptions of the body basic to both the pursuit of health and the pursuit of immortality predated the emergence of Daoism as a formal system of thought.

Among the earliest extant medical texts are those recovered from the

Mawangdui tomb (sealed 168 B.C.E.) in present-day Hunan. The Mawangdui medical texts demonstrate the Han aristocrats' obsession with preserving health, avoiding disease, and living life to the fullest. Many of these texts deal with what Donald Harper has called "macrobiotic hygiene," or *yangsheng*, a word more commonly translated as "nurturing life."[4] *Yangsheng* texts described sexual practices, dietetic regimens, movements, and medicines designed to nurture the vital forces and ensure the proper flow of *qi* within the body. *Yangsheng* was recognized as a separate category of practice from medicine, a set of techniques that were specifically developed to prevent disease, harmonize the body's vitalities, and prolong life. Vivienne Lo has convincingly argued that *yangsheng* texts had considerable influence on the formation of canonical Chinese medicine during the foundational years of the Western Han (202 B.C.E.–8 C.E.). Similarly, Harper has demonstrated that the organized Daoism that emerged between the second century B.C.E. and the second century C.E. adopted *yangsheng* health practices in its program for personal cultivation and salvation, but Daoism did not invent them.[5]

Later on in the imperial period, individual practices for health were often associated with Daoism, but it is important to recall that their origins predated Daoism and did not exclusively belong to a distinctly separate "Daoist tradition." Health practices related to diet, meditation, and self-regulation emerged along with the very bases of Chinese culture, and were diffuse enough to be associated not only with being Daoist, but also with being Chinese. The Daoist textual origin of *weisheng*, however, is significant in this story of the emergence of hygienic modernity. In fact, the Japanese physician who first used *weisheng* to convey European ideas of a state-centered public health claimed to have found his inspiration in Nanrong Chu's ancient quest (see chapter 5).

If our hypothetical nineteenth-century scholar regarded Daoist classics as frivolous distractions and instead spent all his time memorizing texts that would ensure him success on the government's civil service examinations, he would still discover a locus for *weisheng* in the orthodox commentaries to the Confucian classics by the twelfth-century philosopher Zhu Xi. For example, the tenth chapter of the *Analects (Lunyu)* describes the admirable qualities embodied in the personal demeanor of Confucius. After discussing the great master's way of walking, speaking, carrying, and dressing, the passage mentions Confucius's approach to eating: "He did not eat his fill of polished rice, nor did he eat his fill of finely minced meat. . . . He did not eat food that had gone off colour or food that had a bad smell. . . . Even when there was plenty of meat, he avoided eating more meat than rice. Only in the case of wine did he not set himself a rigid limit. He simply never drank to the point of becoming confused."[6]

In one of his commentaries on the *Analects, Lunyu jing yi* (Essential meanings of The Analects, c. 1180), Zhu Xi praised the ancient sages for exercising control over the human desire to consume more than necessary. By leaving the table slightly hungry, not gorging on rich meats, and knowing when to put down the wineglass, Confucius followed the path of "guarding life." Zhu Xi provided a pithy quote that captured the healthy virtues of the sages: "By minimizing their desires, the ancients maximized the Way of Health" *(gu ren yu xin ze gua wei sheng zhi dao ze jin ye).*[7]

The "Path of Guarding Life" or the "Way of Health" *(weisheng zhi dao)* appears in another Song (960–1279) commentary to the *Zhou li* (The rites of the Zhou dynasty). The ancient Zhou (1027–771 B.C.E.) court (the ideal model of rulership) appointed medical officials to oversee the health of the people and the court, including *jiyi* (literally, illness doctors) and *shiyi* (literally, food doctors). The "illness doctors" attended to the sicknesses of the common people, whereas food doctors made sure that court elites ate food appropriate to the system of cosmological correspondences. By steering a course of moderation and balance in their daily lifestyle, the Zhou rulers never got sick and thus avoided the use of "illness doctors" altogether. One well-known explication of the *Zhou li* from the Song dynasty notes that by balancing the yin and yang *qi* of their foods, the Zhou rulers achieved the *weisheng zhi dao:* the Way of Guarding Life.[8]

For late imperial scholars, these classical references would perhaps be more respectable—and more memorable—than the Way of Guarding Life as it existed within a rambling Daoist text. Benjamin Elman has illuminated the ways in which Song commentaries became the intellectual lifeblood for aspiring scholars in the late imperial period: memorized, quoted, and internalized by generation after generation of young men. These passages reflect how a phrase that appears in several texts from the twelfth century—*weisheng zhi dao*—could become part of the cultural repertoire of scholars in early modern China. The Way of Health might be associated with the natural "rippling and flowing" of Master Zhuang's Daoism, but if asked to recall a passage in which *weisheng* appears, a nineteenth-century scholar might turn to the works of Master Zhu and associate the Way of Health with the perfect restraint and moderation practiced by Confucius. In either case, the *weisheng* that appears in all of these texts suggests that curing sickness before it happens requires an ability to discern the underlying patterns of the universe.

NINETEENTH-CENTURY POPULAR PRECEPTS
FOR GUARDING LIFE

Neither the *Zhuangzi* nor the works of Zhu Xi contain information about the practices that were associated with *weisheng*. For this we must turn to the popular collections of medical aphorisms and household health manuals that circulated widely in late imperial China. The late imperial period saw an explosion of commercial printing that facilitated the spread of cheap print beyond urban centers and into small towns. Among the most widely dispersed books (besides copies of the Classics and guides for studying for the civil service examinations) were books that gave advice for daily life: almanacs, household encyclopedias, morality books, medicinal recipe collections, and manuals on preserving health.[9] A glimpse into one such health compilation provides insights into more popular meanings associated with the term *weisheng*.

The *Book of the Immortal Celestials* (*Wan shou xian shu*, c. 1560) is a wonderfully rich combination of advice on the art of preserving health.[10] By the nineteenth century, the book appears in local editions with crudely cut characters and clumsy illustrations, intended for household use on a mass level. The original authorship of the work is somewhat dubiously attributed to the renowned sixteenth-century literatus Luo Hongxian (1504–1564).[11] Whether a brilliant optimus *(zhuangyuan)* in the Ming imperial examinations would have authored such a folksy compilation of health advice is questionable, but Luo was regaled as a famed student of the Dao, and thus attributing this work to him might have helped bolster its image. Authorship in this case is not an entirely applicable concept. The *Book of the Immortal Celestials* is not a coherent treatise but a down-to-earth collection of preventive, curative, and regenerative practices, expressed in hundreds of short essays and easily recited maxims (see fig. 1).

One subsection in the *Book of the Immortal Celestials*, entitled "Precious Precepts for Guarding Life" *(Weisheng bao xun)*, contains the following advice:

- "In the fourth month, the Way of Heaven is moving west, therefore when traveling it is best to go in this direction. In this month, the *qi* of life is in the Earthly Branch *mao*. In sitting and lying down, it is best to face due east."

- "In the morning, eat just one bowl of rice gruel."

- "If in the summer you frequently ate raw or cool melon and fruit, in the fall take two liters of the urine of young boys. Add five betel

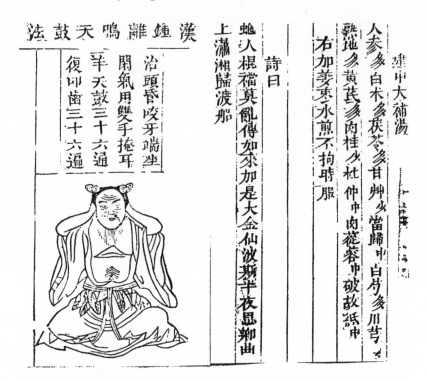

Figure 1. "Illustrations of the Various Immortals Doing Guiding and Pulling" *(zhu xian daoyin tu)* from *Wan shou xian shu* (Book of the immortal celestials [1832]). Each illustration includes an herbal formula (far right), an inspirational poem (center), and instructions for a *daoyin* posture (left). Pictured here is the immortal Han Zhongli demonstrating a cure for dizziness and toothaches. These illustrations are similar to those found in the seventeenth-century work *Wei-sheng zhen jue* (Perfected formulas for guarding life). Reproduced from *Zhong-guo yixue dacheng sanbian* (Great compendium of Chinese medicine, in three parts) (Changsha: Yue lu shu she), vol. 8, p. 827.

nuts, finely sliced and fried. Take eight doses of this, and then take one dose of fresh ginger juice and water from melted snow. This will purge you two or three times, thus expelling the Cool things that you ate in the summer and the water accumulated in your bladder. . . . After purging, rice gruel with Chinese chive and sheep kidney—this is an excellent replenishing medicine."

· "During great heat or great cold, do not give in to lust, and do not enter the chamber when you are full and drunk."

· "One must frequently turn one's vision inside, sink the Heart-

Mind *[xin]* into the Cinnabar Field, and make the Spirit *[shen]* and *qi* firmly embrace the Great Profundity."[12]

This miscellany of advice conveys the major categories associated with *weisheng* as guarding health in the late imperial period: ingestion regimes, sexual economy, and meditative exercises, all done in accordance to a system of correlative cosmology that dictated an activity's time, season, and direction. Each category, considered separately below, contributed to the interrelated webs of guarding life in the nineteenth century.

Guarding Life by Knowing the Right Time and Place

In the fourth month . . . the *qi* of life is in the Earthly Branch *mao.*
In sitting and lying down, it is best to face due east.

This guideline about the proper position for healthful movement and resting encompasses the most fundamental concepts of Chinese thought: *qi* and the system of correlative cosmology. *Qi* is a central concept not only in Chinese medicine, but also in Chinese understanding of the cosmos.[13] I follow Nathan Sivin and leave *qi* untranslated, although other scholars have rendered the term variously as "vapor," "energy," "matter-energy," and "influences."[14] *Qi* is at the same time the stuff that makes up the universe and that which energizes, enervates, or "makes things happen in stuff."[15] It is at times associated with air and breath, and even with visible terrestrial phenomena such as mists. But *qi* is more subtle, more refined and essential. *Qi* both creates and permeates everything in the world, pulsing through the earth in veins discernable to the expert in geomancy. It also fills the human body in many different manifestations, ebbing through *mai*, the circulation tracts known to physicians of Chinese medicine. *Qi* is thus the "shared substrate" between the world of humans and the physical world.[16]

Qi's manifestations occur through qualities that arrange themselves in a complex system of relationships, described by Western scholars as "correlative cosmology" or "systematic correspondences."[17] These correlations/correspondences organize phenomena into categories and then form relationships between the categories. This creates a web of mutual interdependence between the myriad phenomena of the human body, society, and the natural universe.

The initial perceptible qualities and the most fundamental divisions within Chinese cosmology are yin and yang. Yin is associated with darkness, dampness, passivity, the feminine, whereas yang is associated with brightness, dryness, activity, the masculine. *Qi* is further manifested in five aspects called the Five Phases: Wood, Fire, Earth, Metal, and Water. These should not be confused with the Four Elements of classical Greek thought, since the Five Phases describe processes or functions more than they do things.[18] They engender each other (when in balance) or overcome each other (when out of balance) through knowable cyclical pathways. Myriad phenomena in the external world, such as seasons, hours, directions, planets, deities, and even government offices in the imperial hierarchy correspond to the Five Phases and follow their patterns of change. The same is true for phenomena within the human body. Organ functions, acupuncture points, emotions, tastes, smells, sounds, and bodily secretions all correspond to specific phases, and thus correspond to phenomena in the external world. The body as microcosm mirrors the macrocosm of the universe.[19] Health and well-being are achieved when all are in harmony. Illness or misfortune might befall an individual (or a family) who acts counter to these natural patterns.

The famous second chapter of the *Inner Canon of the Yellow Emperor (Huang di nei jing)*, entitled "The Great Treatise on Adjusting the Spirit According to the Four Seasons," outlines the activities one should follow to achieve harmony with the cosmos.[20] In the three months of spring, one should rise early, stroll about in the courtyard, and wear one's hair loose to allow one's emotions and thoughts to develop freely. In the summer months, the *qi* of heaven and earth commingle and the natural world flourishes; therefore one should rise early, not tire one's self out, and avoid anger in order to allow one's *qi* and spirit also to flourish. The consequences of not adjusting one's behavior according to the season is borne by the organ system that corresponds with that season as grouped according to the Five Phases. Going against the way of spring, for example, will result in an injury to the Liver *(gan)* function, since both spring and Liver correspond to the phase of Wood. The illness remains hidden until summer, however, when the Fire phase of summer waxes and Wood wanes, thus exposing its damaged state.[21]

Specialized knowledge of the correspondences could also be used to predict the future of ill health. The cyclical nature of commonly experienced illnesses was apparent to the observers who composed the earliest Chinese medical texts and is a predominant theme in the *Inner Canon of the Yellow Emperor*. The logic of the Chinese divinatory tradition held that such cycles would be knowable through proper application of Five Phases analysis. By the Song, medical thinkers combined the Five Cycles *(wu yun)*, the Six Environmental Influences *(liu qi)*, the Heavenly Stem and Earthly Branch system *(tian gan di zhi)*, and the Eight Trigrams *(ba gua)* to form an elaborate mechanism for predicting both seasonal fluctuations as well as long-term disease patterns, a system rendered by the German sinologist Manfred Porkert as "Phase Energetics." Physicians employed this Phase Energetics system together with consideration of locally occurring unseasonable weather and internal factors in an attempt to predict the course of disease in individual patients. The Phase Energetics system also helped the compilers of almanacs to make their predictions about the coming year's epidemics. By the seventeenth century, many scholars had become skeptical about the usefulness of such overarching cosmological systems. Some physicians, particularly those who became associated with the Warm Factor school, began to think of the causes of disease as random events that could not be predicted by the use of Phase Energetics.[22] Nevertheless, these systems of correspondence still permeated popular culture and were available as a technique for preserving health.

The "Precious Precept for Guarding Life" quoted above is now quite clear. "In the fourth month the Way of Heaven is moving west, therefore when traveling, it is best to go in this direction. In this month, the *qi* of life is in the Earthly Branch *mao*. In sitting and lying down, it is best to face due east." The fourth month is the height of spring, associated with the Wood Phase. The Earthly Branch *mao* corresponds with both this time of the year and with the direction east. The *qi* of life is fullest in this location, therefore, it is advisable to face this direction when at rest to absorb its healthful benefits. When in motion, however, it is advisable to go with its east to west flow; therefore journeys should begin in a westerly direction. Knowledge of the patterns of space and time would allow the individual to guard life by "rippling along" on the same wave with the forces of the universe.

Guarding Life through Ingestion Regimes

In the morning, eat just one bowl of rice gruel.

Frederick Mote once observed that when we consider the Chinese approach to food as "active agents in the cosmic process" we come face to face with the very concepts that ordered Chinese civilization.[23] Knowledge about the medicinal properties of foods is extremely widespread in Chinese culture, whether passed down in the kitchen through tales and aphorisms, or internalized intently by the scholar through study of materia medica *(bencao)* or treatises on healing disease with food *(shiliao, shizhi)*. Works associated with *weisheng* from late imperial China are invariably concerned with questions of ingestion: ingestion of food, ingestion of medicine, and the ingestion of food as medicine. In texts on maintaining health, drink/food *(yin-shi)* and drugs *(yao)* are represented as potent forces, each capable of significantly altering the balance of the human body when ingested. Both can prevent or cure illness: the difference between food and medicine is one of degree alone. Both can cause illness as well: food through overindulgence and improper combination, medicine through inexpert application and unnecessary use. More than anything else, the key to guarding life is the judicial practice of proper ingestion regimes.

In the long history of Chinese texts about food, surprising consistencies occurred as specific classic passages were cited over and over. In addition, all authorities were in agreement about the central role of overall moderation in diet. The simple phrase—"In the morning, eat just one bowl of rice gruel"—epitomizes this principle. Gastronomic excess inevitably led to calamity: volume after volume intoned the same injunction. The stern call to restraint encompassed not only amount, but variety as well. Guarding one's life entailed avoiding unhealthful foods and potentially fatal combinations, no matter how exotic or appealing such delicacies might be in the eyes of the gourmand. An understanding of the properties of food and their proper combination was essential to guarding life.

Flavors, Natures, and the Physiology of Nutrition   The *Divine Pivot* (Ling shu) of the *Inner Canon of the Yellow Emperor* sets out the basic approach to food and digestion that is quoted, elaborated upon, and occasionally challenged in medical texts and pharmacopoeia throughout the imperial period. All vegetables, fruits, meats, spices, grains, herbs, minerals, and animal products that could be ingested possess one or more of the qualities known as the Five Flavors *(wei)*: Sweet *(gan)*, Sour *(suan)*, Bitter *(ku)*, Pungent *(xin)*, Salty *(xian)*.[24] In addition to Flavor, all ingestibles also possess one of the specific "Natures" or "Characters" *(xing)*, namely Cold *(han)*, Cool *(leng)*, Warm *(wen)*, Hot *(re)*, and Neutral *(ping)*.

The process of digestion is one of distilling and dispersing the *qi* of ingestibles. Foods enter the Stomach *(wei)*, which is the "ocean" for all the internal viscera, the marvelous storehouse from whence the viscera receive their proper *qi*. From the Stomach the *qi* of the Five Flavors proceed to the organ/function to which they correspond, or to the one for which they have an affinity. Sour "goes to" the Liver *(qan)*, Bitter the Heart *(xin)*, Sweet the Spleen *(pi)*, Pungent the Lungs *(fei)*, and Salty the Kidney *(shen)*. These entities, sometimes called the Five Depots or Five Viscera *(wu zang)*, are not to be confused with the organs of biomedicine, but refer instead to what Sivin calls part of the "Visceral Systems of Function." In Chinese medicine,

Heart, Stomach, Liver, Lungs, and Kidney store specific bodily vitalities and perform essential tasks but are not always conceived of as specific entities that exist in specific spaces. They are conceptualized more in terms of what they do than what they are, more physiology than anatomy, more function than location. Judith Farquhar, in her lucid discussion of contemporary traditional Chinese medical concepts, defines the Five Viscera as "highly contingent sites at which regular transformations of *qi* take place."[25]

Through the system of correspondences, a food or drug's flavor will indicate which Visceral System of Function it is most likely to affect, and yet the correspondence does not mean that in the Chinese medical imagination the *qi* of the ingested entity simply "goes" to this organ or affects it alone. The human body in Chinese medicine is far too diverse to be reduced to a grouping of organs. It may be approached through a variety of analytical systems, depending on a physician's proclivity and experience, the nature of the disorder, and even the regional locale of the practice.[26] This contingency is also reflected in the descriptions of drug action. Materia medica entries for any particular drug might also refer to its "tract affinity," indicating the circulation tract (sometimes called "meridian") that the drug is drawn to, and thus indicating its usefulness to a physician who chooses to map the phase/location of an illness according to the system of the Six Warps *(liu jing)*.[27] Flavors are also associated with actions that may have a more global effect on certain pathological states. Bitter things will drain or dry disorders that are replete or damp. Sweet things will replenish depletions and boost vitalities. Pungent will move *qi* and Blood and moisten dry disorders. Sour will constrict and contract, preventing loss of vital fluids. Salty releases lumps and drains downward, leading away unwanted accumulations. Both food and drugs have powerful effects on the body, achieved within a system of mutual influence.

Food as Medicine, Food as Pathogen The potent ability of food to affect the human organism is clearly demonstrated by the inclusion of foodstuffs in many materia medica or medical texts. The characterizations of foods from such sources are in many cases remarkably consistent over the centuries, indicating the ability of certain foundational texts to serve as authorities for well over a millennium. In China, the following advice on mutton and crabs rang true from the eighth through the nineteenth century: "The meat of sheep: Flavor: Bitter, Sweet. Nature: Very Hot. Not toxic. Governs being hit by Warmth, young children's illnesses, and sweating produced by the head being struck by Great Wind. Governs Depletion and Exhaustion/Cold and Cool [syndromes], can bolster the Center and benefits the *qi*. Stops pain."[28]

Mutton seems a poor word indeed to describe the ingestible entities associated with the Chinese word *yang*. Not only are different parts of the sheep seen as food/drugs possessed of their own physiological effects—kidney, skin, marrow, brains, hooves, to name a few, in addition to the meat—but different kinds and colors of sheep have widely divergent properties as well.[29] A host of infelicities awaits the person who seasons mutton with vinegar, washes it down with alcohol, or eats it while pregnant.[30] But most sources praise its beneficial warming and vitality-bolstering effects. The meat is particularly helpful for men's various "exhaustions" and can be beneficial to women who are giving birth during the cold of winter.

It is not surprising that mutton came into a sort of medicinal vogue during the Yuan dynasty (1279–1368), when Mongol rulers enlisted dietary experts to codify healthful foods. A great number of the curative recipes collected by the fourteenth-century imperial dietician Hoshoi featured mutton or other parts of the sheep such as liver or kidney, combined with other warming food/drugs such as ginger and pepper.[31] Sheep parts continue to be in favor, especially in north China, well into the late imperial period. The postpurge gruel advised in the nineteenth-century *Book of the Immortal Celestials* gets its curative power from the addition of sheep kidney and Chinese chives. According to Li Shizhen, the great sixteenth-century compiler of knowledge on food and medicine, this combination was perfect for eliminating uncomfortable "swelling and knots" in the abdomen.

> Crabs. Flavor: Salty. Nature: Cold. Slightly toxic. Cures stomach *qi*, aids digestion. Crab with vinegar aids the joints, removes discomforting *qi* in the Five Viscera. The *Inner Canon of the Yellow Emperor* states: "Crabs with eyes that face each other and crabs with mottled legs are harmful to eat. Do not eat crabs or soft-shell turtles in the twelfth month: they injure Spirit and *qi*." The *Inner Canon* also states: "Eating pork together with crab is harmful. Eating crab meat in the autumn with fruits and vegetables shortens *qi*. Drinking alcohol and eating crab . . . gives rise to Cold-Heat syndrome. . . ." Frequent eating moves Wind and causes Sudden Chaos [*huoluan,* acute gastrointestinal distress associated with modern definitions of cholera].[32]

Few foods in Chinese gastronomy seem simultaneously as desirable and as dangerous as crabs. Textual evidence indicates that Chinese have enjoyed eating the crustacean since well before the common era. The healthful qualities of the meat enumerated in various classics might have seemed a pleasant plus for those fortunate enough to dine on it. Yet the earliest mention of crabs in medical texts dwells not on benefits but on the harms they might bring to the unsuspecting gourmand. Even the venerable *Inner Canon* contains numerous proscriptions on crab (as well as the meat of various other shellfish). Some of these warnings specify morphological abnormalities to avoid, but many more emphasize troublesome seasons and questionable cooking methods. These proscriptions are repeated again and again through materia medica and *weisheng* texts for the next two millennia. Besides giving rise to Sudden Chaos, crab that is improperly prepared or eaten out of season can also cause insect infestation, painful accumulations of Cool *qi* in the abdomen, and breech births. Well into the nineteenth century, epidemic illnesses that swept through coastal cities were blamed on the Cold nature of crab (see chapter 5), even as a new discourse of health and disease challenged the precepts of the ancients.

Guarding Life with Drugs

> In the fall take two liters of the urine of young boys. Add five betel nuts finely sliced and fried.

The terms used to describe the properties and action of foods also encompassed the roots, herbs, fungi, minerals, and animal products known as *yao*. Although foods were imbued with the same kind of properties associated with medicines, it was widely acknowledged that drugs worked on a more intense level, with faster, more dramatic effects. One well-known adage describes this difference in degree, not in kind: "The basis of daily well-being is food, but to rescue someone from illness requires the speed of drugs."[33] Drugs too are Hot, Cold, Warm, or Cool, possess one of the Five Flavors, have specific affinities for Visceral Systems of Function and circulation tracts, and perform specific actions. Chinese materia medica list hundreds of drugs, each with their own complex array of properties. Works on medicine and pharmacy include formulas or recipes *(fang)* for combining these drugs into efficacious supplements and cures.

Texts bearing *weisheng* in their title from the late imperial period all have one thing in common: they contain information on formulas. They differ in the means of presentation of the formula: some include detailed discussions of medical theory and diagnosis; other works simply list dozens of formulas categorized according to simple afflictions. Some formulas are simple, combining only two or three basic herbs, others are baroque mixtures of rare and expensive ingredients. Some works present nothing but formulas, and others include formulas as part of a wide range of practices, including divination and yoga. Within this diversity a central theme is apparent: *Weisheng* is as much about curing illness as it is about preventing illness.

To guard life meant to practice basic precepts of disease prevention, but when those failed, guarding life also meant taking pills and potions in an attempt to drive disease away.

Formulas could be used for cure, but they could also be used to prevent illness by boosting vitality or warding off dreaded seasonal disorders. The "Precious Precepts for Guarding Life" in the *Book of the Immortal Celestials* offers a glimpse of this popular approach to preventive medicine. It tutors the administration of a cathartic combination of human urine, betel nuts, and ginger juice in order to clear away the Cool Yin accumulated (through eating cooling foods like cucumbers, watermelon, or crabs) during the summer months. After the drug-induced purge, imbalance could be rectified through the use of medicinal foods. A follow-up bowl of rice gruel with sheep's kidney would restore the Viscera and vitalities to their normal post-purge equilibrium.

Luo Tianyi's (1220–1290) *A Precious Mirror for Guarding Life (Wei-sheng bao jian)*, condemns the popular use of purgative potions, and even goes so far as to attribute epidemics to their use. Luo's work was written in the thirteenth century but was circulated and quoted throughout the late imperial period, particularly by those physicians who shared Luo's tendency to see the Stomach and the Spleen functions as the key to human health and disease.[34] Luo decried the common post-New Year purges of the northern Chinese—a seasonal inverse of the postsummer purges described in the *Book of the Immortal Celestials*. Fearful that winter months spent bundled in coats and eating warming foods might result in the accumulation of internal Fire, with the coming of warm weather, individuals consumed pills made of the Bitter and Cold drugs such as *qian niu zi* (morning glory seeds) or *da huang* (rhubarb). The medicines worked by attacking and "draining" the Heat, an action manifested thorough a catharsis of the bowels. The logic underlying such practices, argued Luo, was entirely counter to the precepts of medicine set out in the classics. If one followed the way of life appropriate for each season (the key to *weisheng*), there would be no need to banish pathogenic accumulations in the body as the seasons changed. Using Cold medicines to purge supposed "accumulated winter Heat" only subjected the Stomach and Spleen to damage from Cold. Since the purging practice was so widespread, the resulting illness was widespread as well. In Luo's estimation, the annual occurrence of spring epidemics *(yi li)*, although they ran through large populations at the same time, were actually caused by the simultaneous erroneous use of medicines by myriad individuals, each purging themselves in the privacy of their own homes.[35]

Formulas were more frequently used not to purge excesses, but to supplement deficiencies. Shigehisa Kuriyama has suggested that *xu*, deficiency or lack, was one of the dominant underlying causes of disorders in Chinese medicine. *Bu*, to nurture, boost, or supplement, was the frequent task of a medicine taken on a prophylactic basis to overcome conditions of *xu*. Such supplements were numerous and appeared in almost any pharmacological compilation. One frequently cited formula from the late imperial period was for a concoction known as *weisheng tang:* Guarding Life Soup. Comprised primarily of angelica *(dang gui)*, dahlia root *(shao yao)*, and rehmannia *(di huang)*, this formula promised to "boost conditions of exhaustion, strengthen the Viscera, nurture Original *qi*, adjust the Pulses, warm the Center, calm the Spirit, and add luster to the countenance." Taken frequently, the formula nourishes the Stomach and benefits the *jing*, the Seminal Essence. Although not specifically designed to boost sexual vitality, *weisheng tang* could perform that function along with many others.

In fact, *weisheng* was frequently, but not exclusively, associated with maintenance of sexual health. In texts that mention *weisheng*, warnings about the harmful effects of sex were second only to advice against overindulgence in eating and drinking. As with eating and drinking, the key *weisheng* precept for sex was restraint and moderation. And as with the issue of self-medication, debates abounded about what exactly constituted proper restraint and moderation in sexual activity.

Guarding Life through Sexual Economy

During great heat or great cold, do not give in to lust and do not
enter the chamber when you are full and drunk.

The warnings about the dangers of sex from the nineteenth-century *Book of the Immortal Celestials* closely mirror concepts found in the earliest literature in the Chinese medical tradition. The locus classicus of such concerns in the medical literature can be found in the very opening lines of the *Inner Canon of the Yellow Emperor*. The Yellow Emperor queries his minister Qi Bo on the reasons the ancients lived to be one hundred, whereas modern men only lived to be fifty. Qi Bo answered:

The ancients who understood the Way patterned their lives [on the
changes of] yin and yang and lived in accordance with the arts of
cosmology and divination. Their eating and drinking was restrained,
their activity and rest were regular, and they did not recklessly tire
themselves out. . . .
    People of today are not like that. For them, alcohol is the preferred
beverage, and recklessness is the norm. They have sex [literally, "enter

the chamber"] while drunk, exhausting their Seminal Essence with desire and scattering their Original [*qi*] with dissipation. . . . In pursuit of their own pleasure, they reject the joys that accompany [the cultivation of] life.[36]

Scholars since the first millennium of the common era have turned to the opening chapters of the *Inner Canon* in order to illuminate the basic principles of guarding life. There it was clear that one of the most egregious violations of health was the wanton enjoyment of sex, particularly for men. The majority of texts related to *weisheng* were addressed to an elite male audience, and for this audience, entering the chamber and not controlling one's sexual expenditure was certain to cause illness. Indeed, for this male readership, the root of "the one hundred diseases" could sometimes appear to lie almost exclusively in the proximity of the penis, and its related internal energy/substance, *jing*.

Jing (Seminal Essence) is central to any discussion of ideas of health and illness in the Chinese context. In some discussions, *jing* takes precedence even over *qi* as the most precious vitality in the body. In one of the Mawangdui medical manuscripts, Ancestor Peng proclaims, "Of man's *qi*, none can compare with penile essence [*jing*]." Ultimately *jing* is but one manifestation of *qi*, but its association with the penis, sex, and procreation make it a unique and very important manifestation. *Jing* is not just the physical entity of semen: it is the body's essential generative aspect, pure, refined, one might say almost sacred. It is the most yin aspect of the male, and thus like all yin it is also the most vulnerable to depletion. Therefore the genitals and the semen appear as the most vulnerable aspects of male physiology. As Ancestor Peng advises, "If there is a calamity for life, it is invariably because yin essence leaks out."[37]

Unlike other aspects of *qi* within the body, *jing* is difficult to nurture or augment through breathing or the ingestion of food and drugs. Indeed, much like the Original *qi* bestowed before birth, *jing* exists within the body in finite quantities. *Jing* is essential for life and health, but one only has so much of it. Once it is spent, it is gone. It seems that one should avoid losing *jing* at all costs, and yet there were obvious forces working against that option. Many medical experts held that sexual abstinence resulted in blockages and infirmities, and thus counseled moderate sexual activity as part of a healthy life.[38] Even Confucius recognized that sexual desire (along with the desire for food) was at the root of human nature, and thus impossible to avoid. Another one of Confucius's dictums held that there was nothing more unfilial than leaving this life without having fathered descendants. Nevertheless, the anxiety over the loss of seminal essence remained. In the words of the seventh-century physician and alchemist Sun Simiao, "When *jing* is reduced, illness results, when *jing* is used up, death results. One can not help but be worried; one can not help but be cautious."[39] One of the crueler paradoxes of male existence, therefore, was the fact that the activity of sex and procreation, so vital to the survival of humankind, inevitably resulted in a loss of that which maintained the individual human life.

This paradox fostered an approach to sex and health that can best be described as an economy. Certainly *jing* was something that needed to be "economized," carefully invested and not carelessly spent. But this "sexual economy" also meant that a careful calculus of inputs and outputs, of benefits and drawbacks, would determine how much sexual activity could be tolerated while still allowing for the maintenance of overall health. For those concerned about depletion, taboo days and inauspicious hours dictated the times when sex should be avoided. More exact advice even dictated the number of ejaculations appropriate for men at different stages of life, ranging from one ejaculation every four days for twenty-year-olds to one ejaculation a month for those over sixty (and then only for those of especially strong constitution).[40] Finally, from the august *Inner Canon of the Yellow Emperor* to the humble *Book of the Immortal Celestials,* the gravest advice warns against entering the bedchamber in a state of intoxication *(zui yi ru fang)*. Sex was a serious business, and one needed a clear mind to keep track of its accounts.[41]

Major shifts in the discourse on health and sex have taken place in Chinese history. Before the Song, sexual advice manuals offered techniques that, although based in ideas of economy, suggested that sex was not a zero-sum game.[42] The male could actually increase his share of *jing* vitalities by absorbing Essence from the female—as long as he did not part with his own Seminal Essence during the course of sex. By the Tang (617–907), a large number of sophisticated techniques for the avoidance of ejaculation had been developed. In the words of Douglas Wile, these "self-defense methods" included "mental imaging, breath control, perineal compression, teeth gnashing" and numerous other techniques.[43] Some were designed simply to stave off the event of ejaculation, whereas others entailed an intentional internal rechanneling of ejaculant. Joseph Needham calls this technique coitus thesauratus and details how its actual practice entails pressing a point in the perineum between the anus and the scrotum at the moment of orgasm. In biomedical terms, the result is that the semen is channeled into the bladder and leaked out imperceptibly in the urine.[44] In Chinese terms, this technique entails putting pressure on the first acupuncture point in the "Conception Vessel Meridian" *(ren mai)*, a point called "The Meeting of Yin" *(hui yin)*.

As a result of this action and internal visualization, *jing* is channeled up the spine and into the head, where it is stored and protected. This technique, called "returning the *jing* to nourish the brain" *(huan jing bu nao)*, is related to the skills of circulating the vitalities and inner alchemy.

This tradition of cheating the tyranny of *jing* depletion seems to have been cut off by the end of the first millennium of the common era. Knowledge of these practices may have continued to spread through oral culture and secret transmission, particularly within Daoism, but by the Song it seems that describing these activities in print was no longer considered a respectable activity. What remained was an understanding of *jing* as a vulnerable, limited resource, and a general "economic" approach to the relationship between health and sexual activity.

More research needs to be done to establish how widespread these understandings were in late imperial society and to what extent they might have actually influenced sexual behavior. Recent work by Hsiung Ping-chen suggests that depletion anxiety was an important factor shaping Chinese private life. The historical demographers James Lee and Wang Feng even hold that that the precepts of sexual economy were partly responsible for the markedly low marital fertility rates experienced in China during the late imperial period.[45] Hugh Shapiro's work on modern syndromes of "spermatorrhea" demonstrate that fear of *jing* depletion lasted well into the twentieth century. Many men in republican-period China claimed to suffer from spermatorrheal exhaustion, a malady exacerbated by the stresses and temptations of modern urban life.[46] Western-influenced ideas on sexual hygiene brought to China in the twentieth century seemed to coincide with some of the moral rhetoric of traditional *weisheng*.[47] Although perhaps the least documented, or least-explicitly commented upon aspect of guarding life, sexual economy certainly formed one of its central themes.

Guarding Life by Circulating the Vitalities

> One must frequently turn one's vision inside, sink the Heart-Mind
> [xin] into the Cinnabar Field, and make the Spirit [shen] and *qi*
> firmly embrace the Great Profundity.

The concept of circulation is one of the most important themes associated with practices of guarding life. The circulation we find associated with *weisheng* in the late imperial period is far removed from that proposed by William Harvey in the seventeenth century: It does not take place along a closed network of specialized vessels within a fleshy anatomy, nor is it a circulation of a singular liquid substance. What circulates is *qi*, although *qi's* manifestation in *jing* is another central entity implicated in corporal circulations. Different manifestations of *qi* flow through multiple routes and in a variety of directions (or no direction at all), through tracts, in spaces between the muscle and skin, within the abdominal cavity, and through internal streams, grottos, and mountain passes. If *qi* is blocked or accumulates in unnatural textures, pathogenic conditions will arise. Like the *jing* that is always in danger of depletion, the natural tendencies of humans to indulge in unhealthful habits renders *qi* highly susceptible to stagnation and blockage.

Most important, *qi* circulation, although ideally natural and spontaneous, can be augmented, controlled, and even rerouted through conscious actions, including breathing, inner visualization, massage, postures, and movement. By the late imperial period, all of these seemingly esoteric techniques had been combined into practical programs for curing ills and warding off the infirmities of old age. Several works associated with *weisheng* are in fact highly syncretic guides meant to popularize methods for the circulation of *qi*.

The *Perfected Formulas for Guarding Life (Weisheng zhen jue)*, attributed to the Ming literatus Luo Hongxian, is one such work.[48] Fragments of this sixteenth-century work appear in the nineteenth-century *Book of the Immortal Celestials.* In the preface to *Perfected Formulas for Guarding Life,* the author reveals how a Daoist immortal presented him with a scroll containing instructions for forty-nine different yoga positions, each one accompanied by a drug formula, an incantation, and a marvelous illustration of the yoga pose. Each position was designed to ensure the uninhibited circulation of the vitalities throughout the body. Luo described the route taken by the vitalities in response to the "perfected formulas" and praises their ability to "conquer the one hundred diseases:"

> Beat the Drum [and it] rides the River Chariot *[hetu]* above the Nine Palaces *[jiu gong]*; [thus] the Wind is born in the Mud Ball *[ni wan]* and the Three Corpses *[san hu]* are eliminated. Circulate [it from the] Smithy Bellows *[tuo yue]* below the Crooked River *[qu jiang]*; thus the waves on the Bitter Sea *[ku hai]* become clear (or settled) and the ten thousand demons are restrained.[49]

The "anatomy" that Luo describes is the inner body of the Daoist imagination. It is a rugged geography of mountains, rivers, and roads, luxuriously populated with palaces and courtyards, furnaces and fires, viscera and deities. Within the head is the Mud Ball, containing nine palaces, some of which house august deities, including the Jade Emperor.[50] Within the throat and leading down into the chest is the "Twelve-story Pagoda." The Viscera lie within the torso, each with their resident deity. If all the visceral deities were represented, a veritable menagerie of phoenixes, turtles, and two-headed deer would crowd the gut. Two animals figure prominently in these internal visions: the Tiger and the Dragon, representing True Yin and True Yang as they come together in the Yellow Court (associated with the Spleen). Beneath the Yellow Court, deep in the abdomen, the Cinnabar Field is a place of perpetual heat. It is the place where the vital Original *Qi* gathers (the Ocean of *Qi*), its fires fanned from below by internal "Smithy Bellows." At the very base of the torso, near the Bitter Sea, the yin vitalities pool, awaiting conveyance via various Chariots up the Marrow Path. The Chariots climb past vertebrae and squeezes through the Three Passes (or Gates) until they reach the Mud Ball . From the Mud Ball the vitalities begin a journey to the central regions of the body. There they will undergo a transformation that is the goal of inner alchemy *(nei dan):* the production of an internal elixir of immortality, symbolized by a representation of a baby boy growing within the belly of the (usually male) adept.

The folksy *Book of the Immortal Celestials* may seem an odd place to find treatises on Daoist anatomy and esoteric formulas for achieving immortality. But the *Perfected Formulas* is at the same time a manual demonstrating simple postures for the relief of backache, dizziness, exhaustion, and diarrhea through the circulation of *qi*. The movements are simple and require little or no exertion. The practitioner may sit in a modified lotus position and rub his belly, lie on his side and press his thigh, or stand with one arm and one leg extended forward. The exertion and skill comes not in the execution of the position itself, but in accomplishing the breathing technique that is part of each exercise. These exercises represent a medicinal form of *daoyin* (literally, guiding and pulling *[qi]*).

Many practitioners may have employed *daoyin* techniques to maintain limberness, unblock *qi*, and provide overall bodily health, but meditative techniques associated with *daoyin* could also be employed toward more transcendent goals. Although *daoyin* offered ways to benefit the circulation of *qi* in its natural directions, *daoyin* could be combined with breathing and visualizations in order to circulate vitalities in directions counter to their natural tendencies. In order to reverse the process of aging, the practitioner must "reverse the way of nature" *(diandao)* and bring together yin and yang, which would naturally be apart. Inner alchemy's theory of countercirculation held that the natural movement of vitalities within the bodies of the average, unvigilant human—the sluggish sloshing of Heavenly Water within the elevated head, the downward leaking of *jing qi* out of the body—led to decline and death. However, disciplined technique could conserve the body's fluids and direct the movement of *qi* through the appropriate crucibles of immortality. Through concentration, visualization, swallowing, and breathing, the adept could cause that which contains yang to descend and that which contains yin to ascend. The two forces converge in the center and their conjoining gives rise to the embryo of immortality.[51]

The practice of circulating inner vitalities during meditation and meditative movements was always linked to the act of breathing air. The breath would be consciously regulated in specific patterns that had to be learned and memorized. Formulas for memorization detailed the number of times one should breathe, the length a breath should be held, and the syllables one should form with one's mouth upon exhaling (making sounds such "shu," "hu," or "ah"). Breathing out in certain syllables was said to expel the *qi* from specific internal Viscera, thus aiding in the elimination of pathogenic *qi* from the body. As an added bonus, by breathing in external *qi*, controlling it, forcing its direction, and controlling its pressure, one also set in motion the circulation of Original *Qi*. Thus the internal circulation of invisible, ineffable *qi* was associated with the workaday process of breathing air. Both actions were related, and both actions could have a curative effect.

During the Ming, an explosion of texts combining techniques of *daoyin*, inner alchemy, *qi* circulation, and breathing become available under the category of *yangsheng*, or nurturing life.[52] It seems that an increasingly leisured yet anxious society increasingly turned to "nurturing life" to stave off old age and counter the effects of affluence.[53] Although the language of these works invoked the complex world of hexagrams, cosmology, and esoteric Daoism, their practical goals were often limited to the quick and ready curing of life's common aches and pains. In the *Perfected Formulas for Guarding Life*, the practical coincided with the extraordinary. The path to health and healing lay along the same road as the path to immortality.

CONCLUSION: CONQUERING THE ONE HUNDRED DISEASES

Texts that discussed *weisheng* in the late imperial period associated the term with at least one of these four things: the choice of the appropriate time and place for life's activities; the maintenance of appropriate ingestion regimes; the practice of sexual economy; and the circulation of vitalities through breathing, movement, massage, and inner visualization. Together these categories more or less describe the sum total of Chinese approaches to health: indeed, in its occurrences from the Song dynasty on, *weisheng* could easily be translated by a word as general and vague as *health*.

There are numerous points of similarity between this sketch of "guarding life" in late imperial China and the holistic traditions of hygiene in early modern Europe. Health had been the responsibility of the individual since ancient times, and texts from classical antiquity informed the creation of regimens in both cultures. Writings on health and longevity in Europe, particularly after the Renaissance rediscovery of Galen, stressed the "regimen of the non-naturals": air, diet, sleep, exercise, evacuation and sex, and the passions. Phenomena inside and outside the body were linked through systematic correspondences. In Europe as well as China, moderation in eating, drinking, and in the emotions were essential to maintaining health, for the body and the soul were in constant mutual interaction. The term *hygiene*, if used in a premodern European sense, is perhaps an adequate approximation of *weisheng*.

However, "guarding life" is an appropriate phrase to describe the preservation of health in a system where the primary vitalities are so susceptible to injury, depletion, and exhaustion. The Spirit, associated with the faculties of human intelligence, sensitivity, and comprehension, could be worn down by extreme emotion and the cares of everyday life. The Original *Qi* bestowed upon a human being before birth declined with age and ceased with death. Seminal Essence, the very essence of life, was spent through indulgence in sex or escaped inadvertently through nocturnal emissions. Its inevitable dissipation leads to premature death and debility. For the Daoist, the infant at birth is a powerhouse of pure energies, able to function at an intense level without tiring, for he has not yet begun the depleting process of living in the adult world of desires and cares. Zhuangzi councils that the "method for guarding life" is to become once again like an infant, brimming with the forces of life. The Way of *weisheng* promises to guard life against depletion caused by the inevitable injuries of living itself.

In order to avoid depletion, *weisheng* calls for constant conservation, moderation, and restraint in all of life's essential activities. Food should be simple and just adequate. Neither joy nor anger should be experienced in the extreme. Physical activity should be moderate. According to some, alcohol and sexual activity should be avoided altogether. Most warned that stern vigilance had to accompany the enjoyment of either. The underlying impulse toward restraint, combined with a belief in the mutual interpenetration of internal and external worlds, led to the development of an economy of health and the body more elaborate than that developed in the European hygiene tradition. The effects of intake/inflow—of foods, medicines, stimulation, and *qi*—needed to be calculated against the effects of output/outflow—of sweat, saliva, emotions, *qi*, and above all, Seminal Essence. This

was obviously not a simple quantitative correspondence of intake to out-
flow, a zero-sum game. The balance sheet could also show harm caused by
too much input, or an input of inappropriate combinations.

Although various adages of *weisheng* tutored a vigilant monitoring of
the bodily economy to ensure health, techniques were always available to
correct the depletions and injuries caused by inevitable lapses. Here the as-
tonishing range of Chinese techniques for health rivaled the complexity of
any European approach. Foremost was the use of foods and drugs to correct
imbalances and bolster the vitalities. Meditation, breathing practices, yoga,
and massage eliminated internal blockages and directed the healing flow of
qi to points throughout the body. Sometimes the ruthless calculus of hygienic economy could be circumvented entirely through the employment
of extraordinary skills. The technique of inner alchemy reversed and re-
combined bodily essences, thereby replenishing the vitalities and reversing
the aging process. For some adepts, the healthful benefits of sexual intercourse could be enjoyed without its attendant depletions through the practice of "returning the *jing* to replenish the brain."

As in European hygiene traditions influenced by Christianity, there is
an unmistakable moral tone to many of the precepts and admonitions associated with guarding life, beginning with Qi Bo's warning about the dangers of wine and women, which opens the *Inner Canon of the Yellow Emperor*. But guarding life also had its earthy side. For all the high moral tone
of some *weisheng* texts, there always seems to be a way out, a sort of practical forbearance for those who falter along the way. For every one admonition against drink, there are two formulas for hangover remedies. For every
lapse that leads to depletion, there are a dozen recipes for replenishing foods
and beverages. The one area that seems to have succumbed to moral sua-
sion over time is the realm of sex. By the late imperial period the goal of
sex is the production of progeny. Formulas and meditations were offered to
nurture sexual energies in order to conceive numerous sons, but *weisheng*
no longer counseled on how to bed multiple partners without depleting "the
jade stalk."

Although not explicitly stated, guarding life is primarily concerned with
the health of prosperous people. Even though the greatest harm to health
comes from internal depletion, depletion is rarely caused by want. Vitalities can be reduced by poor nutrition or deficient living conditions, but this
is not the main concern of most authors who write about *weisheng*. The real
culprit is almost always excess, and excess is a disease of the comfortable.
Anything done greatly *(da)* or in excess *(guo)*, whether it be mental exertion, sensual enjoyment, or even religious sentiment, will result in injury

(shang), scattering *(san)*, depletion *(xu)*, and even extinction *(jue)*. The ultimate anxiety is fear of lack, and yet lack is the result of abundance. In the calculus of *weisheng,* more is always less. Occasionally the sentiment is expressed that when it comes to health, the poor are in fact better off than the rich. They eat simply and avoid overindulgence in life. Since they are unable to afford luxuries, they are less likely to dose themselves with unnecessary medications or seek the advice of local "quacks." In their most ironic moments, learned doctors might comment that the poor's lack of access to drugs and medical advice actually worked to their advantage. As the thirteenth-century physician Li Gao noted, "The poor are better off than the rich in two ways: When they have strong opinions they can't be persuaded to change their minds, and when they get sick, they can't afford to be treated by a doctor."[54] It is clear that if any one group bears the stigma of lack with regard to *weisheng,* it is the elite. They can afford a surfeit of the good things in life, and yet they lack the moral vigilance to enjoy them wisely. *Weisheng* in late imperial China was the product of wealthy, cosmologically confident society whose primary anxiety was that it possessed too much.

.   .   .

A more complete discussion of Chinese paths to hygiene might focus on the thousands of texts dedicated to *yangsheng.* If there was a word that encompassed the practices discussed here into a discrete recognizable category of knowledge, it was *yangsheng,* or nurturing life. "Nurturing life" was in the title of hundreds of books and constituted a separate category in medical compilations. Texts on *yangsheng* and texts that discuss *weisheng* overlap in content: they both encompass *daoyin* exercises, meditation techniques, and dietary guidelines. *Yangsheng,* however, was the far more common term for hygiene in the late imperial period. Computer technology helps provide a crude indicator: a searchable database of the *Si ku chuan shu* (Complete collection of the four treasuries), a massive imperial compendium of texts compiled in the eighteenth century, reveals 6,773 occurrences of the term *yangsheng* in texts ranging from the Confucian classics to medical texts to the collected writings of literary worthies. A search for *weisheng,* on the other hand, only generates 925 "hits," many of which are repetitions of the same phrases over and over: *weisheng zhi dao* (the Way of Guarding Life), the formula for *weisheng tang* (Guarding Life Soup), and the titles of books, especially *Weisheng baojian* (A precious mirror for guarding life). In spite of these differences in frequency, however, it is clear that before the twentieth century, *weisheng* and *yangsheng* overlapped and coexisted within the same matrix of meanings, centered on a cosmology of correspondences, deeply concerned with *qi*.

In his audience with Genghis Khan, Changchun the Perfected One may have boasted that he possessed the Way of Guarding Life, but in general, paths to guarding life in late imperial China were diffuse, intertwined with food culture, projected through aphorisms about time and place, embedded in herbal formulas, hinted at through beliefs about health and sex. *Weisheng* was also diffused throughout the terrain of China's cities, interwoven with the markets, rhythms, and pleasures of urban life. It is to these connections between guarding life and the urban environment that we now turn.

2 Health and Disease in Heaven's Ford

Pan Wei (1816–1894) spent much of his time in Tianjin pondering how he could best avoid illness and death. While filling a lowly post at the city's imperial salt commissioner office, he studied ancient medical texts and culled their best techniques. On the first day of winter in 1858, he completed his compilation, entitled *Essential Arts of Guarding Life (Weisheng yao shu)*. *Essential Arts* begins with this meditation on the importance of guarding the body's vitalities: "Whether a man lives or dies, whether his sickness is serious or light, all depends upon the preservation or destruction of his Original *Qi* [*yuan qi*]. . . . All [things in the body] rely on it—the Viscera, the circulation tracts, Blood and *qi*, the muscles. If you are not careful, evil influences [*xie*] will enter and cause illness."[1]

Pan informed his readers that the harmful effect of external pathogens could be readily avoided if one employed the art of guarding life, which he summarized as follows:

> If every day you concentrate on the Cinnabar Field and intentionally
> cause your body's Water and Fire to mutually embrace, then your
> Spirit will flourish, your *qi* will be full, and evil influences will not dare
> to enter. Instead of waiting for pain and sickness to reach your body
> and then, moaning and groaning, go begging for a cure, it is far better
> to practice this technique for a few brief moments each day and thus
> avoid suffering.[2]

There was good reason to be worried about strengthening the body against "evil influences" in the late 1850s. Epidemics were rife in the area around Pan Wei's hometown of Suzhou. In 1853 the Taiping rebels captured the great southern city of Nanjing. For the next ten years, the modern world's most destructive civil war raged across the lower Yangtze Delta. As

Taiping rebels fought imperial forces and loyalist militias, death and chaos hovered over the Qing empire's most prosperous region.

Tianjin may have been called the "Ford of Heaven," but for Pan Wei, it is quite likely that this northern city lacked the charms of Suzhou, known throughout the empire as "Heaven on Earth."[3] In terms of Chinese urban history, Tianjin was a relative newcomer, a city created for business and bureaucracy in a later dynasty. With an official history only dating back to the Yuan (1279–1367), it was devoid of ancient temples and lacked its own great literati tradition. Tianjin was best known for uncouth things: fast-talking deal makers, crassly wealthy salt merchants, and swaggering hoodlums. Nevertheless, at the height of the civil war, it may have seemed like a safe and desirable abode. Taiping rebels reigned in the Jiangnan region, but the northern advance of their armies had been miraculously turned back just three miles short of Tianjin's walls.

Tianjin would not remain totally unscathed by the chaos that engulfed so many parts of the Qing empire in the mid–nineteenth century. Only a few months after Pan Wei completed his *Essential Arts of Guarding Life*, the city was attacked by an enemy that would prove far more successful than the Taiping. In the summer of 1858, a small fleet of British and French warships battled their way past coastal defenses at Taku and sailed up the Hai River toward Tianjin. After a brief battle outside the city walls, the victorious foreigners set up camp in the grounds of an imperial palace on the banks of the Hai.

Upon their arrival, European observers quickly created an image of the Chinese as a people who were ravaged by disease, lacking in personal hygiene, and devoid of any public consciousness about the preservation of health. By the early twentieth century, some Chinese embraced this image and critiqued their own people as lacking in something called *weisheng*, a term that grew to encompass personal cleanliness, environmental order, and government administration of disease prevention. Most mid–nineteenth century European observers lived isolated from Chinese communities and refused to acknowledge Chinese modes of preserving health. There is no reason for our scholarship to do the same.

Rather than use a twentieth-century definition of *weisheng* as "hygienic modernity" (and thus finding Chinese cities lacking), this chapter considers issues of health and disease in a Chinese city from the perspective of *weisheng* as "guarding life"—the constellation of practices, derived from long-evolving traditions, that guided the preservation of health for many Chinese. It takes seriously indigenous debates about the origin of disease and approaches to disease prevention, and suggests how these may have played themselves out in a specific urban setting. Each city, with its own configurations of land and water, its own assortment of natural assets and social configurations, provides a specific set of challenges to health—and specific resources to meet these challenges. During the tumultuous middle decades of the nineteenth century, the history of Tianjin's bounty and wealth, famines and floods, peacetime contentments and stresses of war, all shaped prevailing conceptions of disease and strategies to preserve health.

A complete consideration of health strategies in Tianjin should also seek nodes of community organization for disease prevention within the social structures of the Chinese city—its temples, its festivals, its religious charities and merchant organizations. A pre-twentieth century definition of *weisheng* would not bring these aspects into consideration: and yet the post-1900 claim that Chinese cities were devoid of public approaches to problems of health needs to be redressed. Before 1900, Tianjin had no government public health bureau. There were no municipal officials charged with the supervision of the city's water, waste, or medical services. This does not mean that these issues were ignored. Rather they were managed in different— and disparate—ways. Before the post-1900 discourse of *weisheng* combined these elements together as a site for the evaluation of the level of advancement of an entire city (or civilization), many of these elements were so tightly woven into the fabric of urban life that they seldom merited separate comment from contemporary observers.

This mode of investigating everyday health practices within a particular urban setting is quite common in the history of medicine in the West. Among its foremost practitioners is Roy Porter, whose many volumes weave tales of the personal experiences of sufferers and healers together with the epidemics, smells, edifices, and institutions of a specific urban environment, usually that of London during the eighteenth century.[4] To create these composite portraits of health and city, Porter made use of the many private diaries and public newspapers generated by early modern British society. If there are far fewer such studies for China, it is in part because these sorts of sources either do not exist at all or are not widely available. To produce a portrait of health and disease in a specific Chinese setting requires the creative synthesis of scattered fragments found in local gazetteers, literati poetry, medical treatises, and the chronicles of war, along with a critical reading of the observations of Europeans. Through these sources we can begin to build a picture of how people in Tianjin explained disease, sought to preserve health in daily life as individuals, and came together as a community to eliminate threats to health in the urban environment.

Chinese sources written before the arrival of Europeans, such as Pan Wei's *Essential Arts of Guarding Life*, tend to present life in Tianjin as healthful and the techniques for guarding life as efficacious. This may be explained in part by the literati physician's tendency—not totalizing, but prevalent—of excluding the poor and diseased from their writings. Certainly the arrival of European critiques based on nineteenth-century conceptions of science and progressive history facilitated the emergence of a Chinese discourse of urban decay. It is also possible that many of the insalubrious conditions associated with the urban environment in modern China—overcrowding, extremes of poverty, unrecoverable degradation of the natural environment, and the spread of devastating epidemics—were exacerbated by (though not entirely caused by) the arrival of imperialism itself. Without the statistics that measure these conditions in modern terms, it is difficult to prove change in a city's health over time. Scholars have detected evidence of increasing anxiety about urban crime, poverty, and overpopulation in the historical record for the late imperial period.[5] Yet in contrast to the specters of death and disease that haunted Industrial Revolution–period European discourse, the discourse of urban poverty in nineteenth-century Tianjin is remarkably muted. Tianjin before the arrival of Europeans may not have been a salubrious arcadia, but one must allow that strategies for guarding life in Heaven's Ford were to a considerable degree effective in preserving health.

TIANJIN'S LAND AND PEOPLE

Before the arrival of Europeans, Tianjin was one of the military and economic centers of north China. Its importance stems from its location between the sea and the empire's capital, Beijing. Tianjin is located approximately ten kilometers from the Gulf of Bohai, on the banks of the Hai River, approximately one hundred kilometers southeast of Beijing and one hundred kilometers southwest of Shanhaiguan, where the Great Wall meets the sea. The area around what would later be the city of Tianjin had been inhabited for thousands of years and grew in importance during the Yuan when Beijing became the capital of the empire. The name "Tianjin," or "Heaven's Ford," dates from the early Ming, when the Yongle emperor (the "Son of Heaven") was said to have crossed the Hai River near the town. Realizing the strategic military importance of this site so near the capital, the Ming established a military garrison, or *wei*, at Tianjin. The elevation of Tianjin to a garrison gave the place its urban status, manifested by the presence of a massive new city wall.

Although the town's identity was shaped by its military and administrative functions, Tianjin's periodic markets grew in size and frequency throughout the Ming, drawing an increasing number of merchants and traders and expanding the city's economic importance in the north China plain. From the mid–sixteenth century on, Tianjin not only guarded the gateway to Beijing from the sea, it also became an important center for the transport of grain and other goods to the capital from the south along the Grand Canal. Finally with the establishment of the Changlu salt administration in Tianjin in the early Qing, the city's economic position as granary, saltworks, transport hub, and credit center for north China was complete (see Fig. 2).[6]

In spite of its economic prosperity and administrative importance, the city of Tianjin did not have a harmonious relationship with its physical environment. Throughout its history, Tianjin waged a perpetual battle with water. The city was located on a flat, low plain that was crisscrossed by a network of nine major rivers and canals. Throughout the imperial period (and well into the People's Republic), Tianjin suffered from the constant threat of floods, and records from the Qing show that a major inundation struck the city once every few years. Even in normal times, water flowed fast by the walls of the city. The Hai River was a stone's throw from the eastern wall, and the Grand Canal wound its way along the city's north wall. To the south and west of the city lay immense marshes where tall reeds and lotuses swayed above the mud. Because of the layout of land and water, the expansion of the city was limited to the higher ground north and east of the walled city. In times of flood, waters encroached upon the south wall and sometimes engulfed entire neighborhoods within the wall. In spite of several major flood control projects undertaken during the Kangxi (1662–1722) and Qianlong (1736–95) reigns, water still remained a major threat to the stability of trade and commerce in Tianjin.[7]

The physical environment in Tianjin placed capricious constraints on the city's economy and greatly affected the lives of Tianjin's people. Yet up until the early nineteenth century, some observers found a certain bucolic beauty in Tianjin's watery world, as expressed in the following lyric that begins with the hearty phrase, ""Jinmen hao!" [Tianjin is excellent!]:

> Tianjin is excellent!
> Everywhere the water makes up our home.
> In the East Marsh, lotus flowers blossom in masses of white,
> By the North River, reeds bend yellow to the sky,
> The ocean tide flows up as far as the three villages.[8]

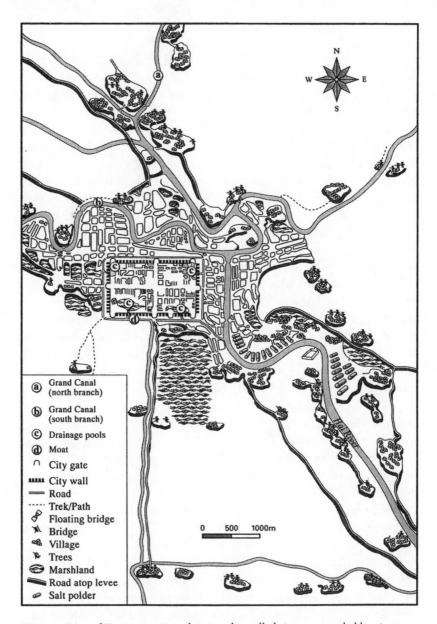

N
W E
S

ⓐ Grand Canal (north branch)
ⓑ Grand Canal (south branch)
ⓒ Drainage pools
ⓓ Moat
∩ City gate
⊥⊥⊥⊥ City wall
═══ Road
----- Trek/Path
Floating bridge
Bridge
Village
Trees
Marshland
Road atop levee
Salt polder

Hai River

0   500   1000m

Figure 2. Map of Tianjin, c. 1842, showing the walled city surrounded by rivers, canals, and wetlands. Note the many salt polders along the banks of the Hai River. From *Remaking the Chinese City: Modernity and National Identity, 1900–1950*, ed. Joseph W. Esherick (Honolulu: University of Hawaii Press, 200), 33.

The author, a native literatus named Fan Bin, wrote a series of one hundred of these lyrics, all of which began with the exclamation " Jinmen hao!" He had been inspired by the poems "Memories of Yangzhou" *(Yangzhou yi)* to write similar lyrics praising his native Tianjin, a city that was sometimes called the "Little Yangzhou" of the north. Indeed the Tianjin that Fan Bin portrays is as picturesque as that garden city of the high Qing, filled with gently swaying reeds, misty landscapes, and happy, prosperous people. Perhaps this pleasant vision of Tianjin was simply the product of a gentry poet's nostalgia. Yet it is possible to envision Tianjin in the early nineteenth century as a city where nature was not terribly strained by the human population, and humans found ways to coexist with nature's vagaries.

According to a census compiled in 1842, a total of 198,715 people lived within Tianjin's walls and in the areas immediately outside the walls—the recognizable urban neighborhoods of the larger administrative unit of Tianjin county *(xian)*.[9] Almost half the population of Tianjin proper, a total of more than ninety-five thousand people, lived within the walled city itself, in a relatively large area of approximately three square miles. The neighborhoods to the north and east of the walled city were home to approximately ninety thousand people; a much smaller number lived in the inhospitable land west and south of the city. The population within and directly around the walled city was approximately the same as that of contemporaneous Edinburgh or Marseilles, and larger than any city in the United States in 1850, with the exception of New York. If one adds the population of the city's outlying villages, then the entire population of Tianjin county in 1842 was 442,342, comparable to the populations of mid–nineteenth century Manchester or Liverpool.

Europeans who sailed to Tianjin in the mid–seventeenth century saw a city possessed of "Strong Walls, twenty-five feet high, full of Watch Towers and Bulwarks, and the place much set forth with Temples, very populous and so full of Trade, that hardly the like Commerce is to be found in any other city in all of China."[10] Sir George Stauton passed through Tianjin with Lord Amherst's embassy in 1816 and was also favorably impressed. He described the city's people as "chiefly well-dressed and of decent appearance, much fairer and better looking than those we had seen upon the coast, and indeed superior to those of Canton." These European observers were struck by the massive Ming-dynasty walls around the city, its parapets and towers befitting a military garrison. They could make out the fact that well over one hundred Daoist and Buddhist temples crowded within the city walls, while an equal number were scattered about in the neighborhoods outside of the walls.[11] What most impressed them was the flourishing commercial activity in the city, including trade in grain, textiles, and above all, salt. The banks of the Hai River were one big salt warehouse, covered with dozens of massive white mounds of salt awaiting packaging and distribution by the merchants of the Changlu circuit monopoly.

By the mid–nineteenth century, European impressions had changed. In 1858, Lord Elgin described Tianjin as "the most squalid, impoverished-looking place we had ever been in," although he was willing to acknowledge that Tianjin's streets were comfortably wide and less odiferous than the streets of southern Chinese cities.[12] What had changed the most between 1816 and 1858 was not so much Tianjin's appearance, but the expectations of British observers. Lord Elgin was particularly disappointed by the lack of grand architecture in Tianjin, citing "a few fantastically carved wooden arches" as "the only ornament of which the town could boast."[13] Elgin's eyes were searching for grand European-style edifices, but he was unable to read Tianjin's cityscape for its own signs of power. Apparently he had either not witnessed or was unmoved by the dozens of towering banner poles erected before Tianjin's many imperial government offices, nor did he realize that the massive stone lions standing before red gates signaled the mansions of Tianjin's wealthy merchants.

In comparison with European cities, Tianjin (like most Chinese cities) was not tall, and its grandeur faced inward, in layer upon layer of interconnected courtyards. Almost all buildings in the mid–nineteenth century were one- or two-story brick or wooden structures, arranged around open gardens, with only a simple facade or a wall facing the narrow streets. But centers of power abounded within the city walls. There were numerous government yamens, including the Tianjin magistrate, prefect, and circuit intendant compounds, the office of the Changlu salt commissioner, the Zhili governor, and numerous military officials. Not surprisingly, the walled city had the largest concentration of degree holders and miscellaneous servants (yamen runners, chair bearers, and so on) of any part of greater Tianjin. The walled city was also home to several of Tianjin's wealthiest families, members of the Eight Great Families (ba da jia) that included the city's leading salt, cloth, and medicine merchants.[14]

The city's commercial center was located north of the walled city, between the north gate and the banks of the Grand Canal. Myriad shops and native banks lined streets with names that signaled their commercial nature: Pot Store Street, Needle Market Street, and Clothes Bargain Street. The stores were filled with the busy negotiations of buyers, clerks, and merchants, while transport workers thronged the alleys, hauling goods to and from the river docks to merchant warehouses along the Grand Canal. At one end of this

merchant's world, outside the northeast corner of the wall, lay the entertainment district of Houjia hou (Behind the Hou family compound), with
its brothels, theaters, and teahouses. At the other end, outside the northwest corner of the wall, lay an area that could be considered the religious
center of Tianjin. This neighborhood was a jumble of Daoist temples, including temples of the City God, the Dragon King, the Immortal Lu Dongbin, Yue Fei and Guan Yi (the Two Loyal Ones) and two of the city's largest
Medicine King temples. The northwest corner was also home to the city's
many Muslims, or Hui people. The center of Hui life was the Great Mosque,
an imposing complex of buildings with sweeping, upturned eaves and multiple spires that dwarfed the more modest City God Temple nearby.[15]

Thriving residential areas spilled outside the city wall to the east as well.
The half-mile between the east wall and the Hai River was a neighborhood
that included the residences of wealthier merchants and degree holders along
with the homes of numerous shopkeepers and commoners. This neighborhood by the river was home to the city's most important temple, the Tianhou gong, the "Palace" of the Empress of Heaven, also known as Mazu, the
patron of sailors. This was one of Tianjin's oldest temples, and was the focus of the richest and most active ritual life in the city. The Tianhou gong
was the center of Tianjin's greatest temple fair, the Huanghui, held once a
year to celebrate the birthday of the Empress of Heaven. During the
Huanghui, the entire city joined in rowdy celebrations, opera performances,
and various street entertainments as the image of Tianhou was paraded
through one neighborhood after the other.[16]

The bustle and hubbub of Tianjin's business and ritual did not extend far
beyond the west or south city wall. The land there was often waterlogged
and not suitable for extensive building. In the mid-Qing some Tianjin gentry built pleasure gardens in the southern and western suburbs, erecting
pavilions, bridges, and cottages among the pools and marshes in an attempt
to create something of a "Suzhou" effect. By midcentury, some of these gardens were still intact but in a state of decline.[17] For the most part, with the
exception of a few temples and ramshackle residences, most of the land outside the west gate was occupied not by Tianjin's living but by the city's dead.
This area was the favorite site for charity cemeteries and individual graves.
To the west and south, unearthed coffins were a frequent sight, as floods
and tides disturbed shallow graves. On one spot of higher ground about one
mile south of the city wall stood the Temple of Oceanic Radiance, or
Haiguang si, one of Tianjin's largest Buddhist temples. This was to become
the site where the Treaty of Tianjin was signed in 1858 after the Anglo-
French defeat of the Qing at Taku. Later in the twentieth century this site

was destined to become the main garrison for the Japanese army in north China. But now, before the arrival of foreigners, the Temple of Oceanic Radiance stood alone in a placid setting of swaying reeds and narrow, sluggish canals.

This was Tianjin at mid–nineteenth century: a city whose economic activity had overspilled its walls and created bustling neighborhoods along the river, while the center of official power and prestige remained within the city walls. No great architectural monuments stood out along its narrow streets. Perhaps the centrally located bell tower or the residence built at the Three River Fork for the emperor Qianlong could be considered among the more distinctive buildings in Tianjin, but essentially there were no great monuments that distinguished Tianjin from other Chinese cities. The Qing officials within the city walls took care of their primary business of maintaining civil order from within yamen courtyards hidden to the outside world. The presence of the government was not signaled by impressive facades. The identity of Tianjin was shaped by its merchants, who kept goods flowing in and out, employed the laborers that thronged the streets, and maintained the homes and shops that made up the greater part of the gray brick and wood cityscape.

DISEASE IN HEAVEN'S FORD

What diseases did Tianjin face in the nineteenth century? Neither Tianjin gazetteers nor the communications of government officials in Tianjin from the period shed much light on the question of disease and epidemics. This lack of systematic coverage of outbreaks of disease makes it difficult to reconstruct even a basic chronology of major epidemics in Tianjin, and even more difficult to discuss the predominant nonepidemic causes of death over the years. It is possible to extrapolate from the historical epidemiological data available from cities in the West and approximate the illness environment of Tianjin, but this is not entirely adequate for two reasons. First, it does not allow for variations in both virulence of disease vectors and resistance to disease in different environments and populations. The greatest problem with such an approach, however, is that imposing categories of disease from biomedicine can distract from the goal of understanding the cultural construction of disease in nineteenth-century China.

Instead of attempting to determine what diseases Tianjiners suffered according to modern biomedicine, the most fruitful approach is to consider how those in Tianjin themselves defined the causes of illness and infirmity.

Sources such as poems, memoirs, unofficial histories, and medical treatises help create an impressionistic sketch of Tianjin's ills as they were experienced by Tianjin's people.[18] By understanding what things were conceived of as points of danger—in the environment, within the body, and in the actions of humans—one can better understand the methods that were employed to guard life against them.

Charles Rosenberg has suggested that explanations for illnesses revolve around two poles: configuration and contamination. The configuration view holds that disease is the result of an abnormal imbalance in an otherwise normally balanced relationship between humans and the environment. Contamination "foregrounds a particular disordering element" in the production of illness: Rather than tracing multiple causes, including imbalances within the body itself, a contamination model conceives of disease as an attack from a particular external agent.[19] Both configuration and contamination models rely on another element, that of predisposition, to explain why certain individuals are susceptible to illness at any given time, whereas others remain immune. Configuration was a predominant explanation for disease in guarding life traditions. Illness arose when abnormalities occurred in the normal, predictable patterns of the cosmos, and personal habits of diet and self-regulation determined which individuals would be predisposed to succumb to the influence of such imbalance.

Later Qing medical treatises from the Tianjin area take a contaminationist approach. They emphasize that disease, particularly epidemic disease accompanied by fever, is the product of unpredictable external pathogenic agents, *li qi,* or pestilent *qi.* This emphasis marks these texts as inheritors of the thinking of the late Ming physician, Wu Youxing (1582?–1652). In modern Chinese historiography, Wu is considered the founder of the Warm Factor school (Wen bing pai). It is commonly thought that Warm Factor physicians distinguished themselves from the Cold Damage school (Shang han pai) by identifying pestilent or heterogeneous *qi (li qi, za qi),* and not seasonal or seasonally anomalous *qi,* as the cause of most epidemic febrile disorders.[20]

For Wu Youxing, pestilent *qi* appeared unexpectedly, causing illness for almost everyone within a certain area. It was impossible to predict its appearance through cosmological systems such as Phase Energetics. It attacked humans by entering through the mouth or nose, not by seeping into the pours as did seasonal *qi.* Pestilent *qi* was not Cold in nature like seasonal *qi,* but caused damage through its abnormally Warm properties. Once inside the body, pestilent *qi* did not follow normally understood channels of movement of seasonal *qi* within the body, so diagnostic techniques based on old theories would not work in treating such ailments.

Wu's iconoclastic text turned much of received tradition on its head. Marta Hanson, in her path-breaking work on the physicians associated with the Warm Factor school, has pointed out that Wu's medical skepticism was in line with the growth of cosmological skepticism in the late Ming.[21] Wu Youxing's work, like the work of many skeptics of his time, presented the natural world as inherently random, unpredictable, and unmeasurable. His work also inspired a general trend toward thinking of regional variety in both physical constitution and in disease causation. The practitioner could no longer rely solely on the classics of the past, but would have to rely on his experience and acumen to treat disease successfully. This was particularly true since bodies varied from place to place, and pestilent *qi* produced diseases "so various there are too many to count."[22]

In the Tianjin area, Hong Tianxi (fl. 1750) and Liu Kui (c. 1735–c. 1805) took up Wu Youxing's challenge to understand local variations of bodies, disease, and treatments. Tianjin native Hong Tianxi sought to fill in the gaps of Wu Youxing's work and tailor it for northern bodies in his *Supplementary Commentary to the Treatise on Epidemic Disease (Buzhu wenyi lun)*. Originally published in the late eighteenth century, it was reprinted again in 1821 and in 1854 by philanthropic Tianjin gentry who wished to celebrate the local physician and popularize his life-saving knowledge.[23] In his *Explication on Epidemics from Pine Peak (Song feng shuo yi)*, Liu Kui pondered the intersections of Warm Factor and Cold Damage theories of disease causation as he saw them manifested on the north China plain. In the process, he catalogued seventy-two different types of "miscellaneous epidemics," their names drawn from the healers and common people of Shandong and Hebei whose approach to disease was decidedly different from that of learned doctors. Together, these works provide insight into how people in Tianjin and the surrounding area may have experienced and named their sufferings.

From Liu Kui's perspective, common north China folk-names for illnesses vividly captured the pains and signs caused by invading pestilent *qi*. In twisted neck fever *(nian jing wen)* the neck and abdomen swelled like the expanding throat of a toad. In toad fever *(jiemo wen)*, the abdomen did not swell, but the throat was swollen and sore, the whole body ached, and grainy tears fell from the eyes. In crab fever *(xiezi wen)*, small bumps grew on the inside of the throat, with red striations emanating out from them like the claws of a crab. Children suffered from the grape epidemic *(putao yi)*, where large and small pustules the dark purple color of grapes broke out over the entire body, and blood issued from the gums. *Fan* illness suddenly turned people over or reversed them, rendering them unable to talk, eat, or even breathe. *Sha* illnesses sometimes entailed loose bowels, violent vomiting, and paralyzed limbs, but sometimes they were characterized by full-body blisters or pains like those caused by contact with blister beetle shell *(ci mao wen sha)*. Other sufferers experienced illnesses that were struggles *(zheng)* named after a variety of animals. These illnesses brought various combinations of headaches, swellings, rashes, loss of sight, and sweating, combined at times with odd behavior such as calling like a bird, running about in the fields like a rabbit, or rolling about in the dirt like a pig.

The modern reader may discern approximations of clinically defined disorders in this list of seventy-two illnesses: smallpox, measles, scarlet fever, meningitis, encephalitis, conjunctivitis, diphtheria, dysentery, stroke. But in Liu Kui's folk catalogue, no one illness has a perfect one-to-one correspondence with a biomedical disease. There are no discrete agents of infection, only (from the physician's perspective) generalized pestilent *qi* or seasonal *qi*. Disorders are distinguished through combinations of symptoms, or they may be almost identical and distinguished primarily by the different cures used to treat them. Psychological disorders by standards of modern biomedicine are not placed in separate categories: many *zheng* diseases include strange behaviors, but an equal number do not.

Absent from Liu Kui's list is anything specifically related to *lao*, a wasting illness that has been associated with tuberculosis by modern scholars. This is perhaps because it was not identified as an epidemic, a sort of sudden onset illness experienced by many in the same region at the same time. Hong Tianxi provides further insights into this absence. For Hong, *lao* was decidedly present in Tianjin, but it was something that needed to be carefully distinguished from Warm Factor illness. The two were often confused, but a misdiagnosis could lead to treatment with the wrong remedies. Drawing on Warm Factor thinking, the Tianjin physician used medicines to nurture yin and repel yang in cases that resembled *lao* but that Hong, through brilliant diagnostic technique, had determined were actually febrile epidemics. He sometimes did so over the protests of the patriarchs of important Tianjin families who were convinced that their teenage children's distressing loss of weight and production of phlegm were sure signs of affliction with *lao*.[24]

Both Liu and Hong agreed that epidemics were primarily produced by impure or filthy *qi (hui qi)*. Liu reasoned that one could tell that filthy *qi* coincided with epidemics because villages where disease raged always contained hundreds of thousands of black flies. Flies love filth, reasoned Liu, and they can smell *hui qi* even when humans cannot. Just as flies swarm around newly excreted human feces, an accumulation of flies indicated a concentration of *yi, xie,* or *hui qi* (pestilent, heteropathic, or filthy *qi*). Neither physician suggested that *hui qi* was the sole cause of disease, or that epidemics were the only form of affliction. Care had to be taken in making diagnosis to distinguish between the underlying causes of disease, which could still include abnormal seasonal *qi,* and imbalances caused by improper behaviors. But Warm Factor fevers afflicted many in times of want, and, as Liu Kui in particular observed, the northern provinces had their share of famine, overcrowding, and poverty.

In the area around Tianjin, individuals suffered from eye afflictions, disorders that manifested themselves through the skin, gastrointestinal disorders, and numerous illnesses that affected the throat and lungs. Children might suffer from terrifying cases of smallpox or measles. Young people in the prime of their lives wasted away from the ravages of tuberculosis, a disease that even attacked the wealthy and well educated. Eyes of young and old alike swelled, became red, exuded grainy discharge, or went entirely white. Sometimes throats swelled, breathing grew difficult, and red clawlike striations appeared. Sudden fevers might be accompanied by uncontrollable loosening of the bowels and vomiting. Physicians who were aware of the latest theories might attribute these symptoms to pestilent *qi,* but this explanation was far from hegemonic. Great shifts in the patterns of the cosmos might bring disease that could sneak in through carelessly open pores, only to become apparent with the change of season. Unwise food choices might upset the balance of the internal organs. Even malevolent spirits might cause mischief with one's health. In nineteenth-century Tianjin, healers and sufferers alike were puzzling out the roles of contagion, configuration, and predisposition in causing "the one hundred diseases."

GUARDING LIFE AND THE URBAN LANDSCAPE

How might a hypothetical middle-aged resident of mid-nineteenth-century Tianjin preserve his health against these threats? The primary locus for disease prevention and cure in China was daily family life. The medicinal properties of foods came into play with almost every meal. Those whose families had adequate incomes could afford to prepare and consume foods in a way that was appropriate to the season and balance the characteristics of foods in a way that fostered bodily well-being. However, Tianjin's local cuisine also provided many opportunities to transgress the guidelines for guarding life with gastronomic indulgences.

Unlike most of Tianjin's poorer denizens, who would content themselves with locally grown barley or corn, a relatively prosperous urbanite could keep his family's larder filled with rice—a commodity imported from the south that passed through Tianjin with reliable frequency. Servants would on a daily basis purchase different varieties of cabbages, spinaches, broccolis, and carrots that were grown in abundance in the countryside around Tianjin. A Muslim resident might wish to use cool yin vegetables to balance the hot yang of frequently consumed mutton, a meat that could be purchased in the northwest area of the city from local butchers who killed the animals in accordance with Islamic law. In the northwest corner, Muslim and Han residents might also stop at one of the many Muslim-run snack vendors and indulge in the more working-class fare of salty dough cakes fried in oil *(jian bing, jian gao)*. Still a Tianjin specialty today, fried cakes were enjoyed as a street snack as far back as the seventeenth century. In the late imperial period, Tianjin was known throughout the empire for its "oily-mouthed" businessmen. Although the adage obviously referred to the adeptness with which Tianjiners' slippery tongues could argue a price, those tongues were already well-lubricated by the abundance of grease and oil found in local Tianjin cuisine.

In the evening, to make up for the Heat of the oily fried cakes, a Tianjiner might order an oil-free and bland *(qing-dan)* bowl of soup with greens prepared for his dinner. He might enjoy several cups of grease-clearing fragrant green tea imported from Jiangsu or Fujian. Or as a special precaution, he may have had a servant brew a medicine to promote digestion. Each of the dried roots and roasted leaves would be individually measured and prepared before being boiled together with water. Medicines were usually simmered until the water content was greatly reduced, resulting in a strong-smelling brew of considerable potency. The bitter taste of this nighttime draught would probably be rendered more pleasant by the addition of sweet (though still medicinal) licorice root, making it a beverage more suitable for evening relaxation.

The family's servants would take care to make sure that the water for tea drinking and cooking had been purified before its use. This took some doing, as household water vats throughout the city were kept full with water from local rivers, typically from the water of the north branch of the Grand Canal. For a small fee, professional water carriers delivered the water from the river directly to the home.[25] Once it was poured into the large covered vats, considerable effort was put into making the water appear clean. Although it is not understood when the practice began, by the mid–nineteenth century, families in Tianjin were clarifying their drinking water through the addition of aluminum potassium sulfate (known as alum, or *fan*). A small amount of the powder would be placed in a bamboo tube that was punctured with small holes. As the tube was swirled in the water vat, the alum would mix with the water and precipitate out particles of sand and dirt. The more prosperous the family, the more vats the household possessed. Wealthier families had as many as three vats. Water was precipitated in the first, then moved to the second vat, precipitated again for extra clarity, and then stored in the third vat. Other water-treatment techniques included the addition of red beans and sesame in the water vats twice a month, or allowing black beans to soak in the water vats overnight.[26] No matter what preliminary water treatments were carried out, water was almost universally boiled before drinking and consumed hot, as cold water could seriously damage the stomach and other internal viscera.

On a quiet evening, the Tianjin resident would retire early with his boiled medicine, ready to begin work even before sunrise the next day. If, however, he had clients to entertain, his evening might take a different course. If the season were right, he might engage a banquet featuring local Tianjin seafood. One dish was sure to be composed of fresh crab lightly sautéed in wine, ginger, and scallions. Other dishes would feature shrimp, jellyfish, or saltwater fish that were plentiful and cheap during the spring and fall. Even visitors from the wealthy south could be impressed by the abundance and flavor of Tianjin's seafood. Once such guest, a Hangzhou man named Jiang Shi, proclaimed that Tianjin's fish "triumphed over that of Jiangnan."[27] He was so moved by Tianjin's aquatic offerings that he composed more than ten poems in praise of them. Jiang even found exotic (and somewhat erotic) seafood adventure when he ate the potentially poisonous *hetun* fish (Japanese, *fugu*) at a Tianjin restaurant. He marked the occasion with the lines: "Swiftly the cleaver cuts the *fugu* / Its center holds the milk of [the famous beauty] Xishi / There is no other taste like it in the world!"[28]

Complex business negotiations or simply the search for continued pleasures might have necessitated a trip to the local entertainment districts. Establishments offered music, wine, opium, and the company of attractive women in simple but elegant settings. Although Tianjin's pleasure quarters never had the reputation of such southern cities as Nanjing or Suzhou, its charms were nevertheless lauded in local literati poetry. In the imagination of the poet, Tianjin's summer evenings resonated with the sounds of frogs chirping after the rain and the plaintive strains of popular airs played on delicate stringed instruments. Perfumed women wearing silk brocades, jeweled hairpins, and alluring curved-sole shoes on their tiny bound feet exchanged amorous glances with handsome young playboys and the occasional successful merchant or aging scholar. Throughout the night, opium smoke formed swirling screens around brothel divans. Even Tianjin's opium pipes were gorgeous works of fantasy, intricately carved with laughing Daoist immortals and beautiful women languidly flying kites.[29]

A gentleman at midlife might have been concerned about declining vigor and the impact it might have on his ability to resist illness. It is difficult to know if Tianjiners intentionally restrained sexual activity for health reasons or practiced coitus thesauratus (returning the Seminal Essence to nourish the brain) when sex was unavoidable. There is no direct evidence of the circulation of such techniques in nineteenth-century Tianjin, nor are there population statistics for the city that might reflect the moderation of fertility that would accompany such techniques.

Whatever the fate of this gentleman's *jing,* circulating vitalities through meditation and movement was certainly common in nineteenth-century Tianjin. From any number of popular manuals, such as Pan Wei's *Essential Arts of Guarding Life,* our Tianjin resident might have begun to learn various postures, exercises, and breathing techniques to circulate healthy *qi* and invigorate the body. All that he would need would be a quiet place within his home and a few quiet moments each day, preferably in the morning, to practice his art. As a guide to practice, he could commit to memory Pan Wei's "Comprehensive Formula for Twelve-Part Brocade," a verse describing the twelve steps of a meditation technique designed to circulate the vitalitites. The "Comprehensive Formula" uses highly allusive language to conjure up a marvelous internal landscape filled with soaring mountains, flowing rivers, and heavenly columns. It describes the practitioner's actions as he controls his breathing, repeatedly swallows his saliva, sways his torso, and massages his head, feet, and waist. He performs these movements according to cosmologically significant numbers: thirty-six teeth gnashings, twenty-four head-knockings, three sets of saliva swallowings. The vitalities, portrayed as leaping tigers and swimming dragons, begin to circulate within the body. The final result is a glowing fire within the abdomen as the vitalities unite and burn with health-giving energy. The verse ends with a praise of the technique's efficacy, and an exhortation to frequent practice: "Continue with diligence, at no point break off with it, / And the myriad illnesses will transform into dust."[30]

IN TIANJIN'S MEDICAL MARKETPLACE

In spite of the urban dweller's best intentions, imbalances within his body might have coupled with external pathogenic *qi* to give rise to debilitating discomforts. What options for cure would be available to him in Tianjin?

> Jinmen is an excellent place!
> Along the river, cloth tents are open for business,
> On red paper men display their salves and medicines,
> Fortune tellers cast the copper coins
> For customers seeking their destiny.[31]

If the sufferer were feeling ill but well enough to walk about, he might seek a cure in the bustling medicine market in the northwest sector of the city, on the banks of the Grand Canal near the northwest corner's Medicine King Temple. There peddlers in herbs set up shop alongside experts in the divinatory arts, men who could consult cosmological charts, read facial physiognomy, or consult the *Book of Changes* for clues to the prognosis of an illness.[32] Some experts in the healing arts might prefer to read pulses and conduct basic examinations before they recommended herbs; others might offer a set of herbs to match specific symptoms.

In general, Tianjin was well-stocked with the herbs, roots, animal parts, and ores used in Chinese medicine because of its central location in the north China medicine market. Ginseng, deer antlers, tiger bones, bear fat, and herbal drugs from Manchuria and Mongolia were transported south to the great wholesale market at Qi prefecture in central Zhili province. Located about 150 kilometers southwest of Tianjin, the market at Qifu (present-day Anguo City) drew buyers from Beijing, Shandong, Henan, and even as far south as the Jiangnan area. After the introduction of steam shipping in the late nineteenth century, Tianjin became the central transport hub for essential northern medicines heading south for large markets in Shanghai and Canton.[33]

If a Tianjiner wished to avoid the common bustle and uncertain products of the Medicine King Temple vendors, he could find a large selection of high-quality raw ingredients and processed medicines in liquid or pill form (*cheng yao*) at one of Tianjin's larger pharmacies. The best known was Longshunrong, located not far away on Needle Market Street outside the north gate. Founded in 1850 by a member of the Bian family, Longshunrong became so successful that the family's profits from medicine outpaced those from their original business in textile trading.[34] In the mid–nineteenth century, the founder of the store, Bian Chufang, was both manager and resident physician. In Longshunrong the Tianjin resident could, in a comfortable setting, consult a doctor of traditional Chinese medicine about his illness, receive a formula, and purchase the herbs all at the same location.

A vast range of individuals identified themselves as doctors of medicine in Tianjin, from men who claimed to be former practitioners in the Imperial court (Taiyi), to itinerant wanderers from the countryside possessed of practical experience and perhaps a few secret family prescriptions. In the nineteenth century, although there was a recognizable hierarchy among doctors, there was no formal definition of qualifications, no medical schools, and no government regulation of medical practice. As a result, the medical hierarchy was constantly contested and reformulated by the sellers of medical services themselves. Holding at least a low-level degree demonstrated an individual's erudition and grasp of the classics and distinguished the practitioner as a "Confucian Doctor," or *ruyi*.[35] The best-known doctors were often those who came from families that had specialized in medicine for several generations.[36] Since medical education was an entirely private undertaking, hereditary lineage spoke of effective transmission of learning, rich accumulated experience, and perhaps the possession of miraculously effective secret family prescriptions that had been passed down from generation to generation.

A doctor of high reputation and scholarly bearing could demand high fees and be selective about his patients. Requests for his services that came from outside his immediate social circle would have to be accompanied by recommendations from prominent citizens. Unless the physician, out of a sense of compassion or social obligation, contributed part of his time to the relief of the needy, it is unlikely that any but the wealthy would benefit from his expertise. As the nineteenth-century Tianjin adage put it, "Palanquin-riding doctors don't call at the door / Of any family that happens to be poor" *(yisheng zuo qiao, qiong jia bu dao).*[37]

Although there is little information from this earlier period about specific Tianjin doctors and their practices, evidence indicates that by the late nineteenth century the central debate among doctors in the Tianjin medical world centered on the nature of febrile disease and epidemics. China experienced its own period of "therapeutic uncertainty" during the Qing. There was increased debate about the nature of seasonal epidemic outbreaks, and sharp disagreements among doctors and in the popular mind about the appropriate methods of treatment.[38] The central question of diagnosis became whether febrile disease was of a Cold Damage or Warm Factor nature. Books on techniques for distinguishing between Cold Damage and Warm Factor symptoms were published and republished by local Tianjin elites and eventually by the Zhili provincial government itself. It was believed that a failure to distinguish between the two types in a diagnosis would lead to an improper drug therapy, which in turn would lead to a swift and certain death.

If a Tianjiner fell ill with a serious "seasonal disease" such as a fever in the early spring or severe diarrhea in the late summer, it would not be surprising if he anticipated the visit of a doctor with considerable dread. A popular adage expressed the consequences of a wrong medical judgment: "A doctor who misinterprets the classics of medicine kills men with an invisible dagger" *(xue yi bu ming, an dao sha ren)*. Accurate diagnosis was crucial, since it dictated the prescription of medicines, and the wrong medicine, in the minds of physician and sufferer alike, could exacerbate illness or even cause death. Just to be sure, the sufferer was likely to call in more than one physician, compare their diagnoses, and then hope for the best. For those who could afford it, the popular wisdom held that "if you're seriously sick, hire three doctors" *(you jibing qing san shi)*.

TEMPLES AND SHAMANS

For many people in Tianjin, preservation of health had a very powerful public element in the form of worship at the city's numerous temples dedicated to healing deities. Temples to Sun Simiao, the deified seventh-century physician known as the Medicine King (Yao wang), were most clearly identified with healing and were among the most common temples in Tianjin. Every neighborhood in the city had its own small Medicine King temple (Yaowang miao); in fact, some scholars have suggested that an area was only considered a neighborhood once it had its own Yaowang miao.[39] The largest Medicine King temple in the Tianjin area was the Mountain Peak Temple (Fengshan miao), popularly called the "Mountain Lair" (Fengwo). Located about one day's walk south of the city wall, this was said to be the most effective *(ling)* Medicine King temple of all in the Tianjin area. A week-long fair was held at the "Mountain Lair" during Sun Simiao's birthday, which was celebrated on the twenty-eighth day of the fourth lunar month. Each spring the fair was extremely crowded with the sick, their relatives, vendors of medicines and foods, and purveyors of rural entertainments. Contemporary witnesses to the festival recorded that the atmosphere inside the temple was thick with incense and the sounds of the ill praying to the deity from their palanquin beds.[40]

Medicine King temples were not the only places where Tianjin residents turned for help when they were sick. Perhaps the greatest concentration of worship associated with healing took place at Tianjin's Empress of Heaven (Tianhou) Temple. The Empress of Heaven, the "patron saint" of China's sailors, had an entourage of affiliated deities who carried out specific healing and disease prevention duties. Married women of Tianjin who desired sons bought small, anatomically correct clay images of male babies from the Tianhou Temple and placed them in their homes in the hope that "Our Lady of Sons and Grandsons" (Zisun niangniang) would grant them their wish. After birth, infants were brought before "Our Lady of Measles" (Banzhen niangniang) to pray for protection from measles and other poxes. The Tianhou Temple also contained an image of the Foolish Brother God (Shadi shen) who helped cure children's diseases, and a statue of Zhang the Immortal (Zhang Xian) who protected children from "fright" *(jing)*. Third Granny Wang (Wang san nainai) intervened in women's disorders, and Our Lady of Eyesight (Yanguang niangniang) cared for the numerous ocular afflictions that plagued Tianjin.[41] Even if the Tianjin gentleman would not have taken recourse in The Empress of Heaven, chances are that some of the women of his household were frequent visitors to Her temple.

Serious illnesses that found no cure elsewhere may have merited the employment of Daoist priests to purify the sufferers' home. The priests would set up an altar within the home and perform ritual movements around it. Less affluent sufferers might frequently turn to Daoist priests, who would, for a small fee, provide a special healing or protecting charm designed to display above a sickroom door. Daoist priests might also write charms on paper for the sufferer to wear on his person, or the sufferer would burn the charm and ingest its ashes. Daoist priests might have particular skill in writing such charms, but charms could also be made at home by consulting instructions found in medical texts or locally produced almanacs.

Some in Tianjin did not only consult Daoist deities formally housed in the city's temples—they sought the direct intervention of spirits with the help of Tianjin's female shamans. Popularly called "aunties," or *guniangzi,* these women conducted semipublic rituals within the sufferer's home that included chanting, incense burning, and incantations to request that spirits descend and possess them for the benefit of the patient. The spirits addressed by these women were the products of local folk beliefs, outside of the formal pantheon of officially sanctioned Daoist deities. The female shamans invoked one or more of five female spirits, collectively referred to as the "Five Great Ones" *(wu da jia),* which included Old Mrs. Bai, Grandma Huang, Auntie Hu, and two other ladies surnamed Liu and Hui. Apparently female shamans did a brisk business in Tianjin's poorer neighborhoods. A disapproving retired Tianjin magistrate observed with scorn that most of the female shamans' clients were "ignorant women," who were drawn to the mediums "like iron to magnets."[42]

Although there were no government bureaus of public health, Tianjin was not devoid of conceptions of social responsibility for the health of the community. Lay associations paid for the upkeep of temples like those of the Empress or the Medicine King, seeing to it that the images inside remained bright, incense and candles remained burning, and the temple space remained open to receive the prayers of the community. Guilds and other organizations collected dues to enable members to make pilgrimages to efficacious Medicine King temples during holidays and in times of illness. Perhaps a definition of "public health" for premodern China should be extended to include the numerous temple associations that provided a basis for collective action and social integration in urban settings.[43]

SALT MERCHANT BENEVOLENCE AND URBAN HEALTH

Another possible locus for finding "public health" in nineteenth-century Tianjin was the charitable endeavors of the city's wealthiest local elites, the salt merchants. Tianjin gazetteers proudly point to the existence of charitable and public welfare institutions going back to the early Qing, when Tianjin was still a small military garrison town. By the nineteenth century, salt merchants ran orphanages, cemeteries, hospitals, and corpse-collecting services for the city.[44] Although many salt merchant families had originally come from the southern provinces of Zhejiang and Jiangsu during the eighteenth century, by the nineteenth century they were considered part of Tianjin's community. Their endeavors to serve the city were seen as a form of local benevolence, conducted in conjunction (of course) with the work of imperial officials, who always hailed from elsewhere.

The increase in charitable activities of local merchants mirrors the increase of merchant involvement in local governance throughout the empire during the Qing dynasty.[45] Scholars of the Qing have noted an expanding zone of local responsibility for local affairs as urban society became more affluent, more complex, and harder to harmonize with the imperial ideal of small government. Later in the nineteenth century, in the wake of post-Taiping reconstruction, Tianjin saw an intensification of salt-merchant involvement in local services. The city also became a center of regional welfare organizations established by merchants from Jiangsu and Guangdong.[46] These organizations functioned with the benefit of imperial government oversight, contributions, and blessings; they were neither independent spheres of private activity nor "public" government office; instead they combined features of both.

An examination of elite charitable activities in Tianjin reveals that many of them either intentionally or indirectly benefited the health of the city. Excluding public works such as bridge and road repair, we find that public cemeteries and burial societies were the favorite undertaking of officials and merchants alike. These projects ranged from simple donations of land for cemeteries by individuals to the formation of corporate organizations that retrieved and buried abandoned corpses.[47] The foundation of public cemeteries and burial societies outnumbered any other form of public welfare work for the eighteenth and much of the nineteenth century. What factors could account for the preponderance of this kind of service?

Simply by virtue of limited space available in a city, the disposal of the bodies of the dead is a serious problem for any urban community. Though often overlooked in studies of public health history, it must be considered a fundamental problem of urban public health management. In imperial China, the proper burial of the dead was one of the cornerstones of Confucian ritual and belief. Funeral rites were one of the highest expressions of *li,* the web of ceremony and proper behavior that ensured stability and cohesion in society and kept *luan,* or disorder, at bay. Providing this most basic rite of burial for the poor was an expression of the ordered humanity of the contributor and of the community he represented.[48]

Another motivation for such a service was the fear that unattended corpses would directly harm the health of the community. There are two related strands that reflect this fear. One is the belief that if burial rituals were not provided or were conducted incorrectly, the soul of the dead would separate from the body and cause illness among the living. In funerals in nineteenth-century north China, as well as those observed in contemporary Hong Kong, caution was taken at several stages during the ritual to ensure that the potentially harmful spirit stayed inside the body in the coffin.[49] The spirits of corpses that have been denied any burial whatsoever might become hungry ghosts that could possibly converge and give rise to epidemics.[50] Thus the dignified contributions of Confucian-minded officials and gentry-merchants to burial societies and public cemeteries protected the public health of Tianjin.

In addition to these undertakings, the officials and gentry of Tianjin also cooperated to form two major institutions that benefited the living. The Yuli tang, or Hall for the Care of the Masses, was founded in 1687 for the benefit of sojourners who came to Tianjin and found themselves sick or seriously injured without a family to provide for them. The complex was located outside of the west gate near the San Guan Temple, on land otherwise devoid of anything save "layer upon layer" of graves. The Hall sheltered some of Tianjin's sick and infirm, providing them with clothes, food, and medicine, and finally coffins when they died. By the mid–nineteenth century the Hall for the Care of the Masses was popularly known as the "Yangbing tang," or Hall for Nurturing the Sick, suggesting that its medical function eventually surpassed its other charitable roles.[51] However, its population of elderly, handicapped, and chronically ill poor were most likely difficult to treat, making the Hall for Nurturing the Sick more like a nursing home than a medical establishment committed to the cure of its patients' ills. In this respect it was analogous to contemporaneous charity hospitals in Europe and the United States, institutions that accepted cases that were beyond the power of medical skill, thus in essence becoming an asylum for the sick poor, an almshouse.[52]

Although Tianjin's one "hospital" was more an almshouse than a center for medical innovation, new medical technologies were disseminated in the city through the activities of local salt merchants. In 1852, the prominent Tianjin salt merchant Hua Guangwei read a book about the foreign method of using cowpox vaccine to prevent smallpox. This technique, developed in England in 1796 by Edward Jenner, was already being used in Canton and other southern cities by the early nineteenth century. Hua decided to try the technique in Tianjin and established a cowpox vaccination clinic (Niudou ju) for the poor in the center of the city. Hua's clinic became popularly known as the "Hall for the Protection of Infants" (Bao chi tang). Branch clinics were subsequently set up in other locations around the city, making this one of the first "public health" institutions consistently available throughout Tianjin to all of Tianjin's residents.[53]

Chinese vaccinators altered the Jennerian technique in accordance with indigenous understandings of smallpox pathology. Clinics offered free vaccinations for two periods during the year, once in the spring and again in the fall, in accordance with the precepts of medical cosmology. The cowpox matter was scraped onto the skin on the upper arm at points on the Lesser Yang circulation tract *(shaoyang jing)*. The Lesser Yang circulation tract is associated with the Kidney system, which is also associated with the Gate of Life, the location where the fetal poison *(taidu)* that gave rise to smallpox was thought to reside. The Lesser Yang circulation tract channeled the vaccine to the Kidney system and also facilitated the drawing out or leading *(yin)* of the hidden poison back out to the surface of the body.[54]

According to one observer, each day during the "vaccination season" hundreds of children received free vaccinations at the clinic. The clinic recorded the names of the children and required them to return three days after the initial vaccination to see if the procedure had been successful. Statistics were kept so that the clinic's success rate could be monitored, and very few children were lost due to unsuccessful vaccinations.[55] These statistics are no longer extant, nor do we know what techniques the clinic may have used to maintain the freshness of the vaccine, a reoccurring problem in nineteenth-century application of Jennerian vaccination.[56] Nevertheless, the Hall for the Protection of Infants proved successful, and its longevity (it continued until 1949) indicated a continued popular demand for its services. The presence of the Hall greatly improved the chances for survival for Tianjin's infants and probably served to increase the average life expectancy of the city's residents. Although it may have begun as a service to the city's poor—and may have even tested the vaccine first on the city's poor to determine its safety—The Hall went on to be the first citywide institution designed to nurture the health of the city as a whole. As such it was a significant element in the history of public health in Tianjin.

The Tianjin cowpox bureau was an example of the speedy assimilation of a recent European medical innovation by Chinese social and medical structures. Within two decades the technique had spread from Canton, with its small but permanent community of Europeans, to a city that by the mid–nineteenth century had seen foreigners pass through only once or twice in its history. The method was adjusted to fit Chinese medical theories and was disseminated by organizations that were well-entrenched in the social fabric of the city. In contrast with the violent introduction of the smallpox vaccination under colonial rule in India, in Tianjin there was little sense that the vaccinations performed at the cowpox bureau were an aspect of an alien European medicine. Acquired in the absence of foreign actors, it was assimilated and adapted by Chinese agents for Chinese society.[57] In the mid–nineteenth century, Tianjin's elites stood in a position of equality and autonomy vis-à-vis Europe, able to pick and chose aspects of the West as they saw fit, without the complication of European personnel or the intrusion of European armies.

CONCLUSION

Tianjin's medical profile was not unique to that city. Tianjin shared many of the same concerns and cures with other cities throughout the Qing empire. Cities from Taipei to Taiyuan had medical marketplaces; millions around the empire were at risk for diphtheria, scarlet fever, tuberculosis, eye disease, and smallpox. Little work has been done on common conceptions and terminologies for disease in late imperial China, but many other places had their share of "grabbing diseases" and "the camel runs." Physicians who aligned themselves with either Warm Factor or Cold Damage debated disease etiology and therapeutics throughout China.

Tianjin's story is perhaps more recognizably a north China story. Warm Factor physicians recommended violent sorts of treatments for their "robust" northern patients more often than they would for "delicate" southerners, treatments that might include "heroic" therapies such as bloodletting and purging.[58] The persistence of more conservative Cold Damage ways of thinking about disease in the north made for particularly sharp debates between physicians. In terms of social practices, the similarities between Beijing and Tianjin are striking. Temples in Beijing had the same deities who dealt with infertility and childhood diseases. Shamanistic healers who invoked the spirits of grannies and animals practiced in Beijing as well. Tianjin pilgrims prayed for health at Beijing's Medicine King temples, and perhaps Beijingers made the pilgrimage to Tianjin's Mountain Lair. Far more work needs to be done to discover regional variations and similarities in healing cultures in China, which, after all, was a massive empire that encompassed more diversity than Europe. Sojourners in business and government such as Suzhou's Pan Wei may have helped to homogenize various parts of the empire: the treatise on guarding life written by this southern gentleman became a best-seller in north China in the late nineteenth century. But whether a picture of regional distinction or integration emerges, one thing is clear: Tianjin in the mid–nineteenth century was a vibrant society whose people strove to achieve health and prevent disease on their own terms.

. . .

Tianjin saw "Western medicine" for the first time in 1858, the same year that Pan Wei published his guide to guarding life. In that year, Western medicine arrived in Tianjin along with invading Western armies who were fighting the Qing in the Arrow War (what Chinese call "the Second Opium War"). In the spring of 1858, French and British forces stormed the Qing coastal defenses at Taku, ten miles east of Tianjin, where the Hai River empties into the Bohai Gulf. The foreign ships cautiously negotiated the twists and shoals of the Hai River and arrived in Tianjin in early June. The "battle" for Tianjin involved a brief skirmish with local forces, which the Europeans easily won. They then anchored at the Three Forks and set up camp at the Ocean-Viewing Pavilion (Wang hai lou), part of a palace complex that had been built for the Qianlong emperor on one of his southern tours. In a large hall within the Temple of Oceanic Radiance complex, the Qing and the British negotiated a treaty that bore the city's name. The Treaty of Tianjin called for the establishment of permanent ambassadors in Beijing, set specific tariffs on opium, and opened six new treaty ports. Oddly enough, the Treaty of Tianjin did not include Tianjin among the cities to be opened.

From the perspective of some Chinese observers in Tianjin, the presence of European troops in their city was a humiliating episode caused by Qing military incompetence.[59] Poorly commanded, the Qing defenses fell too quickly, and the local merchant-led civilian militia was no match for the foreign armies. When they realized that the defenses would not hold, most of the households in Tianjin that could afford to do so quickly fled the city, leaving behind what one American observer called "a beggarly population."[60] Looting was widespread as poorer Tianjiners took advantage of the absence of the wealthy. The elites who remained to try to preserve public order watched with shame as poor Chinese jumped into the Hai River and swam up to the foreign ships, begging for food and other handouts. Tianjin's elites had given the foreigners fine meat and other delicacies as a gesture of peace—and to avoid the chaos that foraging soldiers might unleash in the city. The foreigners in turn threw these gifts overboard into the Hai for the sport of watching the Chinese fight among each other for the spoils.[61]

Chinese chroniclers of the events of 1858 contain many such criticisms of the Chinese themselves, but only a few eccentric observations about the invading British and French. One observer noted that as soon as the British set up camp at the Ocean-Viewing Pavilion, they proceeded to slaughter hundreds of sheep. The foreign soldiers seemed to exist on nothing but massive quantities of fresh meat, and the stench of mutton hung around them wherever they went.[62] Other observers criticized the Qing's lack of organization while praising the kindness and efficiency of the Europeans. Much to the surprise of the townspeople, who expected to encounter a ruthless marauding enemy, the barbarians were not only rather well behaved, they also took in wounded Qing soldiers, treated them with medicine, and then released them to return to their homes.[63]

Chinese sources leave no trace of what kind of medical treatment these men received. Perhaps it was not the medical techniques themselves that seemed surprising, but the manner in which they were delivered. This pattern would continue as the European presence in Tianjin increased through the nineteenth century. Western medicine in the mid– to late nineteenth century was in a state of considerable flux. Some of its theories of disease causation and therapeutic practices would not have seemed so unusual to a Chinese physician. The major difference between Chinese and European approaches to health and disease in the later half of the nineteenth century lay in their social and political context. In the decades that coincided with European conflicts with the Qing, Northern European nations had solidified an unprecedented philosophy that linked the health of a population directly to the economic and military success of the nation-state. National and municipal policies of health quickly became a core aspect of a newly emerging European discourse on progress and civilization. By the end of the nineteenth century, the perceived lack of government involvement in matters of disease prevention would become a powerful symbol of the deficiency of Chinese civilization. In a new world of global imperialism, "guarding life"— *weisheng*—could no longer be left as a responsibility of the individual or the local community, but would have to involve the state, the nation, and the race.

3   Medical Encounters and Divergences

> Of the whole preceding process of civilization, nothing remains in their consciousness except a vague residue. Its outcome is taken simply as an expression of their own higher gifts. . . . And the consciousness of their own superiority, the consciousness of this "civilization," from now on serves those nations which have become colonial conquerors, and therefore a kind of upper class to large sections of the non-European world.
>
> NORBERT ELIAS, *The Civilizing Process*

The year 1842 was an important one in British history. That year saw the signing of the Treaty of Nanking, which ended the Opium War, opened Hong Kong, Shanghai, and other Chinese ports to British Settlement, and signaled the beginning of Great Britain's military dominance over Asia's largest empire, the Great Qing. It was also the year Edwin Chadwick published his monumental *Report on an Inquiry into the Sanitary Conditions of the Labouring Population of Great Britain*. In his report the lawyer, reformer, and utilitarian sought to demonstrate the primary importance of environmental factors in disease. He proclaimed through numbers and powerful prose that the shamefully high mortality rates among Great Britain's poor were caused first and foremost by dirt, stagnant water, and bad air, conditions that the nation's government had the obligation to detect and to eliminate. Within the next few decades the health of cities became a centerpiece of European definitions of their "advanced" civilization. For many Europeans, superiority in medical theory and disease control became the main characteristic that distinguished the "West" from the "Orient."

European confidence in such a "great divergence" in medicine was misguided and premature. I draw the phrase "great divergence" from Kenneth Pomeranz's work of the same title, *The Great Divergence: Europe, China, and the Making of the Modern World Economy*.[1] Pomeranz argues that economic differences between China and Europe were minimal until the nineteenth century, when parts of Europe began to reap the full benefits from accessible fossil fuel sources and armed imperialism. Until that moment of divergence, both sides of the Eurasian land mass labored under the same demographic and environmental constraints and developed equally successful strategies to address those constraints. Although Pomeranz's theory has stirred considerable debate, such questions of similarity and divergence can meaningfully be applied to other areas where Europe claimed an early advantage. Theories of disease causation and disease prevention in China and Europe did not manifest great divergence for most of the nineteenth century, in spite of the congratulatory self-evaluation of Europeans as they established their military superiority over the Qing empire. What did differ was the political and social organization of disease prevention, and this very recent divergence fueled the most contentious medical encounters between Chinese and Europeans at midcentury.

A sanitary revolution was sweeping Britain's cities, but this recent interest in government-organized methods of disease prevention was not the result of medical innovation. It was instead the product of a unique set of trends in the economy, society, and philosophy of England in the mid–nineteenth century. Reforms in the political organization of health and medicine were reactions to shocking deficiencies that were revealed in the course of battling epidemics at home and fighting wars abroad. Great Britain's successful simultaneous prosecution of industrial production and imperial expansion rested on the health of its two national forces: labor and the military. Trial and error in the laboratories of the city and the empire produced meaningful divergences between Europe and China that emerged later in the nineteenth century, divergences that would fuel the creation of a discourse of Chinese deficiency centered on hygiene.[2]

Arriving only a few years after the publication of Chadwick's report and the contentious beginnings of national public health reform in Great Britain, the British soldiers and civilians who came to Tianjin in 1858 nevertheless brought with them a well-established sense of medical and sanitary superiority. Once they landed on Qing soil, British military officers and civilians seemed to forget that their home country still had high infant mortality rates, increasing rates of tuberculosis and dysentery, and was still susceptible to devastating epidemics of cholera and typhus. The Industrial Revolution that had produced the military might needed to defeat the Qing and other foreign powers had brought disease to an increasingly impoverished domestic populace. The British medical profession was experiencing a period of uncertainty about the efficacy of their therapies, and British practitioners possessed diverse ideas about what caused disease.

The diversity of understandings about disease and therapy held by the British physicians who came to Tianjin (and the sometimes surprising similarities between the approaches of British and Chinese practitioners) demonstrates that at this point there was no single "Western medicine" that was different from and dominant over "Chinese medicine," and no single view of Chinese as unhygienic and unfit. When they first arrived in Tianjin, the British changed the city's landscape and established hospitals in the name of health, but it would be another forty years before shifts in science and an intensification of imperialism would join these practices under the hegemonic construct of a hygiene that distinguished modern from non-modern, a distinction embodied in the twentieth-century meaning of *weisheng*. This lack of hegemony came in part because the diversity in British practice was accompanied by no small measure of error. For all their sense of civilizational and hygienic superiority, the British in Tianjin were not immune from sanitary blunders or eccentric medical theories. Like the Chinese around them, they were susceptible to the ravages of epidemic cholera. And in Tianjin, Great Britain was not even immune from military defeat at the hands of the Great Qing.

This narrative of medical encounters and divergences begins amid the Arrow War, as Western medicine entered the Hai River and sailed toward Tianjin aboard HMS *Coromandel*.

BLOOD AND WATER IN THE BATTLE FOR TAKU

In mid-June of 1859, the newly appointed British minister to the Qing court, Sir Frederick Bruce, arrived off the north China coast near the Qing fortifications at Taku. Accompanied by a large fleet of British and French gunboats, Bruce planned to sail up the Hai River from Taku to the city of Tianjin. From Tianjin, Bruce was to travel overland to the imperial capital of Beijing. There his task was to present the Qing court with the ratified version of the Treaty of Tianjin that his brother James, the Eighth Earl of Elgin, had negotiated in that city the year before.

As the British fleet prepared to approach the Taku forts, Dr. Walter Dickson, surgeon of Admiral James Hope's flagship HMS *Chesapeake* and head medical officer of the fleet, prepared a small hospital aboard HMS *Coromandel*.[3] Dr. Dickson's preparations were thorough but calm. The British did not expect many casualties. Given the ease with which Lord Elgin's smaller fleet had defeated the Qing at Taku the year before, the fleet's commander, Admiral Hope, was confident that this year's mission would meet with little military resistance. Dr. Dickson did note that in spite of the anticipated ease of the military mission at Taku, his ship had been excellently stocked with medical supplies, from bandages and quinine to dried beef and brandy. This medical abundance for the China Station had also been noted the year before by Lord Elgin, who described the generous provisioning of medicines and "oceans of porter, soda water, wine of all sorts and delicacies . . . for the military hospitals" in Hong Kong, and correctly concluded that his pleasant situation was the result of the "fearful memories of the Crimea which were too close for anyone to count the cost."[4]

Lord Elgin was referring to the Crimean War of 1854–56, an event that demonstrated to the British empire the central importance of sanitary services for its armies. The British force of over 97,000 troops lost only 2,255 men at the hands of the enemy, but suffered 17,225 casualties from disease. French losses were even more horrific: of a total of 68,065 casualties in the war, 59,815, or 88 percent, were the result of disease.[5] Cholera, dysentery, and fevers swept through entire regiments, in some cases striking seventy-five out of every one hundred men.[6]

Contemporary observers blamed these woeful disease rates on the inefficiency and inadequacy of the Army Medical Department. Reports in London newspapers exposed numerous problems in the staffing, supply, and management of battlefield medical hospitals. Among the Medical Department's most outspoken critics was Florence Nightingale, the British nurse famous for both her selfless service to the wounded and her ability to mobilize public opinion. Reports in the British press from Nightingale and others made the state of military medicine a cause for national shame. An article in the *London Times* in January of 1855 lamented that the sad conditions of the hospitals and medical care in the Crimea would earn for the British "the title of the 'European Chinese,' incapable of anything but the merest routine, unequal to the slightest emergency."[7] It was through the efforts of Florence Nightingale and other critics that a Royal Commission on the Health of the Army was founded in 1857. Thus the medical debacle in the Crimea had resulted in improvements for medical personnel aboard ships in the China Station.[8]

Dr. Dickson's first journal is lost. Perhaps he, like many of his fellow medical officers in the Royal Navy, had filled his first medical journal with detailed observations about the atmosphere and environment at various points along the China coast. Medical officers had good reason to be vigilant about the Chinese climate, for the medical theory of the day held that many illnesses could be attributed to the actions of the air on the human body. European bodies were believed to be particularly vulnerable to the effects of "exotic" or "tropical" climates. By the mid–nineteenth century, British physicians had lost their earlier enthusiasm about the ability of Europeans to adapt to the climates of Asia. The "acclimatization" of the European body to exotic environments was an unlikely possibility. For whites, diseases caught in the colonies seemed to be more intense than the same disease at home, and tropical locales seemed to produce their own unique set of devastating infirmities.[9] Each colonial locale produced its own particular geo-medical configuration, and medical observers had to be vigilant in mapping out the miasmal terrain. This was a difficult challenge for medical officers aboard navy ships, since their vessels might be exposed to a number of different torrid zones on any particular journey. For ships in the China Station, a mission to sail from Hong Kong to Tianjin was, in terms of climate, like crossing the oceans from Bombay to Portsmouth. South China's waters may have threatened with tropical vapors, but north China's cool waters offered the danger of tropical disease without the tropics.[10]

Dickson began the second volume of his journal in mid-June 1859, with his ship's arrival in the waters off of Taku. After pausing for a few days to make ready, on the afternoon of June 25 the chief military officer of the expedition, Admiral Hope, ordered the ships to proceed into the mouth of the Hai River to begin their journey to Tianjin.

The Qing court had no intention of signing Elgin's treaty and issued orders to repulse the invading forces before they reached the capital. British gunboats broke through the chain barrier that the Qing had placed at the mouth of the river and proceeded upstream in direct line with the great Taku fort on the left bank of the river. To the astonishment of the British, the Qing fort opened fire with a salvo so accurate that it immediately crippled the lead ships. Unable to pass, the British forces attempted to storm the fort at low tide, but they had to wade across an open plain of five hundred yards of wet mud with no cover against the Qing fire. Qing muskets and cannons opened on the British with deadly precision as the hapless soldiers staggered in the muck.

Near the fighting on the Hai River, the U.S. Navy steamer *Toeywan* watched as the British troops fell beneath the Qing guns. The United States had proclaimed neutrality in this episode of the Arrow War, but the sight of Anglo-Saxon sailors being killed by an "Asiatic" enemy was too disturbing for the *Toeywan*'s captain, Josiah Tattnall. In a violation of official U.S. neutrality, Tatnall ordered his flat-bottomed steamship to tow the British launches back to their fleet. As he made this order, Tatnall reportedly let out a ringing cry that expressed his racial affinity with the wounded British and galvanized his men into action. "Neutrality be damned!" Tatnall exclaimed in a now oft-quoted phrase, "Blood is thicker than water!"[11]

Anchored some distance away from the fighting, Dr. Dickson awaited the outcome of the battle as darkness fell. He described in his journal the trauma and confusion met by his well-stocked hospital on the *Coromandel* when the hundreds of wounded finally arrived. By midnight, Dickson estimated that the number of wounded had reached more than 360. Surgical supplies ran out; Dickson noted that his assistants preformed numerous amputations without the aid of chloroform. The surgeons worked late into the night, treating the wounded liberally with opiates and alcohol in an attempt to "alleviate the great sum of misery" that lay before them.[12]

After the traumatic assault on Taku, Dickson and his assistants managed as best they could the fevers and wound infections still under their care. The treatment of wounds illustrated one of the basic underlying concepts that guided Western therapeutics: an overheated body must be aided in ridding itself of the poisons that cause disease. Light cold-water dressings and catheters helped drain off pus. Such treatment may have led to infections and gangrene, but the principles of antisepsis were not well known until later in the nineteenth century, long after anesthesia was commonly used.[13] Chemical and herbal drugs were also administered with the goal of helping the body expel poisons. Many illnesses, particularly inflammations and fever, were believed to be caused by an overstimulation of the system. The purges and sweats that resulted would drain away heat and produce a calming of overexcited organs.[14] Emetics such as tartaric acid compounds and ipecacuanha helped purge the patient's stomach, whereas mercury, usually in the form of calomel (Hg_2Cl_2), produced increased salivation and purged the bowels.[15] Aboard the *Coromandel*, the postoperative high fevers and excited pulses of wounded soldiers were treated with oral doses of mercuric chloride, a therapy that may have only served to hasten their all-too-frequent decline to death.

If a sailor survived the trauma of wounds, amputations, and postoperative infection at Taku, it was likely due in great part to his possession of a hearty constitution. However, one should not minimize the contribution made by the skill of the surgeon. By the 1860s, the most useful advances in British medical techniques had been in the field of surgery. New methods of managing wounds, setting bones, and staunching bleeding were making amputation less of an automatic response to severe wounds.[16] The surgical skill of Dr. Dickson and the inherent resilience of the body helped many British sailors survive their ordeal at Taku.

The last element that should not be overlooked in the relative success of British medicine was the role of organization. Post–Crimean War reforms had ensured the proper stocking of nutritious foods for the sick, along with bandages and bedclothes to provide for their comfort. Medicines were requisitioned through regular channels within the military command. Although no British nurses were employed aboard ships in the China Station, wounded soldiers were treated by a regular and increasingly professionalized staff of medical personnel after they returned home. The sailor wounded at Taku would be returned to England for convalescence at one of the Royal Naval hospitals, perhaps at Portsmouth or Greenwich. There he would find himself in the company of other British amputees from stations in far-flung, exotic lands.[17]

The accounts from Dickson's journal provide a vivid description of Western medicine as it was practiced in the late 1850s, when Western doctors and Western medical concepts first entered Tianjin. Unlike the experience of many other cities in China, Western medicine was brought to Tianjin not by benevolent medical missionaries, but by the military surgeons who accompanied belligerent British forces in the Arrow War. Medicine increased the efficiency of the army and aided the objectives of the expanding British empire, particularly after the debacle of the Crimean War. Although his medical journal narrates the human suffering accompanying a military failure, the very presence of Dickson and his skilled assistants at Taku clearly demonstrates the British state's employment of medicine to further its interests and secure its goals.

It is this political aspect of Western medicine in the mid–nineteenth century that most distinguished it from healing and medical thought in the Qing. British physician's theories of disease and the therapeutics they used to cure them were not inherently superior, more complex, or more scientific than Chinese approaches to healing in the mid–nineteenth century. There actually existed many points of similarity between the medicine of British physicians in Tianjin and that of Chinese healers, particularly with regard to their conceptualization of disease etiology. Western expertise in surgery (in contrast with Chinese approaches) is well documented, but in terms of internal medicine, particularly approaches to febrile epidemic diseases, Western medical superiority was far from evident. Most British physicians, like Warm Factor physicians in China, blamed disease on miasma, or a combination of miasma and invisible fermenting agents that rose from the soil or climate of a region. At this point in history, British and Chinese medicine were distinguished by divergences in sensibilities and divergences in action. For example, both British and Chinese observers feared miasmas, but unlike the Chinese, the British were obsessed with *smelling* them out. Once they had identified the effects of miasma on health, Qing medical thinkers planned preventions for individuals, whereas the British countered miasma through sanitary engineering. Organization and action, rather than underlying premise, provided the main divergence between the Qing empire and Western Europe.

THE BRITISH NOSE COMES TO TIANJIN

In the summer of 1860, Britain had its revenge on the Qing for the 1859 defeat at Taku. The British command learned from their fatal mistake the year before and took the Taku forts from the rear instead of launching a frontal attack from the sea. A force of more than two thousand men occupied Tianjin while the rest of the joint Anglo-French force went on to Beijing and the fateful burning of the Summer Palace. The Qing was forced to sign the Peking Convention, which enacted the terms of the Treaty of Tianjin. Almost as an afterthought, perhaps in light of how fierce the resistance had been at Tianjin in 1859, the Peking Convention also mandated that Tianjin be open to foreign settlement.

The large garrison left at Tianjin included Irish cavalry, several hundred Cantonese laborers from Hong Kong, British engineers, and a medical staff of several doctors.[18] Part of the occupation force set up camp at the Temple of Oceanic Radiance (Haiguang si), the large Buddhist temple where the Treaty of Tianjin had been negotiated two years before. Another camp was set up in the Ocean-Viewing Pavilion, the palace that had been built for the Qianlong emperor's visits to Tianjin. From these headquarters in the north and south, teams of British soldiers took daily forays around the city walls and into the city itself. Some teams searched out food and supplies, while others made maps and drawings of their surroundings, recording the appearance and location of temples, the government buildings, the dwellings of the people.[19] A bit later, British military and civilian personnel brought their surveying equipment to a location southeast of the walled city and began plotting out the boundaries of what would become the British Settlement in Tianjin.

Colonel G. J. Wolseley, quartermaster to the British forces, recorded his impressions of Tianjin and the surrounding area in his journal. His visual observations of the land and the people were augmented with frequent comments about potent, unseen forces: the unknown emanations that rose from this foreign land and permeated the atmosphere around him. Wolseley was a direct inheritor of the anxiety over putrefaction that gave rise to early modern Europe's obsession with "the foul and the fragrant."[20] Even though Wolseley expressed considerable doubt about "those wild theories" of disease and the "twaddle about sanitary arrangements" that were prevalent in the post-Crimean British army, he was deeply worried about the foul vapors that frequently offended his nose.[21] It seems that the olfactory aspects of China detracted from its ocular pleasures. At an otherwise picturesque temple, he was repulsed by and somewhat fearful of a nearby pile of coffins awaiting an auspicious time and place for burial. According to Wolseley, "The musty odors prevalent there detracted much from the charm of the scene, and rendered a frequent application of the pocket-handkerchief to one's olfactories indispensable."[22] Later while passing through a rural district he noted: "There is no part of the world to which distance lends more enchantment to the scenery than in China. When actually amongst the highly-manured fields of that empire, the olfactory organs are so rudely assailed by the variety of stenches . . . that a second trip across the fields is seldom taken."[23] Wolseley had stumbled upon one of the secrets of Chinese agriculture: the use of human waste to fertilize fields, a practice that, at least from Wolseley's perspective, was more unpleasant than the bird guano or crushed bones that the British used to fertilize their fields back home.

But Europeans were not the only ones intrigued by new odors during this Sino-British encounter: It seems that smells and vapors were among the first topics of discussion that Wolseley shared with the Chinese. Entries from his journal and fragments of Chinese writings give some sense of the combination of mutual prejudice and good-natured curiosity with which the two peoples observed each other, a curiosity that included interest in the odor of the "Other." In what seems to have been a fairly jovial conversation, Wolseley somehow conveyed to his Chinese audience that he found their country olfactorily offensive. The Chinese responded in kind, informing Wolseley that they found the British to be a particularly odoriferous race. Wolseley was willing to admit that the British might have "a national odor" easily distinguishable to the Chinese, but he claimed that his Han Chinese informants found his British smell less objectionable than the boiled-mutton smell they attributed to the Manchus and Mongols.[24]

Wolseley and his fellow British officers were convinced that the smells and vapors they sensed rising from the Chinese landscape were not harmless but had the potential to inflict severe illness, particularly if the vapors were emanating from a groundwater source. One of the first engineering tasks the British forces undertook in Tianjin was the elimination of stagnant water from the area around their camps. The worst offending spot was the moat that ran the entire course of the city wall. Convinced that vapors from the moat would visit pestilence upon the troops, the British (or rather, the Cantonese laborers employed by the British) moved tons of soil from higher ground and used it to fill in the part of the moat that stood between the city wall and their headquarters at Qianlong's Ocean-Viewing Pavilion.[25]

Unfortunately, the British had failed to realize that the moat was an essential part of the walled city's drainage system. Normally, runoff from the walled city's water collection pools poured into the moat and was flushed away into the Hai River by summer rains. Their engineering feat may have temporarily made the British more confident of their surroundings, but by the middle of the winter, water in neighboring Chinese residential areas on both sides of the city wall was a foot deep. Rather than alter their drainage plan, the British troops simply moved to higher ground within the city walls and took up residence in the Temple of the Empress of Heaven. The temple had large courtyards and spacious buildings perfect for storing munitions and housing soldiers, but the British found them cluttered with a large variety of odd statues and altars. To make room for troops and supplies, the British removed the statues from the temple and destroyed them. According to one observer, the people of Tianjin watched in anger as the foreigners smashed their most beloved deity and all her accompanying deities, including the Holy Mother of Mount Tai, Our Lady of Sons and Grandsons, Our Lady of Measles, and Our Lady of Eyesight. Tianjin was now devoid of the gods that guarded the city's health.[26]

THE GREAT DIVERGENCE: "A HYGIENE OF THE PUBLIC"

British troops filled in the city moat and destroyed the Tianhou Temple in part because they brought to Tianjin a different way of approaching the health of communities. This approach found the cause of disease within the environment, not within individuals, and it saw the environment as inherently malleable. To prevent disease, it turned not to the individual body, but to the very structure of the environment. "Public health," as it became known much later, was a product of the Enlightenment, the Industrial Revolution, and imperialism. This product of late-eighteenth and early-nineteenth-century Western Europe represented one of the greatest divergences between the Great Qing and Great Britain.

Writing from Paris in 1790, Jean Noel Hallé, a professor of physiology and hygiene in the newly reorganized Royal Academy of Medicine, noted a change in approaches to health that had been evolving since the seventeenth century. According to Hallé, two important divisions of hygiene had emerged: "*Public hygiene* and *private hygiene*, depending on whether one attends to man collectively or in society or whether he is viewed as an individual. It is in the *public hygiene* that the philosophic physician becomes counsel and spiritual guide to the legislator."[27]

This new public hygiene was at once expansive (rethinking the meaning of government and people) and parsing (counting, dividing, calculating). In

England, Germany, and France, physicians, state counselors, and amateur scientists counted populations, calculated death rates, and diagnosed the health of groups, particularly the poor. The French Revolution added salubrity to the state's obligations to its citizens. But as the poor were studied, they became a "race apart," a barbarian within. The question became how to provide for their salubrity so that their ill-health would not compromise the health of the nation.

This new understanding of the relationship between the state and its population, together with the combined crises of cholera and the Industrial Revolution, brought a full-fledged sanitary state in England. During the cholera epidemic of 1832, the mortality of the laboring poor in Britain's overcrowded, dismal cities shocked utilitarians into thinking through the knotty problem of how to reduce poverty and eliminate disease without creating a class of dependent poor. After the cholera epidemic, Edwin Chadwick, author of the 1834 New Poor Law that incarcerated the poor in workhouses, conducted a massive survey of Great Britain's major cities. The resulting *Report on an Inquiry into the Sanitary Conditions of the Labouring Population of Great Britain* correlated occurrences of filth, fever, and poverty. Chadwick's solution for this problem was for the government to remove filth—and the miasma it produced—through a comprehensive program of public works: sewers, drainage, water supply. By improving the urban environment through engineering, Chadwick reasoned, the government could reduce poverty and reduce its resulting economic loss to the state, all without eliminating the role of individual culpability.[28] Some physicians countered that the diseases of the poor were caused not so much by dirt, but by predisposing factors such as poor diet, insufficient clothing, overcrowding, and the other deleterious effects brought on by unemployment, low wages, and poverty. Some went so far as to suggest that the best way to eliminate disease was to have the government guarantee a basic, healthful standard of living to all its citizens.[29] But for Chadwick, "disease was smell."[30] Eliminating smell through the sanitarian path of state-mandated public works was the most economical and rational way to eliminate disease.

This new political emphasis on the role of miasma in producing disease inspired a surge in drainage projects, the building of sewers, and a reconfiguration of water supplies throughout England. New awareness and anxiety over bad air, decomposing matter, and "sewer gas" increased as town authorities negotiated with water companies, debated the costs of sewer systems, and struggled to hire qualified civil engineers who could—with soil, shovels, and science—eliminate the swamps and cesspool that covered the British landscape.[31] Overseeing these projects were municipal sanitary boards staffed not by physicians but by lawyers, clergy, and other political elites. By the 1860s, the elimination of marshes would become a hallmark of advanced civilization. Thanks in part to Chadwick and the rise of sanitarianism in nineteenth-century Britain, the "wilderness of marshes" found in and about China's newly opened treaty ports would not be tolerated for long by their new landlords.[32]

The development of public health regimes was not entirely a domestic story. The European discovery and management of "the barbarian within" was achieved simultaneously with the discovery and management of indigenous populations in the colonies. Colonial administrations provided numerous opportunities for the enumeration of populations, the study of disease, and the examination of poverty. Suspicions of miasmas in the colonies simultaneously stemmed from, and fueled suspicions of, miasma in the metropole. Some scholars have suggested a direct connection between reports on the climate and health of India and Chadwick's development of a miasmal approach to disease among England's poor.[33] European urban elites discovered noxious smells everywhere, from London to Lahore, but in the popular imagination, miasma somehow seemed to smell worse in Asia. The arrival of Colonel Wolseley's nose in Tianjin and the subsequent filling of the city moat represented an outpost of British sanitarianism in the Qing empire, but it also represented how the presence of Britain in these "outposts" in turn shaped the prejudices and aspirations of domestic administrators in London, Manchester, or Liverpool.

THE BIRTH OF THE CLINIC IN TIANJIN

Another unique element in the European organization of health was the institution of the hospital. In January 1861, the British established the Hospital for the Treatment of Sick Chinese, Tianjin's first institution of Western medicine. The immediate function of the hospital was to meet the medical needs of the hundreds of Cantonese laborers that the British had brought north with them from Hong Kong. The motivation for making medical care available to the Chinese is suggested in the comments of Colonel Wolseley, who observed that "a single coolie was actually of more general value than any three baggage animals; they were easily fed, and when properly treated, most manageable."[34] Eventually the services of the hospital were extended to the Chinese residents of Tianjin, although little is known about the number of locals who availed themselves of British medicine during the hospital's brief existence. The only extant information is from the perspective of the British, who were convinced that the Chinese elite would be both puzzled and impressed by this benevolent institution, created by the victors for the benefit of the vanquished.[35]

The British newspapers described the army hospital as an institution established for the benefit of the Chinese, but the clinic promised to provide very specific benefits to the British as well. Since the eighteenth century, hospitals had increasingly become a forum for medical advancement and education. The effectiveness of various treatments could be measured quantitatively, injecting the rigor of numbers into a profession that had previously only relied on the accumulated impressions of isolated practitioners. In case of the failure of treatment, hospital facilities for autopsy enabled physicians to link internal changes revealed within the bodies of the dead to the external signs of disease observable during life. The export of the hospital to the corners of the empire allowed clinicians to observe, tabulate, and dissect in remarkably varied foreign climates and among (from the perspective of the practitioners) remarkably varied foreign bodies. Hospitals in the colonial outpost as well as in the metropole became loci for the emergence of modern biomedicine.[36]

From another perspective, the hospital can be used as a window into the specific practices that constituted Western medicine at the point of contact between European and indigenous groups. Although the Hospital for the Treatment of Sick Chinese only lasted for a year and a half, it served as the city's first introduction to Western doctors, diagnosis, drugs, and, most important, to the distinct social environment of the hospital itself. A fragmentary glance at the hospital's brief history demonstrates that Western medicine was not an inherently superior, monolithic science, but was filled with theoretical debates and questionable therapies. In the mid-nineteenth century, Western practitioners and Chinese physicians struggled with many of the same phenomena: the causes of febrile epidemics, the possibilities for treating smallpox, and the nature of the relationship between the body and the environment.

DOCTOR RENNIE'S CURE:
WESTERN THERAPEUTICS AT THE POINT OF IMPACT

One of the practitioners of medicine at the British hospital was a Scottish physician, Dr. David Rennie, who had long been part of the British empire's expansion around the globe. His first assignment was as a doctor to a "convict establishment" in Western Australia. He then moved north to serve the British army in Hong Kong. By 1860, Rennie was serving as surgeon to the British army's 31st Regiment, one of the units that stayed behind in Tianjin as others moved on to more high-profile tasks in Beijing. The doctor made good use of his time in Tianjin by discovering what he considered to be nothing less than the cure for smallpox, a feat that in his words was "of the greatest importance, not just to the British army but to the world at large."[37]

During the winter of 1861, smallpox was "very prevalent" among the British soldiers stationed in Tianjin. Rennie believed that smallpox (and indeed, all other febrile diseases) was caused by the presence of "a latent material in the blood." This latent material lay dormant until it was acted upon by environmental influences, such as "atmospheric changes, electrical states, or currents in the air." Thus stimulated, the now-poisonous material caused fevers and attacked specific parts of the body. It could cause internal suppuration and production of pus, for example, or attack the lining of the intestine and cause dysentery or typhoid fever. The different stages of illness, such as the sweating followed by chills in malarial fever, or the "hot and cold" stages of dysentery, were manifestations of the poisonous material being transferred from one part of the body to another. That was why in cases of dysentery the fever seemed to subside after the onset of diarrhea, since the poison had moved on to the intestines and was then discharged through a "watery flux from the bowels or elsewhere." The different stages of disease was a manifestation of nature's search for a site for "the elimination of morbid material." The key to all therapeutics, Rennie postulated, was to "guide" this elimination "to its most innocuous site."[38]

With this understanding of the nature of the disease, Rennie devised a new method of cure for smallpox. It consisted of rubbing a preparation of one part tartrate of antimony, one part croton oil, and seven parts lard onto the chest of the smallpox victim. The combination of antimony and croton oil raised welts on the skin, which Rennie cultivated with repeated applications of his preparation. Not only did this prevent the outbreak of pustules on the face (the original goal of the treatment), but it also resulted in the complete recovery of all of the Chinese and British smallpox victims treated in the hospital. Rennie held that the effect was not due to "counterirritation," a therapeutic mechanism widely employed in European and American medicine at the time. Rennie was more modern and scientific in his thinking. He postulated that the croton oil and antimony actually produced an electric current, "which," as Rennie explained, "on portions of the blood coming within its influence, wherein morbid matter is held in solution, causes its separation from the vital fluid, and deposit on the surface of the body, by a process probably analogous to chemical decomposition."[39] Thus the external application of irritants caused internal chemical changes that made the smallpox poison separate from the blood. The welts raised on the chest by Rennie's cure were a manifestation of the smallpox poison as it escaped from the body.

Rennie argued that this treatment could work for any number of ailments, since most "diseases" had the same root cause. Rennie saw little sense in the medical profession's recent attempts at creating discrete disease categories: what he called "the mania . . . for the conversion of symptoms into special maladies." Just as this "profusion of nosologies" was unnecessary and confusing, Rennie held that the modern profusion of drugs and treatments was superfluous. He looked forward to a time when the electrochemical effect produced by the tartrate and croton oils could be replicated by some sort of easily used electronic apparatus. Rennie was confident that his discovery of the mechanism of "electroprecipitation" would soon be recognized as an almost-universal method of cure for all diseases.[40]

Rennie professed faith in modern scientific chemistry and physics, but he was much more skeptical about modern advances in public health. The recent trend toward state involvement in England's health had led to such things as massive drainage and landfill projects and compulsory smallpox vaccination. Rennie was convinced that these "advances" had actually worked to the detriment of his nation's well-being. He called for a halt to smallpox vaccination with cowpox variole on the basis that it did not in fact provide immunity. According to Rennie, Jenner's smallpox vaccination technique only served to make holes in the skin through which the pox could travel both in *and* out. If an individual already had an internal predisposition to disease in the form of morbid matter, then the cowpox would only settle within the body, rendering the individual even more susceptible to virulent outbreaks of smallpox. In fact, Rennie postulated that the increase in deaths in England due to tuberculosis and dysentery were the result of the increased use of smallpox vaccination. Morbid material in the blood had to be eliminated. A mild case of smallpox could release internal poisons through surface lesions and provide a certain amount of immunity to other disorders. A decline in the common childhood disorder of smallpox simply meant an increase in other diseases. Following the same reasoning, Rennie criticized such public health measures as the draining of swamps, a move that had left city dwellers with "no more intermittent fever to catch." With the decline in what Rennie called "common ague" came a rise in the frequency of a whole host of more serious diseases.[41]

The impact of Rennie's "discovery" on Western medicine beyond Tianjin is unknown. Rennie proclaimed that his theory and treatment of small-pox had been "invested with due importance and brought prominently under the notices of the highest military authorities in England."[42] Nevertheless, it can be said with certainty that while he was in Tianjin, his brand of therapeutics defined Western medicine for the Chinese who experienced treatment at his hands.

Rennie's ideas about morbid matter in the blood and the need for the body to cast it off were widely held—albeit widely debated—opinions in the medical profession at midcentury. His notion that morbid material was already lurking within the body, awaiting atmospheric influences to "activate" it, resembled somewhat the zymotic theory of disease that was influential throughout the nineteenth century. Yet the zymotic theory held that disease was caused when *external* seeds of disease entered the body and triggered fermentation within the blood, and was used to explain how miasma caused diseases like cholera and typhus.[43] Rennie's approach resembled beliefs held since the ninth century, when the Persian physician Rhazes postulated that smallpox was caused by an innate fermentation hidden within the blood. Rhazes' ideas were questioned in the sixteenth century by the Italian physician Fracastoro, who held that the action of smallpox, like all other infections, was similar to putrefaction, but this putrefaction was transmitted by particles that passed directly from person to person or through intermediaries such as clothing or air. The influential seventeenth-century figure Thomas Sydenham emphasized the role of atmospheric changes as an "exciting cause" of smallpox outbreaks. But by the eighteenth century, the increasing use of inoculation and the trend toward more discrete nosologies of disease had pushed the "innate seed" theory of smallpox further into medicine's backwaters.[44] Rennie, it seems, had combined fairly "modern" theories about disease causation with long-lived traditional explanations for smallpox. For him, the results of this synthesis were cutting edge, even though they were based in part on medical theories held since the Middle Ages.

The nature of the atmospheric emanations that caused disease and their mechanism of operation was one of the most actively debated questions in medicine at the time. Physicians in the mid–nineteenth century sought to add scientific rigor to the received knowledge that epidemic fevers were caused by the decay of "vegetable matter" found in marshes and low-lying land. In their attempt to refine medical knowledge, they drew upon a wide range of new knowledge, from observations of the natural environment in India, Africa, the Caribbean, and Asia to recently published experiments in chemistry and electricity. Some physicians suggested that decay and putrefaction produced "sulphureous emanations" or other harmful gases such as carbonic acid, nitrogen, ammonia, or various forms of hydrogen. Others held that "living vegetables," and not the dead and decaying, were responsible for epidemics. The assumption that the putrefaction of organic matter was the cause of febrile disease fueled Chadwick's crusade for sanitary reform, yet none in the medical profession could claim to understand the mechanism whereby miasma worked its pathological influence.[45]

Rennie's eccentric, or old-fashioned, approach to medicine was characterized by three positions: his disappointment at recent sanitary reforms, his resistance to the "profusion of nosologies" advocated by his colleagues in Great Britain, and his suspicion of smallpox vaccination. Although many physicians—particularly those active in the Poor Law medical system—may have protested Chadwick's disregard of poverty as a cause of disease, few would have objected to the sanitary reforms such as improved drainage brought about by Chadwick's report. Although shortcomings in technology made the realization of cleaner, drier streets a difficult task, the goal was generally held to be advantageous to health.[46] Rennie's complaint that the draining of swamps left the population more prone to illness was decidedly a minority opinion.

Rennie's belief that a little swamp ague was good for the body was linked to his general theory of disease. Since all complaints stemmed from the same underlying cause, namely, the venting of morbid material from the blood, deliberate exposure to a light affliction was the best way to avoid the devastation of more serious manifestation of "venting." Here Rennie found himself both partially allied with and opposed to two major trends in European medical thought. Chadwick and the sanitarians would agree with Rennie's approach to the environmental cause of disease: Miasma somehow gave rise to fevers. Yet Rennie's unified theory of disease was at odds with the more recent trend, begun in French clinics and adopted by British and mainland European practitioners, that specific diseases had specific causes. Whether conceived of as specific chemicals, poisons, parasites, or fungi, the "fermentation" characteristic of a number of diseases was caused by individual zymotic agents, each of which gave rise to specific lesions within the body.[47] A new generation of physicians would abandon the idea that "a little ague" could stave off an attack of dysentery.

Rennie's approach to smallpox vaccination places him in a small minority of medical dissenters from recent trends in British public health. Nevertheless, Jennerian vaccination was not without its problems in Britain. It had been introduced in the closing years of the eighteenth century, yet vaccination for infants in Great Britain had been made mandatory by law only in 1854. Vaccination was far from a consistent practice. Multiple variations existed in the preparation of vaccine and the technique of application; inconsistencies sometimes resulted in ineffective or dangerous vaccinations. Many in the working class, suspicious of the technique and the elite physicians that practiced it, avoided the procedure, and in the early 1860s it was still just being introduced in the more rural areas of the United Kingdom. One did not need to travel to India to find a population suspicious of, and resistant to, smallpox vaccination. The arrival of the Poor Law vaccinator was for many in Scotland and Ireland their first personal contact with the government. But although preachers, herbalists, feminists, and libertarians railed against smallpox vaccination, those within the more established medical profession who doubted its basic efficacy were few. Rennie seemed to base his aversion to the technique on his own clinical experience with smallpox patients (who may have been inadequately vaccinated), but ultimately the doctor neglected to alter his theory to match his practice.[48]

MEDICAL ENCOUNTERS I:
DOCTOR CHANG AND DOCTOR LAMPREY

If Dr. Rennie had had the opportunity to sit down and talk with a Chinese counterpart, he may have discovered some striking similarities between their conceptions of the etiology of smallpox. Both hypothesized the existence of an internal predisposition to the disease, fetal poison *(taidu)* in the Chinese case, "morbid material" for Rennie. Both were convinced that the disease was triggered by an external influence, whether evil/heteropathic qi *(xie qi)* or atmospheric emanations of an electrical nature. Rennie (along with many other British physicians as well) was struggling to explain the reasons for the puzzling sequence of symptoms of febrile disease by locating the movement of poisons through various organ systems. Fevers that alternated chills with sweats with extreme heat, dysenteries that were accompanied by large quantities of evacuated feces, others that were not, or that moved from one type to the other—both Chinese and European physicians in the nineteenth century explained these patterns through a spatialization of disease. For Rennie, morbid material might first attack the brain and circulatory system, resulting in high fever, and then move on to the intestines, producing loose and frequent evacuations. In one widely disseminated Chinese view of smallpox, fetal poison moved from the Gate of Life through various visceral systems and was finally expressed through the skin. Chinese physicians (particularly those of the Warm Factor persuasion) explained the progress of febrile symptoms by pinpointing the advance of heteropathic *qi* through visceral systems, membranes, and circulation tracts.

To be sure, spatialization of disease for the anatomy-grounded European was a different matter than spatialization for the Chinese physician, with his network of correspondence and flexible frameworks for conceptualizing the body. Nor did the Chinese physician peel back the layers of the body in search of an internal lesion to mark the seat of disease as did the European. Finally, it may be said that the precise spatialization of disease at a specific point in time actually had more implications for therapeutics for the Chinese physician than for the practitioner of medicine from the West. With the specific spatiofunctional actions of his elaborate materia medica well established, the Chinese physician was confident that he could affect with great precision any one of the visceral systems, circulation tracts, or any of the other function zones of the body. Although some medicines in the British physician's cabinet were linked to specific actions on specific organs, many organs remained out of the reach of his medicine; many other medicines operated on a more global level, working to stimulate or calm the state of the body as a whole.

In the mid–nineteenth century, Chinese and Western medicine were seeking answers to similar questions, and in some matters seemed to be arriving at similar answers. The language in which these answers were expressed, however, remained a zone for contention between "East" and "West," where medical meanings were charged with the burden of expressing the essences of civilizations. One such encounter in this zone took place at the British Hospital for the Treatment of Sick Chinese, when the hospital's head physician, Dr. Lamprey, was approached by a "native practitioner" by the name of "Doctor Chang." Doctor Chang wished to volunteer his medical services for the hospital. Lamprey interviewed him to see of what use he might be.

It is not known if Lamprey or Chang communicated through interpreters with any knowledge of the two modes of medical expression, but that would probably matter little. Lamprey dismissed Doctor Chang forthwith. Lamprey found his "absurd notions of attributing diseases to wind, breath, water, or sweat" laughable and dangerous. The British doctor pronounced the Chinese doctor to be "such a mass of deceit and imposition that I could not tolerate him for a moment." Lamprey was unwilling to interpret *feng* as anything but wind, when it could have as easily been draft or chill, or even miasma. He was apparently entirely ignorant of the concept of *qi*, and the poor translation of the word left the British doctor wondering how "breath" could cause disease. It is even possible that the word interpreted as "water" *(shui)* was actually the word indicating heteropathic forces *(xie)*.[49]

Thus the first recorded attempt at cooperation between Chinese and Western doctors in Tianjin ended in a debacle of bad translation and British reluctance to find common ground. Lamprey even imagined that the stage had already been set in the city for a competition between Chinese and Western medicine. Lamprey had noticed that the number of Chinese patients coming to the hospital had declined. Rather than querying the effectiveness of his cures or the appeal of the clinical setting for Chinese patients, Lamprey asserted that a reduction in the numbers of patients coming to the hospital was the result of "sabotage" conducted by "jealous local doctors and merchants of medicines."[50]

By the spring of 1862 the bulk of the British and French forces had pulled back to Taku, and the hospital that had served both Chinese and European civilians in Tianjin was dismantled. The removal of the military hospital brought some alarm to the British settler community of fewer than fifty, who felt they were being abandoned to an uncertain and unhealthy Chinese environment. The British Consulate requested that the medical officer of the hospital relinquish whatever medicines they could spare to the concession's civilian doctor. The consul was particularly anxious as medical supplies had not arrived from England, leaving the tiny British community to face the rapidly approaching "unhealthy season" unaided and alone.[51]

MEDICAL ENCOUNTERS II: CHOLERA AND CATHOLICS

In 1862, China was hit by a cholera epidemic that had begun in India in 1861.[52] Cholera moved along the network formed by the British empire. Spread by vessels from India to Hong Kong, it moved from Hong Kong to the area around Nanjing in the spring of 1862 at a moment when fighting between joint Qing/European forces and the Taiping rebels was particularly intense. Cholera reached Tianjin from Shanghai via Taku by the midsummer of 1862. There are few detailed accounts of the situation in Tianjin, but it seems that mortality rates were highest in the crowded walled city and eastern suburbs. Chinese accounts tell of high mortality without giving specific numbers. European observers estimated a death toll of four hundred per day, spread out over the course of a month.[53]

British naval physicians in China struggled to reason through the causes of cholera. Dr. W. E. O'Brien of HMS *Acorn*, like most European medical men of his time, was convinced that exposing the body to extremes in weather would result in gastrointestinal disorders, but he puzzled over the strange symptoms his patients suffered in the China Station.[54] In his treatise, entitled "Practical Remarks on Periodic Fevers, Dysentery and Diar-rhoea As They Occur on the China Station," O'Brien attempted to explain the simultaneous appearance of fever and diarrhea symptoms in his patients. He also speculated on the reasons why some patients experienced severe ab-dominal pain but produced few feces, whereas others vomited and evacu-ated their bowels in copious quantities. He attributed acute dysentery in sailors to the exciting causes of lying out on the open decks or otherwise exposing the abdominal surface to cold air. The cold resulted in an inflam-mation of the mucous membrane of the large intestine. The development of organ pathology in the eighteenth century had given physicians the knowledge that certain changes in tissues occurred with certain diseases, thus encouraging them to seek the seat of disease within a specific organ rather than an overall system. But the exact cause of such changes, and how such localized lesions might give rise to the puzzling symptoms of disease, was still a topic of considerable debate.

O'Brien's detailed observations and attempts at understanding the rela-tionship between different symptoms did not result in the development of any therapies that diverged from the accepted norms in Great Britain. Dur-ing his time on the China Station he remained "painfully aware of the inef-ficacy of all modes of treatment" for dysentery.[55] In cases of "dry cholera," he recommended treating the patient with saline purgatives to relubricate the intestine. He also recommended immersing the sufferer in a hip bath morning and night, in water as hot as could be withstood. When not in the bath, the abdomen should be wrapped up in flannel soaked in oil of turpen-tine or iodine to provide a warm external counterirritation. His treatments mirrored standard treatments in the West, which similarly focused on rein-troducing warmth into a system that had been attacked by cold. Victims of cholera from New York to London—and most likely, Tianjin as well—were wrapped in tight flannel girdles or given frequent hip baths in hot water. Brandy or other spirits were administered to further warm and stimulate the system. Finally elixirs containing opium helped to calm the patient and re-lieve the terrible pain that accompanied the final stages of the disease.[56]

There are no extant writings that describe how cholera was treated by Chinese doctors in Tianjin. Some healers may have been familiar with the writings of the Jiangnan doctor Wang Shixiong, whose brief *Treatise on Cholera* (*Huoluan lun*, 1838) aided the practice of physicians who faced in-creasingly common epidemics of "sudden chaos" (*huoluan*), a syndrome that included cholera, but may also have included many other biomedically differentiated gastrointestinal illnesses.[57] Wang's *Treatise on Cholera* pre-sents ten cases of *huoluan* that he himself treated during the 1830s, when epidemics of febrile diseases accompanied by vomiting and diarrhea swept through the Jiangnan region.[58] Wang argued that without the proper distinction of the stage and nature of the syndrome—whether Hot or Cold, caused by external influences or internal imbalance, lurking just beneath the skin or located deep within the yin regions of the body—deadly mistakes might be made in the selection of formulas.

In Wang's own cases, he carefully noted the age, sex, and sometimes the class background of the patient. In accord with diagnostic techniques common since Zhang Ji's third-century *Treatise on Cold Damage* (Shang han lun), Wang noted whether the sufferer's body and limbs were cold or hot and whether or not they were thirsty, for this gave clues to the nature of the illness. Wang went beyond simple considerations of Hot and Cold to detect the possibility of latent imbalances:

> A person [male] by the surname of Qian came down with *huo luan.*
> Since he had been sweating, his limbs were cold and his pulses weak.
> He generally ate cool things and drank cold beverages, so everyone
> said this was a Cold Syndrome and wanted to treat it with extremely
> Hot medicines. Then I examined him. Although his face was white,
> it was sunken and crimson red along the periphery. He was extremely
> thirsty and had a severe headache. It could not be that the cold and
> cool had become an illness. [Those who argued for treating this with
> Hot drugs] had not detected the hidden Summer Heat within him.[59]

Although this case was caused by an external illness factor, Wang's next case was of a young man whose cholera was the result of internal imbalances caused by inattention to the rules of guarding life:

> A young man, of plump constitution and hot stomach, with an
> extreme personality. On a hot afternoon he laid naked on a mat placed
> on a brick floor and stuffed himself with several pounds of watermelon.
> That evening he felt his head grow heavy, and a Cold malaise filled
> his body. Later that night he began to vomit and excrete feces in great
> quantity. His limbs were stiff. He sweated lightly. Occasionally he would
> become extremely agitated. His pulses were sinking and weak.[60]

Wang treated the first case of invading Summer Heat with cooling drugs, a Five-Herb *Poros cocos* Fungus Formula *(wu ling san)* with added cooling ingredients such as magnolia bark, quince, and broad beans. He treated the second case with warming drugs such as cassia bark, dried ginger, and aconite. In all of his cases, Wang shows the same ability to diagnose the nature of an illness, demonstrating dexterity in moving back and forth between Warm Factor and Cold Damage, or combining a variety of approaches in a creative synthesis.

In certain severe cases of cholera, Wang suggested the use of vigorous rubbing or scraping of the skin *(guasha)*, a therapy similar to that employed by Dr. Rennie in the British hospital at Tianjin. Wang's technique involved rubbing the limbs with saltwater or alcohol, or scraping the skin with an earthenware blade dipped in sesame oil. The logic behind both the Chinese and Western treatments was similar: scraping allowed the release of poisons that lurked within the body. But while Rennie identified the blood as the carrier of poison, scraping on the chest simply in order to prevent pox from reaching the face, Wang directed the scraping specifically to the back of the knees, elbows, the back, and the bottoms of the feet, areas that coincided with acupuncture points along circulation tracts associated with the Five Viscera. Rennie had looked to new evidence from laboratory science to explain the curative action of his therapy. For Wang Shixiong, the validity of his technique was justified by its inclusion in ancient texts and its success rate in practical application.[61]

The cholera epidemic of 1862 demonstrated that the diversity of approaches to disease was not only the preserve of elite physicians. To focus solely on the ruminations of learned doctors would miss entirely the healing options to which most individuals turned. As in Europe and America, the cholera epidemics that swept across China in the nineteenth century inspired religious responses. American ministers urged their congregations to pray that cholera might pass. Europeans sought charms blessed by priests to protect them from the malevolent vapors of cholera. Similarly, many people of Tianjin sought cures not from learned doctors but from an increasingly diversified field of spiritual specialists.[62]

Many sufferers in Tianjin turned to a Buddhist monk who offered healing at the San Guan Temple near the city's western gate. The monk would take mud, bless it, and make it into pills, or he would lay his hands on the sick and cure them with the power of the Buddha. His most effective cure against cholera, however, was a magical elixir that consisted of water that he had blessed. People crowded into the temple carrying water bottles and pitchers so they could carry his magical water back home. The ill for miles around flocked to the temple and pitched tents in and around the grounds, waiting for the monk to lay his hands on them or distribute his holy water cure. So much water was needed that hundreds of members of Tianjin's water-carrier guilds hauled water from the Grand Canal to fill the temple's tank. All along the route, thousands of people stood banging gongs and cheering the volunteers' benevolent contribution.[63] This concentration of large numbers of sick and dying in pitched tents with no facilities, drinking river water from one communal tank, quite likely assured a rapid entrance into the next life for many of the faithful.

In their desperation, some of the people of Tianjin were willing to turn to a new and exotic source for protection from cholera. Only a few days before the epidemic reached its height, fourteen French and Belgian Sisters of Charity of the Order of Saint Enfance arrived in Tianjin. They set up residence in a small compound outside the city's east wall. The people of Tianjin, now perhaps accustomed to the sight of British soldiers, were perplexed by the arrival of the nuns. There was uncertainty about their national identity and even their gender. In the eyes of Tianjiners, the nuns seemed to resemble women, but their long plain gowns (which constituted masculine attire in China) and their habit of walking about unescorted through the city streets made many think that the sisters were actually men.[64]

The sisters had brought a few medical supplies with them for their own purposes and as a benevolent supplement to their conversion activities. They did not anticipate that a week after their arrival in the summer of 1862, hundreds of Tianjin's poor would crowd into their compound courtyard, looking to the nuns for a cure for cholera. When they first arrived, the nuns had taken in a laborer who had collapsed of choleric symptoms on the road in front of their compound and nursed him back to health. Word spread quickly of the nuns' success, and within a few days relatives of the sick were lined up at the Catholic compound with a bowl in each hand, waiting for some sort of medicine to be distributed. The nuns did the best with what little they had: in one bowl they placed some nourishing soup, and in the other they placed some camphor. They also distributed simple mustard poultices to use as counterirritants on the abdomen. The Catholic nuns, like the Buddhist monks at the San Guan Temple, prayed that their simple remedies would be bestowed with miraculous effectiveness.[65]

This new element in the healing diversity of Tianjin would soon be imbricated in the tragic Tianjin Massacre. The hospital that the nuns founded had none of the pretenses to medical experiment and scientific advancement possessed by the previous British army hospital. Still it became another site of contact, a representative of foreign medicine, combined with foreign religion, in the local Tianjin setting. Peculiarly modern European ways of delineating space—keeping meddlesome family members out of the hospital, or barring curious and undisciplined crowds from the church—combined with the mysterious Catholic practice of baptizing dying infants to fuel the suspicion that burst forth in the violence of 1870. Convinced that the foreigners had been "stealing the souls" of hospitalized converts and kidnap-

ping (and then killing) Chinese babies, Chinese crowds killed sixteen foreigners, including the Sisters of Charity.[66]

CONCLUSION

The Tianjin Massacre was the event that first placed "Tientsin" on the map
for most Europeans and Americans. It was used as evidence to confirm what
many nineteenth-century European and American observers had already
suspected: China was a place of superstition, confusion, and benightedness,
unwilling to accept the advances of Western civilization, whether in the form
of religion or medicine. The incident was quickly assimilated into a larger
discourse that envisioned a clash of diametrically opposed civilizations. An
impoverished, chaotic East, whose government was unable to provide for
its population, stood in contrast with a wealthy, orderly West, with its sanitary commissions and boards of health. A charitable, Christian West had
attempted to provide medicine for a selfish, heathen East, but had been
grossly misunderstood. A healthy and robust West had come to the aid of
a sickly East and was met with ingratitude.

An examination of midcentury encounters between "East" and "West"
at a local level dissolves such stark dichotomies. The British navy managed
to ensure adequate provisioning for sick and wounded soldiers in the China
Station because of the medical catastrophes experienced during the Crimean
War. While British commanders made tactical blunders upon entering Tianjin's waters, physicians on board puzzled over the reasons for the preponderance of fevers and dysentery among the troops, noting the same kinds
of symptoms and diagnostic problems that Chinese physicians were struggling with at the same point in history. The doctors practicing at the first
hospital of Western medicine in Tianjin professed theories of disease etiology that were not altogether different from those held by Chinese physicians, and even employed similar therapies in treating febrile syndromes.

In 1860, the British sense of smell may have detected much cause for concern in Tianjin's atmosphere, but a walk through streets in any number of
London's neighborhoods would have produced similar anxieties. England's
sanitarian movement had just begun, sparked by Chadwick's 1842 report.
This massive trend toward the government administration of urban health
had not been motivated by a breakthrough in medical science, or even by
an agreement on the part of the medical profession about miasma as the
predominant cause of disease. It was instead the product of a particular set
of trends in British political philosophy. Followers of Jeremy Bentham's util-

itarianism had lobbied for a wide variety of government reforms, from prisons to Poor Laws. The sanitarian movement and the rise of British public health was a political movement that complemented laissez faire economic policies and overemphasized the extent to which the medical profession attributed disease to smells. And finally, it was the product of an expanding empire that was contending with massive famine, economic depression, and the increasingly evident immiseration of its urban poor at home. If there was a great divergence arising between Great Britain and the Great Qing at midcentury, it was primarily political, and not medical, in nature.

.   .   .

In spite of the existence of common medical ground, in the post–Tianjin Massacre climate it was difficult to find any Western observers who found similarities between the two healing traditions or virtue in Chinese health practices. The confidence in medical superiority voiced by European observers in China, though misplaced, was almost universal. It was the rare commentator who even perceived the existence of a Chinese tradition of nurturing life or guarding life *(yangsheng, weisheng)* and credited it with keeping the population healthy.

John Dudgeon (1837–1901), a missionary and long-time resident in Beijing and Tianjin, was such a rarity. Dudgeon was an astute observer of the habits of Chinese daily life, not just among the poor, but among the scholars and merchants of the cities. He was even something of a scholar of Chinese meditative healing movements, which he called "Chinese Gymnastics." Dudgeon collected and studied books on the subject, and had even plumbed the complexities of Pan Wei's *Essential Arts of Guarding Life*.

Based on his studies and observations, Dudgeon concluded that Chinese daily life abounded in healthful habits. They universally drank boiled water. The Chinese were vigilant in keeping off drafts, which Dudgeon held to be the major cause of liver disease. They limited their bathing in order to avoid drafts, and wore long robes and layered tunics. He criticized European men for their short-cut jackets and women for their revealing décolletage, noting that "our chests and abdomens are not half so well protected from sudden cold as those of the Chinese."[67]

According to Dudgeon's observations, what truly distinguished the Chinese as a healthy race was their moderate lifestyle. Chinese were almost universally "temperate" and sober, the result being that drunkenness, "which is the common disfigurement of life in our cities and towns, is a rare sight in China." He noted the increase in opium addiction in China, but blamed foreign influences, for "wherever European civilization has gone, intemperance among the native races has followed." Finally he suggested that the relative absence of heart disease and aneurysm was due to the "phlegmatic and unexcitable nature" of the Chinese. Unlike many other commentators of his day who attributed this "unexcitable nature" to the inherent insensitivity of Chinese nerves, Dudgeon suggested a cultural reason. In what was a rare criticism of a prevailing European racist notion of the time, Dudgeon observed that Chinese "insensitive" stoicism during operations without chloroform "is not to be accounted for, as is often done, so much by a less acute nervous system, but rather by moral training."[68]

This "moral training" led the Chinese, from Dudgeon's perspective, to lead calm lives and work at a steady but measured pace. In a lightly veiled indictment of modernity and its attendant stresses, Dudgeon noted that "the Chinese are always struck with our activity in everything—we can not even walk slowly, although we have enough of time and money." In contrast to the Chinese, "We have carried industry and competition to an extreme." The result, in Dudgeon's eyes, was a European society that was increasingly wealthy but also increasingly unhealthy.[69] Dudgeon's opinions about the "essential nature" of Chinese civilization provided him with a basis for criticizing his own civilization:

> The great strides made by European nations, and ourselves in particular, in trade and international intercourse with the ends of the earth, by virtue of our discoveries and inventions, whatever else may have been done in adding to the sum of human happiness and comfort, have not tended, either among ourselves or nations lower in the scale of civilisation, to longevity or the diminution of disease, but rather the reverse.[70]

In spite of his unique opinions about Chinese health practices, Dudgeon, like myriad European observers before and after him, condemned Chinese civilization as universally dirty. Individual Chinese exhibited "a want of personal cleanliness, no body linen, and wear the same garments day and night." Like Colonel Wolseley, Dudgeon proclaimed that "China is, par excellence, the country of bad smells," and the nation as a whole was "totally destitute of sanitary science."[71] Dudgeon's observations of China's hygiene confounded both his middle-class European sensibilities and his medical understanding of disease causation. He struggled to comprehend the apparent conceptual paradox that a people could, in his eyes, be so lacking in hygiene (cleanliness) and yet lead such hygienic (healthy) lives at the same time. Dudgeon was particularly puzzled by what he perceived as a general lack among Chinese of the acute fevers that plagued his native England, even proclaiming that the "disgusting habits" he had observed among people living along the

Grand Canal in Tianjin "would almost unsettle one's ideas of the connection between typhoid fever and polluted water."[72]

Dudgeon's perceptions of the lack of epidemic disease among Chinese may have stemmed from a common nineteenth-century belief in racial immunity, the idea that resistance to disease was a hereditary characteristic that rendered "natives" less susceptible to diseases that would otherwise devastate the "tender frames" of Europeans.[73] Dudgeon's notion that the Chinese were not suffering from fevers may have been anecdotal, stemming from what Warwick Anderson has called nineteenth-century Europe's "vast ignorance of the actual distribution of disease in colonial populations."[74] Certainly his observations of health and disease in Tianjin were inextricably intertwined with his own perceptions of European society. The supposed calm and measured habits of Chinese contrasted with the frenetic and hedonistic nature of whites, and provided Dudgeon with a platform for the promotion of temperance in his native Great Britain.

Nevertheless, Dudgeon's observations marked one of the last moments that a European would condemn Chinese "lack of sanitary science" yet simultaneously praise Chinese approaches to healthful living. Dudgeon thought that disease was caused by many different things: cold air, intemperance, miasma, modernity, and perhaps, although not certainly, by germs. This multiplicity of disease origins allowed Dudgeon to entertain multiple approaches to the preservation of health. "Sanitary science," defined primarily as the elimination of smells and the ordering of the environment, was not the only measure of medical advancement. Dudgeon validated Chinese techniques of guarding life, and did not view hygiene solely as a signifier of Chinese deficiency.[75] His position would become virtually untenable in the twentieth century.

At the time that Dudgeon was contemplating the seeming paradoxes between "private hygiene" and "public hygiene" in China, no word existed in Chinese to describe the latter, and no concept existed that linked the two. During the last quarter of the nineteenth century, translators in China began to render certain British and American texts on health preservation under the rubric of *weisheng*. Medical diversity, combined with the political conditions of late Qing treaty ports, allowed Chinese to adopt, alter, or reject the content of this translated *weisheng*. Changes in medicine, health administration, and military organization in Western Europe rapidly eroded this diversity, and set the stage for a far more decisive divergence in the twentieth century.

4 Translating *Weisheng* in Treaty-Port China

Beginning in 1880, new treatises on *weisheng* appeared in China's treaty ports. A few curious Chinese readers in Tianjin would have noted their arrival. The basic content of these works was the same: Each informed the reader that chemistry dictated the proper path to health. The word *weisheng* on the cover signaled that these works contained wisdom on how to strengthen the body and prevent disease. But beyond the title page, readers encountered a world far removed from correlative cosmology, yin and yang, Hot and Cold. Here air, soil, water, and food were composed of specific combinations of discrete chemical elements. Understanding how the human body thrived by transforming these chemical elements was the key to guarding life.

These texts, British and American popular science tracts translated by an Englishman and his Chinese associates in Shanghai, marked the beginning of an altered set of meanings for *weisheng* in China. *Weisheng* still meant "guarding life." It still signified what the individual should do in order to be healthy, without reference to social or political context. This *weisheng* did not mark a race or a people as fit enough for modernity, it did not exclude Chinese from membership in "civilization" due to habit or health. However, with these translations, the basic concepts associated with *weisheng* began to shift away from an entirely Chinese context and moved to embrace an authority generated by the laboratories of Europe. The phrase "the Way of Guarding Life" *(weisheng zhi dao)* might still conjure up tales of Daoist masters and maxims from the Yellow Emperor's *Inner Cannon,* but now it was also used to convey the proper consumption of proteins and the use of chemicals to remove odors. By providing a new set of explanations for eating, drinking, excreting, and even breathing, translated *weisheng* carried with it the possibility of becoming an alternative logic for the ordering of daily existence.

The content of early translated *weisheng* texts reveals how the meanings of the word may have shifted at this early juncture. Translations of Western science were produced in Shanghai and circulated in treaty-port cities such as Tianjin. Ultimately *weisheng* as "hygienic modernity" had a tremendous power to shape political and social realities in China, but it was imbued with this power only after the turn of the century, when new terms of habit and being were enforced by occupying armies. In order to understand the production, through translation, of an altered textual tradition for *weisheng,* it is essential to sketch out two contexts: the nineteenth-century "science" of hygiene in Europe and the United States reflected in the original texts, and the conditions for dominance, association, segregation, and influence in the early treaty-port worlds of Tianjin and Shanghai.

Scholars have long ceased to think that the translation of science involved the simple transfer of ideas from one culture to another. Questions of power relations and the impact of imperialism have come to the fore in the study of translation between Europe and the rest of the world. Some studies of science translation in the colonial context have highlighted the ambivalent role of the native translator: He must convey knowledge that he has enthusiastically embraced, even though this knowledge often dictates the conditions of his inequality. At the same time, language and translation have provided a vehicle for thwarting a colonial vision of unobstructed domination. As Gyan Prakash has observed for scientific translations in India, the hegemony of Western science "could not be established through imposition" but was a possibility only through the generative participation of Indian translators who figured science into their own terms. The shifts, challenges, and hybrid forms produced through translation resulted in "the undoing of dominance with the establishment of dominance" by creating an elite who questioned the logic of colonialism itself.[1]

Lydia Liu would question whether such conditions of dominance were established at all in China. In the process of translation under conditions of imperialism in China, Chinese became a "host language," a medium of considerable power that invented its own meanings within its own environment and eventually created its own modernity, a modernity that was "not necessarily un-Chinese."[2] This was made possible by the semicolonial environment of China. Since colonial domination was not total and since Chinese in China never switched to conducting their lives in English, linguistic and intellectual space was present in greater abundance and was infused with less ambivalence and anxiety than in India.[3]

It is difficult to generalize about the translation process in treaty-port China or to attribute its distinguishing characteristics to a static state of semicolonialism. Conditions of foreign imperialism and domination—actual and potential—changed dramatically according to the time, geographical place, and the specific sector of life and ideas under consideration. They varied as different languages—particularly Japanese—entered the translation process. Analysis of translation in China becomes particularly complex when one considers that many of the most influential scientific translations of the late nineteenth century were not produced by Chinese alone, but by collaborations between Westerners and Chinese who were working to spread the gospel of science for their own particular purposes. The conditions under which translated *weisheng* was produced and encountered in treaty-port China were as complex as the conditions of imperialism itself. A consideration of cultural production and circulation of an altered *weisheng* must begin with a glance at the institutions and settings in Shanghai, where *weisheng* was reconfigured, and in Tianjin, where its content would soon be contested.

THE CONTOURS OF COLONIALISM
IN TIANJIN AND SHANGHAI

If one were to approach the city of Tianjin from the south in the late nineteenth century, a strangely disjointed scene would meet the eye. On the right, a very thin line of European-style brick edifices rose along the bank of the Hai River. In front of these buildings, looming over the flat, empty plain, stood a massive gothic castle called Gordon Hall. With its huge towers and parapets, Gordon Hall looked like the fortress of some medieval European king. It was, in fact, the home of the solidly bourgeois British Municipal Council, a small group of men who made decisions for the five hundred Europeans and several thousand Chinese who lived in the British Settlement. To the west of Gordon Hall, separated by a mile and a half of marshes and scattered low dwellings, rose the spectacular walls of Tianjin. Within the walls, hidden from outside view, lay a city of more than 150,000 subjects of the Qing empire, along with the offices of the empire's most powerful officials. The physical separation of these two different Tianjins—the Chinese and the European—set the stage for the production of new cultural meanings for that city in the late nineteenth century.

Tianjin came late to the treaty-port world. By the time European buildings began to rise on the banks of the Hai, Shanghai had already been a treaty port for twenty years. By the 1880s, Shanghai was larger and possessed a more active economy than Tianjin. There was also considerably less distance, both literally and figuratively, separating the foreign settlements from the Chinese. The French Concession shared a border with the "Chinese city," and the International Settlement (a combination of the British and American Concessions) was in close proximity to centers of Chinese population. More important, in 1860, thousands of Chinese entered Shanghai's foreign concession to seek refuge from the Taiping rebellion. From that moment on, Chinese residents of the concessions always greatly outnumbered foreigners. Numerous Chinese guilds and native place associations were located in the International Settlement. Residents and offices of wealthy Chinese who worked with foreign firms—the compradors—lined the streets of the foreign settlements. By the late nineteenth century, Shanghai was home to a host of sites of Sino-foreign interaction: schools, hospitals, arsenals, newspapers, and businesses.[4]

Located at the juncture of the wealthy Yangtze River delta area and the Pacific Ocean, Shanghai was advantageously positioned for the making of money, and much of the association between foreigners and Chinese revolved around this pursuit. Tianjin, however, was advantageously positioned vis-à-vis the center of imperial power, and much of the interaction between foreigners and Chinese focused on the workings of diplomacy and the court. By 1870 Tianjin had become the base of operations for one of the Qing empire's most powerful officials, the "Viceroy" Li Hongzhang. One of the leading self-strengtheners of the late Qing, Li orchestrated the establishment of modern steamship companies, military installations, mines, and telegraph networks along the Chinese coast. He interacted with the foreign community to an unprecedented degree, consulting with foreign consuls and customs officials and granting frequent interviews. Li seemed to make the affairs of the foreign concessions his own. He even attended the opening ceremony for Gordon Hall, an architectural paean to British imperialism, named after General Charles "Chinese" Gordon. According to European observers, the opening ceremony moved Li Hongzhang to tears because it reminded him of his dear old friend, General Gordon, who had helped Li defeat the Taiping rebels outside Shanghai thirty years before.[5]

Li Hongzhang and other Qing officials in Tianjin realized that careful interaction with foreigners was essential because foreigners simultaneously threatened and helped maintain Qing sovereignty. Foreign mercenaries may have helped Li defeat the Taiping rebels, but from his offices in Tianjin, Li Hongzhang managed one crisis after another involving the threat of foreign incursion: the Tianjin Massacre, the Margary Affair, Japanese annexation of the Ryukyus and possible moves in Korea, and a war with France over the possession of Vietnam. At the same time, Qing officials had to deal with natural disasters on a massive scale, disasters that severely challenged Qing mechanisms of domestic governance. The worst crisis hit in 1877–79 when a tremendous famine resulted in the deaths of an estimated nine million people across a wide swath of north China.[6] The fragility of Qing sovereignty—and the threat that foreign imperialism presented to it—was becoming more and more apparent throughout the nineteenth century, even as Li Hongzhang enjoyed tea and scones in the comfortable homes of Tianjin's European elite.

The threat of foreign imperialism was constant and looming, but locally, on a day-to-day basis, the Qing government and their subjects were not in a position of subordination. Members of the European community did not always persevere in conflicts between Chinese and foreigners. Interactions between foreigners and Chinese were often managed through wealthy and powerful officers of native place associations. In conflicts, these men and their extensive networks were frequently able to thwart foreign attempts to enter Chinese markets or take over Chinese land.[7] In late-nineteenth-century Shanghai and Tianjin, the foreign presence could not entirely constitute a manifestation of "colonial domination." The actual number of foreigners was negligible. Foreigners and subjects of the Qing frequently collaborated, and sometimes the outcome was to the detriment of parts of the foreign community itself. However, these tiny settlements were conceived and born through violent imperialism, and more important, they existed within a cultural and political field constantly charged with the potential for more violence and more strident manifestations of colonial domination. Qing officials and leaders of native place associations alike did not need to function with some sort of divinatory foresight of things to come in Chinese history in order to feel that they operated on a slippery slope: each had their own reasons for anxiety about an encroaching imperialism. Certainly, Qing officials in Tianjin and wealthy Chinese businessmen in Shanghai might have felt different levels of anxiety about the future. But all Chinese moved within an environment where foreigners worked within assumptions about racial hierarchy and where "Western learning" increasingly set the standard for knowing the world.

"FU LANYA" AND TRANSLATING THE SCIENCE OF HEALTH

It was in this complex treaty-port world that new meanings were given to *weisheng* through the collaborative translation enterprise of a British schoolteacher and a group of Chinese chemists. In 1880, a few readers in

Shanghai and Tianjin would have noticed the publication of a treatise that presented foreign ways of thinking about preserving health. That year, the *Chinese Science Magazine (Gezhi huibian)*, published in Shanghai but distributed in other treaty ports, began to carry a serialized work entitled *Huaxue weisheng lun*. The title of this work might be understood as *Treatise on [the Applicability of] the Study of Transformation [to] Guarding Life*, or, perhaps, more simply, *Chemistry and Hygiene*. The magazine was published by John Fryer (1839–1928), a Englishman who was a key translator of Western books for the Jiangnan Arsenal, one of the Qing government's major centers for military modernization in the late nineteenth century and a major site of intellectual collaboration between Chinese and foreigners in Shanghai. An initial perusal of the content of *Huaxue weisheng lun* would reveal an eclectic array of information. With these translations, Fryer sought to establish Western knowledge as the guiding principle for the preservation of health and the organization of daily life.

By the end of the nineteenth century, the name "Fu Lanya" (John Fryer's Chinese moniker) had become almost synonymous with translations of "Western knowledge" in China. After an unsuccessful stint as a missionary educator, Fryer began his translating career in 1868 at the Jiangnan Arsenal.[8] In 1876, Fryer founded the *Gezhi shuyuan* (literally, the Academy for the Investigation of Things, known in English as the Shanghai Polytechnic), which, after a shaky beginning, became one of China's best-known centers for the public demonstration of science. Fryer edited the Polytechnic's affiliated journal, the *Chinese Science Magazine*, which published a variety of essays on subjects ranging from botany to engineering. Fryer also established a book marketing network, the Chinese Scientific Book Depot *(Gezhi shushi)* in Shanghai and several other treaty-port cities, including Tianjin. Finally, his work in the production of missionary school textbooks ensured that a generation of Chinese children learned basic sciences from Fu Lanya primers.

In spite of Fryer's reputation as a popularizer of Western learning, Fu Lanya translations were never solely the product of one British mind. Fryer's limited education in both Western science and the Chinese language made it impossible for him to act independently as a translator. Fryer's Chinese collaborators were far more capable in the classical Chinese idiom; several of them, including the practicing scientists Xu Shou, Xu Jianyin, and Hua Hengfang, were better versed in Western science and mathematics than their Western collaborator.[9] A Fu Lanya translation was always produced in concert with these Chinese colleagues. However, Fryer dubbed these talented intellectuals his "assistants" and warned foreign readers that any mistakes contained within his translations were attributable to Chinese ignorance. Many of Fryer's works—including all translations bearing *weisheng* in the title—do not even credit a Chinese cotranslator, although one (or more) certainly existed.[10]

One of the primary interests of Fryer and his Chinese colleagues was the translation of Western texts on chemistry. Xu Shou and others who worked with Fryer had long been interested in chemistry and were conducting experiments well before Fryer arrived on the scene. In addition, Fryer brought with him to China a mid-nineteenth-century European enthusiasm for chemistry as the most demonstrable, most portable, and most useful of sciences.[11] Fryer felt chemistry would appeal to the Chinese, who had a long indigenous tradition of alchemy. Chemistry could be done at home: Chinese scholars could tinker with chemical reactions in their own studies. In the demonstration hall, the color changes, bubbles, and miniature explosions that accompanied experiments offered maximum entertainment effect. Most important, Fryer, like many others of his day in Europe, held that chemistry revealed the underlying truth about the processes of life. Of all the sciences, chemistry was the one that could give man the power to control his environment. Chemistry could offer a complete set of knowledge that could replace Chinese "superstitions" about the nature of the cosmos and the interactions between man and his environment.

The books through which Fryer presented Western techniques of *weisheng* were fundamentally chemistry texts. They show how the world is composed of a finite number of elements that were rendered visible and knowable through laboratory experiment. In these texts, chemistry explains how the human body interacts with its environment. Chemistry could even eliminate pathogens in the environment through its remarkable powers of transformation. Overall, the *weisheng* presented in these translations, although it rested on an entirely different approach to cosmology, still maintained valences of meaning exceedingly familiar to Chinese readers. It warned against the consumption of alcohol. It tutored readers in the proper components of a healthful diet. It was founded on the premise of individual knowledge and individual moral action. In Fryer's *weisheng* texts, an understanding of chemistry is the foundation for the preservation of health and the prevention of disease—but only for the individual who is willing to master this knowledge and act according to its precepts.

These similarities to Chinese hygiene traditions existed not because translation produced a uniquely Chinese hybrid form of *weisheng*, but because Fryer chose to translate original texts that were themselves part of a Euro-American tradition of hygiene based on individual morality and personal behavior. Chinese translators did not simply take a preformed set of dominant "Western" knowledge and render it interestingly into an exotic indigenized Chinese idiom. What constituted science, particularly the science of hygiene in late-nineteenth-century Europe and the United States, was itself in considerable flux, and individual texts reflected specific facets of a very fluid situation. While tracing the outline of what *weisheng* might have meant in late-nineteenth-century treaty ports, one must understand the forces that produced the original texts and examine the sometimes controversial knowledge they transported to China. To understand the *weisheng* that emerges in treaty ports in the late nineteenth century requires a transnational synchronization of analytical lenses, each focused on two moving targets on opposite sides of the world.

Huaxue weisheng lun *(1880): Chemistry as the Key to Health*

Huaxue weisheng lun was one of the first major texts in Chinese to present Western learning under the rubric of "protecting life."[12] The entire work is a celebration of chemistry as the basis for human existence, human health, and human prosperity. The original text, *The Chemistry of Common Life* (1855) by the Scottish agricultural chemist James Finlay Weir Johnston (1796–1855), reflects a particular moment in British science and society. In this two-volume work, Johnston enthusiastically presents chemistry as the key to unlocking the secrets of God and Nature, a science that is capable of eliminating disease and bringing prosperity to mankind.[13] At the same time, the text uses racialized ethnography as scientific data, advocates the use of mind-altering drugs, and obsessively seeks to refute the philosophy of temperance advocates. Fryer and his associates approached this text with a combination of enthusiasm and caution. Like Johnston, they embraced chemistry as a path to wealth and power, but they sought to separate the scientific from the moral in Johnston's rhetoric. In the process of translation, Fryer produced a text at once enthusiastic about and ambivalent toward the possibilities of a Western *weisheng*.

James Finlay Weir Johnston was a Scottish student of Berzelius who was best known for his work on the chemistry of agriculture.[14] Toward the end of his career, Johnston became active in the popularization of scientific knowledge, and published several handbooks on the practical application of chemistry to farming and food processing. His works were widely read in the England, the United States, and Europe, and even found their way onto the natural science reading list of Karl Marx.[15] First published in Edinburgh in 1855 and in New York City in 1859, *The Chemistry of Common Life* was Johnston's magnum opus. A six-hundred-page combination of chemistry textbook, botanical treatise, and anthropological adventure tale, *The Chemistry of Common Life* provided up-to-date information on chemistry, but it was also clearly fashioned to convey a very specific social message.

The Chemistry of Common Life begins with an explanation of the chemical components of air, water, and soil. It then details the chemical nature of the plant and animal matter consumed by man. It breaks food down into constituents such as gluten, proteins, sugars, and starch, and lays out how the body derives energy and building material from these substances. The knowledge catalogued in *The Chemistry of Common Life* stemmed from attempts, made by European chemists and physiologists in the eighteenth and early nineteenth centuries, to unlock the nature of plant and animal life. Beginning with Antoine Laurent Lavoisier's early experiments on respiration, European scientists extracted and named the chemical constituents of food and pondered what the body did with food, medicines, and toxins. By the mid-nineteenth century, chemist Justus von Liebig could boast that science "no longer has any difficulty in understanding the different actions of aliments, poisons, and remedial agents—we have a clear conception of the causes of hunger, and of the exact nature of death."[16] *The Chemistry of Common Life* conveys this sort of confidence about the mastery of science over the processes of nature and attempts to transmit this confidence to a popular audience.

Johnston's work reveals itself as far more than a simple "popular chemistry" textbook; a surprisingly large section of the second volume is dedicated to an analysis of what Johnston classifies as narcotics: opium, coca, hashish, thorn-apples, and "the Siberian Fungus," or hallucinogenic mushrooms. History and anthropology are very much a part of the reasoning in this chemical review. Ultimately Johnston wishes to show that the consumption of mind-altering substances is an inevitable outcome of the progress of human civilization. By breaking down both nutrition and addiction to their chemical constituents—glucose, alcohol, caffeine, nicotine, morphine—and showing that humans around the world naturally sought out the pleasures of these chemicals, *The Chemistry of Common Life* attempted to present a rational, "scientific" counterweight to Victorian England's moral and religious debates over alcohol. While teaching laymen the basics of chemistry—or, perhaps, under the guise of teaching laymen the basics of chemistry—*The Chemistry of Common Life* strongly advocates the consumption of alcohol (in moderation), and suggests the possibility of a rational approach to the use of other mind-altering substances.

With its frank exploration of drug use, *The Chemistry of Common Life* is a highly interesting choice for a former missionary to translate as China's introduction to the Western way of "guarding life." Fryer's choice makes more sense if one views *Huaxue weisheng lun* not as a text on health, but as a continuation of Fryer's general work on the translation of chemistry.[17] *The Chemistry of Common Life* is an encyclopedia of knowledge about the chemistry of the everyday world. Moreover, Johnston's original text presents—and Fryer's text translates—chemistry as the key to a wealthy and disease-free future through manipulation of the elements of nature.

Chemistry and the Power to Transform Qi   The Chemistry of Common Life* suggests that chemistry can eliminate disease, not through the development of pharmaceuticals, but through the transformation of air. John Fryer's translation shares this hope, but takes extra steps to get the message across. Air is a foundation of *The Chemistry of Common Life.* The text begins with a discussion of the chemical composition of air, informing the reader of the height of the atmosphere and introducing the concept of air pressure. Although this discussion is retained in the Chinese translation, Fryer and his cotranslator first preface this information with a definition of air itself, giving their readers a name for air that would distinguish it from other conceptualizations of *qi.* Thus the very first line of the *Huaxue weisheng lun* reads, "Human life can not exist without breathing in a certain type of gas *[qi]* and this type of gas is known as the *qi* of the void *[kongqi]*." For Fryer, the first challenge of writing about *weisheng* in Chinese is to distinguish between gas (translated as *qi*) and *qi* (the basic stuff of the universe in Chinese cosmology).

With this opening line, Fryer and his cotranslators briefly revisit terrain covered by Jesuit missionaries to the Ming court, including Matteo Ricci, who felt it necessary to dislodge Neo-Confucian understandings of *qi* and replace them with an understanding of the elemental makeup of the universe.[18] The primary problem for Fryer was not that Chinese readers would have no conception of "air," but that they would associate the word *qi* with meanings that spread beyond a narrow correspondence with the English word *gas.* A nineteenth-century Chinese reader might understand the first lines of *Huaxue weisheng lun* to suggest that empty *qi (kongqi)* is a subset of that *qi* which is the fundamental energy-stuff of the universe. What Fryer emphatically wants to convey is that that air *(kongqi)* was a combination of elemental gases *(qi),* the separate existence of which could be demonstrated through laboratory experiment.

Johnston's work reflects the common nineteenth-century European belief about miasma. Air sustains life, but it is also the primary cause of disease. Air contains within it deadly pathogenic gases from a variety of sources:

factories, sewers, "the steaming marsh," volcanoes, and decomposing corpses. *Huaxue weisheng lun* translates the smelly gases given off by rotting plant and animal matter as *chouqi* (literally, stinking *qi*) and styles the invisible and scentless malarial steam of the marsh as *huiqi* (literally, filth *qi*)— vocabulary familiar from Chinese Warm Factor discourses on the causes of epidemics.[19]

For Johnston, chemistry not only has the power to identify the components of miasma, it also has the miraculous power to eliminate miasma as a cause of disease. Chemistry can identify the specific chemical composition of poisonous gases; they are not mysterious influences, but specific compounds such as hydrogen chloride, "sulphuretted hydrogen," ammonia, and phosphorus. By mixing these dangerous gases with other compounds, the chemist can transform their chemical composition and thus eliminate their pathogenic nature. Johnston particularly praises the ability of charcoal to filter out and transform harmful gases and suggests that scientists distribute charcoal masks to farmers throughout the world. With florid urgency, Johnston proclaims that charcoal masks "may . . . even prove a safeguard and health-preserver in many of those inhabited parts of the world where rich crops are dearly bought at the expense of rarely absent fevers, aguish fears and tremblings, debilitate frames, and short, unhappy lives."[20]

Fryer and his cotranslator share Johnston's excitement about chemistry's ability to eliminate malarial fevers and debilitating epidemics. The miraculous power of chemistry to render air harmless is made particularly clearly through a creative use of the Chinese language. In Fryer's translation, Western knowledge has unlocked the true nature of almost all the forms of *chouqi*. Through application of the knowledge of *huaxue* (literally, the study of transformation), the poison *(du)* of pestilent gases *(liqi)* can be eliminated by transforming *(hua)* their elemental makeup and thus changing their nature *(ling zhi hua fen er bian qi xing)* or creating entirely new substances through combinations *(yu zhi hua he er cheng xin zhi)*. In Fryer's text, the Western science of transformation *(huaxue)* becomes a key to guarding life *(weisheng)* because of its ability to alter the composition of noxious gases.[21]

Since the arrival of Westerners in treaty ports, Chinese had attributed to them an ability to effect remarkable transformations of physical materials. Missionaries were suspected of taking the eyes and blood of Chinese and transforming them into powerful medicines. In a less sinister mode, some Chinese believed that foreigners' tremendous power and wealth came from their ability to turn baser metals into silver.[22]

In *Huaxue weisheng lun*, however, belief that Western science could transform the very nature of the atmosphere was not the product of the Chinese imagination, but came instead from the hopeful aspirations of a British chemist. Fryer may have chosen to translate *The Chemistry of Common Life* into Chinese exactly because it preserved an early-nineteenth-century exuberance about the ability of chemistry to solve the problems of the world.

By 1880, the time that *Huaxue weisheng lun* appeared in Shanghai and Tianjin, hope in the power of science to eradicate disease stood poised to be passed on to the bacteriological laboratories of Europe. Microbes, however, hardly appear at all in Fryer's *weisheng* translations, and when they do, their association with disease is tenuous. It is clear from Fryer's overall output of medical translations that he is not concerned about bacteria or the threat they pose to health. Fryer instead identifies opium addiction as one of the worst health problems facing late-nineteenth-century China. It is on the question of opium and addiction that the translators contest the scientific authority of *The Chemistry of Common Life.*

The Anthropology of Addiction Johnston's text delights in the ingenuity exhibited by man in his quest to derive pleasure and profit from the earth's bounty. This unrestrained enthusiasm for chemistry as human ingenuity is at the center of Johnston's argument against temperance. His description of the science of brewing is filled with wonderment: He calls the chemical process that produces the dry ales of Prussia or the stouts of Scotland "beautiful" no fewer than four times.[23] Besides having a beautiful chemistry, alcohol has a virtuous role to play in the sustenance of the human race. Alcoholic beverages can warm the body, provide energy, assist digestion, and lift the spirits—in short, liquor is a sort of liquid bread, capable of nurturing life. With this flattering evaluation, Johnston specifically calls into question the reasoning of temperance advocates who portrayed liquor as a poison, a substance with no nutritional value, harmful in all doses and in all cases.

This same embrace of moderate consumption continues as *The Chemistry of Common Life* considers various plant products that it classifies as narcotics—including tobacco and opium. Here, however, the logic of chemical analysis gives way to the logic of clinical anthropology. Johnston is able to name the active compounds in most of these botanical substances but confesses that the laboratory has not yet determined the mechanisms through which they produced their distinctive psychotropic effects. In order to "illuminate the nature of narcotics scientifically," Johnston relies on ethnographic observations culled from travelogues, missionaries, and colonial administrators. This data includes information on the suitability of specific drugs for specific human types: hashish for the Arab camel driver, opium for the Chinese coolie, and tobacco for the German philosopher (who, "with the constant pipe diffusing its beloved aroma around him . . . works out the profoundest of his thoughts").[24] His catalogue of clinical observations thus complete, Johnston reaches a surprising conclusion: "Narcotics" are used so universally, with so little detriment to their respective societies, that when consumed within their appropriate cultural context, their effects on the human body may not be as disastrous as commonly thought.

At the bottom of Johnston's argument is the belief that different races possess radically different constitutions and thus react to drugs in different ways. Alcohol, for example, only poses serious harm when it is imbibed by the more "excitable" races, such as the American Indian, the Malay, or the Irish.[25] Johnston's discussion of opium highlights his use of ethnographic rhetoric and his racialized views of human bodies. To convey the effects of opium on the British constitution, Johnston turns not to the laboratory but to literature, quoting at length the delights and tortures narrated by Thomas De Quincey in *Confessions of an English Opium Eater* (1822). Johnston then selectively quotes the observations of Protestant missionaries about the benign effects of opium use in China.[26] Comparing the two sources, Johnston suggests that the Chinese have developed both a constitution and a culture suitable to opium use, and are thus able to escape the torments that more sensitive European users experience with the drug. After comparing the effects of alcohol in England and opium in China, Johnston asks, "Is opium necessarily deleterious?" He concludes that for the Chinese, the effects of opium are "not worse than those which are produced among ourselves by fermented liquors." In an interesting twist to common nineteenth-century theories of racial immunity, Johnston proclaims that the Chinese constitution is as well suited to opium as the Anglo-Saxon constitution is to dry ale.[27]

Johnston's rhetoric about race and addiction echoes similar discussions from the early nineteenth century about race and "acclimitization." In the pre-twentieth century colonial context, European observers investigated the interactions between racial constitutions and regional environments in order to explain what they believed were the natural immunities of indigenous populations to certain disease that otherwise felled normal Europeans. European scientists "resurrected Hippocrates" by linking doctrines of "airs, waters, and places" to explain the attributes of peoples, thus producing racial typologies that mirrored geography and climate. Although others noted that body types were the perfect product of environment, Johnston maintained that cultural habits were perfectly suited to specific body types, which were in turn distributed according to distinct geographical divisions.[28] Chinese were not immune to this way of thinking: Marta Hanson, Frank Dikötter, and Laura Hotstatler have all shown that medical thinkers and government administrators in late imperial China also associated specific climates with specific body types, and created hierarchies of body and culture during "colonial" encounters with non-Han peoples.[29] The impulse to critique European racism clashed with Chinese propensities toward thinking in racial categories in Fryer's translation of Johnston's text.

Translation as Evaluation   In *Huaxue weisheng lun*, John Fryer and his Chinese colleagues rejected Johnston's racial logic—but only as it was applied to China. The translation maintains statements about the relationship between Arabs and hashish or South American Indians and coca, but it directly refutes Johnston's conclusions about opium: "There is no doubt that opium truly causes harm to all those who use it. Among those who use it or those who do not use it, there are none who do not know this. It is regrettable that there are ignorant people in the West who frequently speak untruthfully [and give rise to all sorts] of baseless stories about opium."[30]

The translation then conveys all of the points about opium use found in *The Chemistry of Common Life* but refutes the veracity of each point, one by one. The translators find particularly objectionable the various ways Westerners tried to lessen the harm of opium by comparing it to alcohol use in the West. Such comparisons inevitably concluded that "alcohol was far more harmful than opium" because it resulted in more crime, more public violence, and more domestic abuse. Fryer and his associates found any attempt at comparing alcohol to opium in this manner extremely misguided:

> The harm from both of these things [alcohol and opium] should be considered extremely great. It is difficult to judge which of the two is worse. [Dealing with the problems of alcohol and opium] is like encountering two vipers on the path: there is no need to kick or poke them to test which one is less poisonous. Better to avoid both of them immediately—and the further away one retreats the safer one is.[31]

The translators' meaning is clear: the chemistry of the West might "enrich the country and benefit the people," but Western scientists did not understand the effects of substance abuse in China. *Huaxue weisheng lun* directly refutes the science of the original by offering its own set of clinical and social observations.

Through its critique, *Huaxue weisheng lun* claims the equivalence of Anglo-Saxon bodies and Chinese bodies—both are equally susceptible to the pains and tortures of addiction. Fryer's translation stops short of a denunciation of imperialism. It remains silent on the West's trade in opium, and does not accuse the West of inducing addiction among the Chinese people. But in refuting aspects of Johnston's racial logic, it does—as Gyan

Prakash has said about translation in India—directly "call into question the terms of colonial dominance," particularly the conditions that allowed the imposition of colonizing ideology on the science of human physiology. The example of *Huaxue weisheng lun*, however, complicates binaries between colonizer and colonized, between dominant and subjected. The ideology of racial immunity is questioned not by a Chinese, but by a white foreigner and his Chinese collaborators. It is only questioned insofar as it is applied to the Chinese and the opium problem; the overall basis of the ideology and its applicability to other "races" are not questioned.

Huaxue weisheng lun celebrates chemistry's ability to improve China's health by recategorizing the building blocks of nature, defining the health-giving properties of food, and eliminating the poisons of the atmosphere. However, in this translation it is obvious that the science of chemistry alone could not displace moral reasoning and personal observation as the basis of good health. It was not until later in the century that Fryer found a series of English-language texts where science upheld both the equality of Chinese and Western bodies and the moral message of temperance.

The Weisheng bian *Series (1893–96):*
Temperance as the Key to Health

In the mid-1890s, as the Qing empire entered its disastrous war with Japan, John Fryer and a Chinese collaborator, Luan Xueqian, translated three American children's hygiene books for use in China's missionary schools.[32] The original texts, published in the United States between 1888 and 1890 with the deceptively benign titles *Health for Little Folks, Lessons in Hygiene,* and *First Book in Physiology and Hygiene,* were actually at the center of a stormy American controversy about health, science, and society.[33] These texts were part of a now-forgotten American mass movement called Scientific Temperance Instruction (STI). Spearheaded by the Woman's Christian Temperance Union (WCTU), this education program invoked the authority of science in its quest to prove that alcohol was the cause of all ill-health.

By selecting these books, Fryer introduced a large Chinese audience to a definition of hygiene that was at the same time being intensely debated by scientists, politicians, and activists in the United States. Although they were translated with the juvenile titles of *Haitong weisheng bian* (1894), *Youtong weisheng bian* (1895), and *Chuxue weisheng bian* (1896) (literally, Hygiene for children, Hygiene for young children, and Hygiene primer), the organizational clarity and encyclopedic nature of these texts made them popular reference works for Chinese scholars (see Fig. 3). Their benign titles belie the important influence they had on formations of *weisheng*'s modern

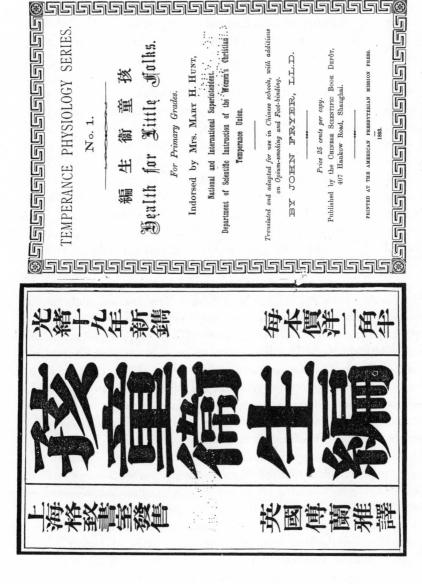

Figure 3. Title page of *Haitong weisheng bian*, John Fryer's 1893 translation of the WCTU Scientific Temperance Instruction textbook, *Health for Little Folks*.

meanings. An examination of the social contexts that produced these texts and their translations reveals that the meaning of hygiene was far from being fixed, either in the West or in China. Through translation of temperance textbooks, treaty ports took part in a cultural movement that was navigating the globe. By translating STI textbooks, Fryer and his Chinese colleagues took Protestant New England's obsession with individual moral behavior and merged it with China's individualistic traditions of guarding life.

Sober Science   In order to understand the creation and reception of Fryer's *Weisheng bian* series, one first has to consider the phenomenon of the temperance movement, one of the most widespread and influential social movements in nineteenth-century Europe and the United States. In the United States, the most influential and ultimately most politically powerful temperance organization was the WCTU, founded in 1874 and led for most of the late nineteenth century by the indomitable feminist Frances Willard. Willard's "army of women" attacked their enemy alcohol from many angles, with tactics ranging from the circulation of temperance pledges at local church meetings to lobbying the U.S. Congress for a total ban on alcohol sales.[34]

Scientific Temperance Instruction was a particularly powerful weapon in the arsenal of the WCTU.[35] A brainchild of New England educator and WCTU member Mary Hannah Hanchett Hunt, STI was an education program that used science to spread the WCTU's message to children in the U.S. public school system. Although the temperance movement had always claimed moral and social authority, with scientific temperance it presented its moral position as a truth verified by the sciences of chemistry, physiology, and anatomy. To spread its vision, STI produced textbooks, trained teachers, and lobbied Congress for nationwide adoption of its program in public schools. By 1892, STI education was mandatory for all the public schools in the United States. Jonathan Zimmerman estimates that by 1919, one out of every two adults had received their basic hygiene education from an STI textbook. Through STI, the WCTU set the stage for Prohibition by educating a generation of Americans in the evils of drink.[36]

Under Mary Hunt's firm and expert editorial hand, all STI textbooks consistently voiced the same main point: According to the wisdom of science, alcohol is poison, not a food. The textbooks begin by expounding the chemistry of good nutrition, explaining the components of healthful foods (gluten, sugar, fats, minerals) and describing their part in maintaining the health of the body. Chemistry is then invoked to expose the real nature of the fermentation and distillation of alcoholic drinks. Through fermentation and distillation, fruits and grains were "decomposed" in a process likened to the detestable and wasteful rotting of wholesome food. Since they were the product of chemical decomposition, alcoholic beverages could not be classified as foods or beverages but were instead poisons that destroyed human health. The chemical transformations that Johnston lauded as beautiful and ingenious became a putrid and sinister conspiracy in STI texts.

STI textbooks most likely came to China in the trunks and suitcases of crusading members of the WCTU. As Ian Tyrrell has observed in his magisterial work *Woman's World/Woman's Empire,* the "zeal to fight against all brain poisons" sent representatives of the WCTU across the Pacific to China. In Hong Kong, Shanghai, and Tianjin, WCTU members lectured foreign sailors on the evils of alcohol and spoke to churches about China's own particular scourge of intemperance, opium.[37] Little research has been done on the influence of the WCTU in China, but from Tyrell's scholarship we know that the cause of the WCTU was energetically taken up by missionaries of various denominations who had already established long-term residence in Shanghai, including Mary Jane Farnham of the American Presbyterian Mission.[38] Perhaps it was through Farnham and the Presbyterian Mission (whose press published General Missionary Conference textbooks) that STI was brought to the attention of John Fryer.

Stale Buns and the Poison of Fermentation: Translating the Message of Scientific Temperance Instruction   By translating the STI series, Fryer hoped to use its strong anti-alcohol message to attack the scourge of China's health, opium. *Weisheng bian* translations begin by portraying opium and alcohol as the commensurate crises of Eastern and Western civilizations. The preface of *Youtong weisheng bian* even quantifies this commensurability, stating that alcohol is responsible for 80 to 90 percent of all the physical and social problems of the West (*Xiguo*), while in China, opium is responsible for an equivalent 80 to 90 percent of the nation's woes. However, in spite of the promise that the texts would be altered to address China's problems, opium never displaces alcohol as the primary enemy of good hygiene in the *Weisheng bian* series. STI's overwhelming anti-alcohol message is maintained, if not enhanced, in the Chinese translations, and the *Weisheng bian* series read entirely like primers in temperance physiology.

The *Weisheng bian* series begins with advice on healthful nutrition. It breaks down foodstuffs into laboratory artifacts: sugars, starches, fats, gluten, and protein. It also instructs Chinese youth that the Anglo-American diet is superior to all others. Wheat is superior to rice, beef is the best of all possible meats, and everything is most healthful when boiled into a soft pulp. Occasionally foods like rice and tofu are added to the list of healthful ingestibles in the Chinese translation, but in general, Fryer's missionary textbooks make little accommodation to Chinese (particularly southern Chinese) ways of eating. Occasionally texts give advice on a scientific diet that includes grainy, stale steamed buns mixed with milk. Inclusion of these discussions of the healthful benefits of "graham" bread was not surprising—one of the authors in the STI series was diet and temperance guru John Harvey Kellogg, inventor of the dried breakfast cereal.[39] However, the choice of the word *mantou*—the Chinese steamed bun made of slightly sweetened, highly refined white flour—to translate the English word *bread* was rather unfortunate. The translation would have conjured in the minds of Chinese readers the unappetizing image of a course brown bun, several days old, crushed, mixed with steaming warm cow's milk, and eaten for dinner. It is unclear whether missionary schools actually subjected their Chinese students to such culinary disasters in their attempts to provide nutritious, "modern" food. Certainly Fryer and his Chinese collaborator provided no qualifying suggestions for this recipe, and simply presented this concoction to the Chinese as the West's most scientifically advanced meal.

Another important translation proved to be far more elegant and meaningful. STI's main contention, that alcohol is a poison, is powerfully expressed in the term that was used to translate alcohol (C_2H_5OH). Instead of *jiujing* (literally, the essence of wine), they used the term *niangdu* (literally, the poison of fermentation). The "scientific" nature of the argument is emphasized: the term *niang* reflects the chemical process that produces alcohol. At the same time, each instance of the word reminds the Chinese reader that the substance is a poison *(du)*. This novel translation uniquely captures the essence of STI and transmits it with every mention of the word for "alcohol" in the Chinese text. Thus STI's message is rendered even more persistently in the Chinese translation than in the English-language originals.

STI's message that alcohol was bad for the health would certainly have been familiar to Chinese readers. Classical texts beginning with the *Inner Cannon of the Yellow Emperor* warned that indulgence in wine would result in physical infirmities and even death. Absent from these American textbooks for schoolchildren was the connection, frequently made in Chinese hygiene texts, between alcohol consumption and debauched sexual activity. Although a prohibition against alcohol was familiar from Chinese health literature and was a particularly strong admonition in Buddhist traditions, the reason for wine's ill-effect was usually linked to the behavior of a drinker under the influence: Mindless indulgences in pleasures of the flesh after a night of carousing debilitated the body and led to disease. STI offered a direct, scientific, and sexless connection between alcohol and disease by illuminating the pathological physiology of alcohol metabolism.

Science, Translation, and Authority STI texts, both in the original and in translation, frequently invoked the authority of science, yet the validity of its science was fiercely debated in the United States. The debate revolved around the nutritional identity of alcohol itself. Was it, as STI claimed, a type of "brain poison," or was it, as some claimed, a form of food? Did it warm the body and provide sustenance, or did it only cause degradation of the body's tissues? At first few scientists actively lobbied against the STI message. It was not until STI received the blessing of the federal government that scientists mobilized to reclaim the "scientific truth" about alcohol from the hands of a crusading laity.

Alarmed that STI had become mandatory fare in public schools, in 1895 a group called the Committee of Fifty to Investigate the Liquor Problem convened to establish "a consensus of competent opinion on the subject of alcohol." Its physiology subcommittee was chaired by the founder of the National Library of Medicine, John S. Billings, and included as members the Harvard physiologist Henry Bowditch, the Yale chemist Russell Chittenden (a student of James Johnston), Johns Hopkins pathologist William H. Welch, and Wesleyan College physiologist Wilbur O. Atwater. Atwater was particularly zealous in his pursuit of data that would counter STI's claims. After two years of experiments conducted with expensive and elaborate apparatus, he conclusively proved that alcohol produced energy in the human body and was thus a food, not a poison. Much to Atwater's disappointment, his work failed to displace STI from its position in U.S. public schools.[40]

The texts that traveled to China in the trunks of Christian women embodied one of the most highly contested currents of American hygiene. In spite of the controversies that raged over STI in Boston, New York, and Baltimore, STI represented—for the treaty-port reader of Fryer's translations— the most advanced science available in the entire Western world. All of the Chinese volumes proclaim that their content was in accordance with *gezhi zhi fa*—the laws of science. The preface to *Haitong weisheng bian* even makes the exaggerated claim that its classroom use has been made mandatory by law in all the nations of the West. To read the *Weisheng bian* series was to understand that the enlightened governments of the West, as a matter of course, turned the laws of nature into laws that governed the affairs of men.

The *Weisheng bian* series entered the missionary classroom (and the minds of curious Chinese scholars) bearing the authority of Western governments, yet its main message was about individual responsibility. From the perspective of STI, the state had the responsibility to educate, but it was not responsible for providing, sustaining, or monitoring health. Health itself was the health of individuals: there was no discussion of the health of nations, no mention of the collective altering of environments in order to ensure a collective health. John Fryer's Western *weisheng* was an altered approach to a familiar goal. It claimed the laboratory as the new basis of appropriate knowledge about the body, but saw human moral will as the appropriate basis for guarding life.

Juzhai weisheng lun *(1880):* Sanitary Engineering to Cure the Poor

One exception to Fryer's focus on individual health is a little-known translation entitled *Juzhai weisheng lun* (The hygiene of residences). *Juzhai weisheng lun* appeared serially and was never published as a separate book.[41] As a result, it seems to have garnered less attention than Fryer's other translations on health. Adding to its obscurity is the unknown origin of the original text. As with most translations that appeared in *The Chinese Scientific Journal,* Fryer did not credit the original author of *Juzhai weisheng lun*. With its frequent allusions to London and its brief suggestion of the possibility of a germ theory of disease, it is most likely a British work from the 1870s.

Juzhai weisheng lun stands in striking contrast to Fryer's other *weisheng* translations. The environment, and not nutrition, is the main focus of concern. Engineering, and not chemistry, is the science that provides answers to the problems of health. The novel names provided in *Juzhai weisheng lun* are not the chemical building blocks of nature—oxygen, proteins, sugars—but the material building blocks of Western domestic and urban architecture: creosote, lead, porcelain, macadam. Illustrations reveal not the internal anatomy of the human body, but the internal anatomy of a Western house or a Western sewer system. Guarding vitality is achieved through a built environment that maximizes ventilation, conveys clean water, and removes wastes.

In surprising contrast to Fryer's other *weisheng* translations, *Juzhai weisheng lun* places the ultimate responsibility for human health squarely on the shoulders of government. Government needs to provide for human health, the text argues, because it is simply an economically efficient way to deal with the poor. Employing a classic utilitarian argument, the author uses aggregate statistics to demonstrate the economic logic of public health.

Every year there were 140,000 unnecessary deaths in England, whereas 280,000 people were unable to function properly because of illness (here the Chinese translation uses a phrase usually reserved for machines and rarely applied to human beings: "unable to function" is *bu neng caozuo*). Deaths due to fever in one area in London alone, over a course of five years, cost a total of 650 million *liang* (here the monetary value of the lives was not recorded in British pounds, but in units of Chinese silver currency). By taking the forty million *liang* that it spent each year on poor relief and using it instead to fund sanitary engineering, the government would not only recoup the investment after a few years, but would also be able to reduce the tax burden placed on the middle class.[42]

In the Chinese context, *Juzhai weisheng lun* is most remarkable for its divergence from the individual-centered models of *weisheng* presented in Fryer's other texts. This is perhaps the first time that this Chadwickian utilitarian approach to the health of peoples had been publicized in Chinese. In its disdain of direct poor relief, its belief in the power of urban engineering to eliminate disease, and its all-encompassing role for the government, it is radically removed from a Qing understanding of statecraft. But *Juzhai weisheng lun* escaped attention because it offered little information of practical use to an individual Chinese reader. With its words of caution directed at the British government and its elaborate blueprints for expensive public architecture, *Juzhai weisheng lun* spoke more to the European urban planner or the English parliamentarian than to the Chinese scholar in his studio. With their focus on food, beverages, and moral behavior, *Huaxue weisheng lun* and the *Weisheng bian* series fit well into preexisting Chinese models of preserving health. The specific content was radically different from Chinese models, but the actions required were the same: equipped with specialized knowledge, the individual contemplated the properties of food, weighed the dangers of wine, and worried about the unhealthy *qi* that lurked in the environment. The Western "Way of Guarding Life" that John Fryer translated was at once alien and at the same time comfortably familiar.

THE RECEPTION OF TRANSLATED *WEISHENG*

Liang Qichao

Although several translations on Western medicine and anatomy were available by the late nineteenth century, the systematic structure and comprehensive nature of Fryer's *weisheng* texts made them favorite reference works on human biology for reform-minded Chinese. There existed, however, no single consensus on the meaning or significance of this translated knowledge. Some began to find within it a new explanation for the superiority of the West and the national woes of China. Other readers took elements of this foreign *weisheng,* evaluated their usefulness, and added them to what they considered to be an equally valid (and even superior) body of Chinese knowledge about health. The lack of a single, unified program in the translated texts ensured that no dominant understanding of *weisheng* emerged in the late-nineteenth-century Qing empire.

One Chinese reader who studied Fryer's hygiene texts was the influential reformer and political thinker Liang Qichao. In his survey of translated texts, *On Reading Books of Western Learning* (Du xixue shu fa, 1897), Liang praised *Huaxue weisheng lun* and *Youtong weisheng bian* for their exposition of the scientific Western approach to nurturing life (here Liang uses the term *yangsheng,* not *weisheng*). In spite of the explicitly individual-focused message of these translations, Liang characteristically placed them in the context of national crisis:

> China's massive population is first in the world. Yet in the past thirty years, Europe's population has grown in leaps and bounds, whereas China's population has remained at four hundred million for the past one hundred years. This is due in part to the deleterious effects of floods, drought, and wars. But it is also because [the Chinese] have not yet perfected the Way of Nurturing Life *[yangsheng zhi dao]* and many die an early death. Recently Westerners have used the principles of science *[gezhi]* to deduce the essential principles of Nurturing Life. [As a result, Westerners] stress [these scientific principles] in all aspects of daily life.[43]

Liang directly linked personal hygiene with national survival. Although the problem is national, the solution is individual. Liang calls upon the Chinese to adopt healthier personal habits and thus exert themselves in perfecting "the Way of Nurturing Life." Here the health of the nation is not the responsibility of the government, but the responsibility of the citizen as he eats, drinks, and orders his daily life.

At the end of his consideration of health and the nation, Liang urges the gentleman who loves life to pay attention to the message of Fryer's *weisheng* translations. Exactly what this would mean for the average Chinese in his daily life is not clear. Would Liang advocate the consumption of boiled beef or *mantou* in milk as the basis of a healthy diet? Was it sufficient to renounce alcohol and opium, or would Chinese also have to replace concern about yin and yang with consideration of gluten and starch content? And if a general concern for heteropathic *qi* should be replaced by a fear of "sulphuretted gases" in an atmosphere made up of oxygen, carbon dioxide, and nitrogen, then how was the individual to act on such knowledge in his daily life? Here Liang reveals himself as a thinker far more concerned with the abstract questions of nation than with the lives of individual Chinese. Interestingly, as Liang shapes the message of Western hygiene to fit the needs of the nation, he simultaneously creates a picture of deficient Chinese bodies. By creating an ideal West that "stresses scientific principles in all aspects of life," he creates a deficient China that is mired in superstition and disease.

In spite of Liang's nationalistic moves, Fryer's texts did not offer a totalizing—or colonizing—program for modernity. Nation, government, and regulation were absent from the texts. The information on healthful living was diffuse, diverse, and at times contradictory. Ultimately the individual was left to adopt or reject elements from Western learning in the pursuit of living a healthier Chinese life. Also strikingly absent from these texts was the suggestion that *weisheng* was a quality that Chinese lacked or a skill that Chinese were incapable of accomplishing. In the social and political context of the late-nineteenth-century Qing empire, elite readers could not only question the advice presented in translated *weisheng*, but could even challenge the validity of the science behind the advice. One such skeptical reading of the science of hygiene came from one of the late Qing's most ardent enthusiasts of technology, Zheng Guanying.

Zheng Guanying and Zhongwai weisheng yaozhi

Zheng Guanying (1842–1922) is best known for his participation in the "foreign affairs" *(yang wu)* movement of the late nineteenth century. Born in Guangdong in the year the Treaty of Nanjing was signed, Zheng studied at Shanghai's Anglo-Chinese school and served as a comprador at the British shipping firm of Butterfield and Swire before he went on to create his own business empire. Zheng was a central figure in several Qing government-sponsored business enterprises, including the China Merchants Shipping Company and the Kaiping Mines. He advocated the official adoption of steamships, telegraphs, and railroads, and advised the Qing court on diplomatic and military affairs. His *Sheng shi wei yan* (Words of warning to an affluent age) was widely read at the turn of the century for its accurate information on the workings of Western capitalism and its urgent call for the Qing to undertake practical economic reform.[44] Zheng was also a frequent denizen of Tianjin, where the Cantonese native interfaced with the inner-Asian world of the Qing court via the person of Li Hongzhang.

Few who encounter Zheng Guanying in his guise as comprador and technocrat realize that he was also an ardent student of Daoism. A surprising portion of the essays in his collected writings are on meditation, visualization, and the nature of the Way. Zheng seems to have taken up Daoism seriously around the age of forty, after suffering physical debilitation during his frequent travels to Southeast Asia on behalf of his emperor and his businesses concerns. He turned to Daoism to seek practical answers to his physical malaise, and, it seems, to seek a remedy for spiritual emptiness in a life spent pursuing profit and modernity. Zheng studied longevity techniques with Cantonese Daoist masters and maintained correspondence with a network of devotees of the Dao across China from the 1880s until his death in 1922.

Zheng's identities as comprador and Daoist come together in his remarkable compilation on preserving health, _Zhongwai weisheng yaozhi_ (Chinese and foreign essentials of hygiene, 1890).[45] The shape of modern Chinese historiography dictates that Zheng's political and economic writings are far better known than his writings on health. However, in its judicious weighing of both Chinese knowledge and Western translations, _Zhongwai weisheng yaozhi_ provides more insights into Zheng's vision of a Chinese modernity than his more well-known writings on reform and steamships. In this consciously constructed "East-West" compilation of advice on health, Zheng holds two points of reference at the same time. Knowledge of Western science does not supplant his understanding of the Dao, nor does his love of the Dao hinder his appreciation of science. But in the end, the Dao proves to be a more fundamental criterion of truth. Zheng frequently marshals the Dao to counter Western science, but science can never undermine the hygienic wisdom of the Chinese ancients.

Zheng's text is a bricolage of translation, original texts, and commentary. He presents entire treatises from Chinese authors such as Wang Shixiong alongside entire translations of texts by Western authors, including John Fryer's translation of Charles de Lacy's _How to Prolong Life_ (1885).[46] Throughout the texts, Zheng interjects commentary (structurally indistinguishable from the original texts), sometimes as a scientific observer, sometimes as a Daoist master. He follows a discussion on the medicinal qualities of the dew waters from rice shoots, lotuses, chrysanthemums, and peonies with an introduction of Western public water-supply technology. He presents ancient taboos on eating the meat of horses or sheep of different colors together with the chemical composition of muscle fibers and plant protein. Aphorisms on the cultivation of the Spirit through meditation and the circulation of inner vitalities through Chinese yoga coexist with discussions of

Western municipal public health, magnetism as a cure for illness, and a brief mention of clitoridectomy as a cure for abnormal female sexual desire.[47]

"Western learning" and "Chinese learning" seem to be balanced, offered as equal options side by side. Zheng praises Western hygienic science for its ability to discern the actual nature of food substances. Zheng admits that Chinese knowledge does well in determining which foods cure particular illnesses, but does little to describe the actual composition and function of food. Zheng goes on to praise Western learning for its ability to analyze and quantify:

> More than one hundred years ago, famous doctors one after the other began to develop the method of chemistry. They used microscopes in order to investigate the composition of all things [in order to deter-mine] how much oil, sugar, starch, and protein [various substances] contained. Not only could they determine whether a food was bene-ficial to health, but [they could also determine] how much benefit [a food possessed]. Western Learning is also able to determine how much food goes in [to the body] and how much comes out in the form of sweat, urine, and feces.[48]

Zheng may have confused the laboratory techniques of chemistry, physiology, and microbiology, but he demonstrates that he has absorbed the message of translations such as *Huaxue weisheng lun* and their attempts at recasting the structure of the natural world in terms generated by the laboratory.

Still, in Zheng's vision, it is the Dao, and not the laboratory, that is the ultimate arbiter of truth. Daoist meditation is presented as the most prac-tical and effective method to preserve health. Health for the body is achieved by calming the Heart and Spirit, looking inward, reducing desires, and main-taining a placid demeanor. Through meditation, the individual prevents the kindling of internal fire, the main factor in precipitating any disease. The man who wishes to guard life practices a concentrated moderation in every-thing: looking, hearing, walking, sleeping, eating, ejaculating, standing, sit-ting, thinking, laughing, and speaking. If one practices such moderation, Zheng suggests, then even if an epidemic disease is raging within one's own house, there is no need to worry, since the body's surface defenses are con-centrated and its internal vitalities are strong.[49]

Western science has its merits, Zheng suggests, but Chinese knowledge contains a universal truth that had yet to be included within the boundaries of science:

> Western science, although it cleverly seeks the Way of *weisheng*, does so entirely on the basis of investigating form and material composition [*xing zhi*]. It does not understand the marvelous [ability] of non-matter

to give rise to matter, or the ability of the formless to give rise to form [*wu zhi sheng zhi, wu xing sheng xing*]. . . . Will Western physicians ever understand this? Even though they know about it, they do not believe in it and only find it laughable. I can only hope that as Western science progresses, in the end it will be able to comprehend the Way of the Immortals. Those who perfect the [Chinese] art [of self-cultivation] earn merit and virtue and enter the abode of the Immortals. Those who practice it even imperfectly can still avoid calamity and illness and live to an advanced age. Is this not a wonderfully felicitous thing for the entire world?![50]

The quintessential comprador and late Qing modernizer Zheng Guan-ying both embraced science and kept it at a critical distance. When embracing science, he supplemented Chinese medical and spiritual knowledge with useful items, presenting them as schemes that China might consider adopting in the future. By keeping science at a distance, Zheng refused to allow it to unseat the Dao as the ultimate arbiter of reality. Science was ultimately a peripheral knowledge, practical in its ability to parse and measure, but inferior to the Dao in its ability to guard life.

Some might see Zheng's presentation as a typical *ti* (Chinese knowledge as the essence) versus *yong* (Western knowledge for usefulness) dichotomy, but this is not entirely accurate. In Zheng's formulation, Chinese knowledge is as capable as Western knowledge of solving the "technological" problems of preventing disease: it is both *ti* and *yong* at the same time. It is also difficult to see Zheng's work as a hybrid that was produced by yet simultaneously subverted conditions of dominance. In *Zhongwai weisheng*, borders between "Chinese" and "foreign" are not porous; there is little mutual reflection or influence, no crossing of borders. Zheng's work is primarily a list, not a narrative, with little connection between separate translations or between quotation and commentary. Zheng offers "Chinese" and "foreign" options on separate menus of hygienic possibilities, with his own strong recommendation for the finest choices. Nor does Zheng's compiling of Chinese knowledge represent the creation of a "tradition" as a refuge of inner cultural identity vis-à-vis the dominance of the foreign in the outer world.[51] Chinese *weisheng* is not presented as a revived "tradition" but as a constantly present and still vibrant way of living life as a Chinese. Indeed, it is difficult to see conditions of colonial dominance at work at all in Zheng's *weisheng* compilation. Elsewhere Zheng issued "words of warning" to his compatriots about the dire threat that the West presented on economic and military fronts, but somehow, for Zheng, in 1895 the Chinese body—and the techniques for ensuring its health—stood firmly in the Dao.

CONCLUSION

The first Chinese translations of foreign *weisheng* and their reception reflected a specific moment in the history of science, health, and imperialism in China. The violence of invading armies allowed Europeans and Americans to create treaty ports. But in the last quarter of the nineteenth century, the actual foreign population in places like Shanghai or Tianjin was miniscule, foreign troops were few, and the day-to-day exercise of power between Chinese and foreigners at the local level was often negotiated, not forcefully imposed. Within this negotiated environment, however, the initial violence of foreign incursion and the threat of future incursions imparted an underlying tension and implicit hierarchy to Qing-foreign interactions. Within this threatened environment, to an increasing number of Chinese, the secret behind foreigners' ability to dominate lay in "Western learning," particularly in the sciences that facilitated the naming and manipulation of nature for profit and power.

John Fryer and his Chinese associates collaborated under these complex early treaty-port conditions of simmering hierarchies, perpetual negotiations, and latent horizons of violence. Fryer could not work without his Chinese colleagues, yet he often viewed them not as colleagues, but as supplicants of a Western knowledge that Fryer possessed by virtue of his identity as an Englishman. Although their work was itself conducted in an atmosphere of racial hierarchy, Fryer and his Chinese associates challenged the racial premises of nineteenth-century Western science.

Both Fryer and his Chinese colleagues were dedicated to the spread of "Western learning" as a superior alternative to Chinese approaches to the natural world. Their translated *weisheng* sought to replace yin and yang manifestations of *qi* with chemical elements and compounds. In spite of the novelty of these suggestions, Fryer's *weisheng* texts nevertheless projected a persistent emphasis on correct individual behavior, an element prevalent in Chinese approaches to health. By selecting specific European and American texts on "scientific hygiene" and not on "sanitary science," Fryer produced a certain harmony between the moral emphasis of *weisheng* and the moral strains of some nineteenth-century Euro-American approaches to hygiene. With the exception of the lesser-known *Juzhai weisheng lun*, all of Fryer's translations about health ignored government, law, nation, or collective action. Also absent from Fryer's translations was any suggestion that Chinese as a people lacked the ability to be "hygienic." All that was necessary was accurate scientific knowledge; the individual could then act upon that knowledge to lead a healthful life. *Huaxue weisheng lun*, the *Weisheng bian* series, and *Juzhai weisheng lun* represent the beginning of an important shift in meanings of hygiene in China. They suggest that the "basic rules for guarding life" come not from the Yellow Emperor's *Inner Canon* or the works of Master Zhuang, but from the laboratories of Europe and the United States. The translated *weisheng* that appeared in 1880 called upon Chinese to use laboratory science as a guide for daily existence.

Yet the particular environment of late-nineteenth-century China enabled Chinese to question the superiority of Western hygienic science. Even members of the elite who were central to the adoption of steamship, telegraph, and mining technologies could draw the line when it came to technologies of the body. Zheng Guanying's *Zhongwai weisheng yaozhi* plumbed the Chinese literature on preserving health and presented it side by side with essays and translations on Western water supply, public health regulations, physiology, and nutrition. After this exhaustive cataloguing activity, Zheng concludes that Western approaches to guarding life are occasionally helpful, but in no way superior to Chinese technology and knowledge. The body represents an untouched zone for Zheng, not only an inner zone of private Chinese profundity, but a zone of sound and useful technologies to employ publicly in daily life.

Zheng Guanying's *weisheng* writings suggest that in the late nineteenth century, foreign colonialism in China was devoid of the power to "colonize the body."[52] Here I employ David Arnold's term to point out two important aspects of late-nineteenth-century colonialism in China. First, foreign settlement governments did not have the resources to employ administrative mechanisms of disease control that "touched the body"—inspection, quarantine, and forced hospitalization of the indigenous population. Foreigners had no immediate jurisdiction over native areas. In Tianjin, in particular, the majority of foreigners and Chinese lived separate lives. The vast majority of Chinese lived more than a mile away from the white settlements. The British and French Concessions operated on small budgets and tidied up their few square blocks, thankful that the "squalid" Chinese city was out of sight. In Shanghai's International Settlement, home to far more Chinese than Tianjin's settlements, health officers accomplished little that had direct impact on the majority of Chinese lives. They tried, with varying success, to push through various reforms of the International Settlement's drainage system, and spent years in managing one small "lock hospital"— an experiment in policing prostitution that was a dismal failure.[53]

This is not to say that a desire to regulate and segregate indigenous populations did not enter into foreigners' management of concession life.[54] Evidence of a fear of indigenous contagion was generated by controversies over the use of public parks. Robert Bickers and Jeffrey Wasserstrom have excavated the exact wording behind the mythical "Dogs and Chinese Not Admitted" sign at Shanghai's Public Garden.[55] There was in fact no specific phrase equating Chinese and dogs in the park regulations, and yet Chinese, with the exception of servants accompanying employers, were indeed excluded from the park from 1894 to 1928. Anxieties underlying such exclusion can be seen in Tianjin, where, as in Shanghai before the 1880s, Chinese deemed "respectably dressed" were allowed access to the British park. British observers in Tianjin suggested that the long robe of the Chinese gentleman might hide a host of hygienic sins that could threaten the health of the white population. Some complained that "fat mandarins" were frolicking on the children's swings, raising the specter not only of contagion but of indecorous behavior as well. The porousness of boundaries in Tianjin and Shanghai reminded Europeans of the incomplete nature of their power in China. Foreign concession authorities eventually exerted the power to restrict access to parks, but they could not police native populations outside of concession areas, and limited resources made regulation of Chinese even within concessions boundaries an impossibility. Later, in the beginning of the twentieth century, anxieties about contagion between Chinese and European bodies lay at the foundation of a foreign "will to power," a potential, but potent, desire to expand authority over territory and people in order to prevent contamination. Still, as late as 1894, Chinese and foreigners still rubbed shoulder to shoulder in public parks, and there was little that foreigners could do about it.

The foreign presence in treaty-port China in the late nineteenth century was also without the means to colonize the minds of Chinese with the superiority of "Western medicine." Numerous studies have shown how Chinese availed themselves of the skills of Western surgeons, but the idea that the West possessed a superior "sanitary science"—and that this was a standard gauge to measure the modernity of individuals and civilizations—was not apparent to most Chinese. In Tianjin, for example, it seems that Chinese observers did not readily discern that health and hygiene played any particular role in the local governance of the foreign settlements. This was in part because as late as 1890 the concessions did not yet boast a municipal water supply, underground sewers, or extensive public medical services. Zhang Tao, long-time resident of Tianjin and chronicler of local history, did note that the concessions hired workers who swept the streets and carted away garbage. He extolled the virtues of this policy with a little poem:

> They clean the streets so that filthy airs can not accumulate
>   and ferment, and thus they prevent the spread of disease.
> The benefits are extremely great—what joy is like it?
> Carts half full of rubbish, half full of ash,
> Filled up in the south, down to the north and back.
> A law most excellent, a method one can trust,
> The workaday Kingly Way, cleaning up the dust.[56]

Zhang Tao saw the municipal sanitation workers in the foreign concessions as a down-to-earth yet very effective way to prevent epidemics. His
understanding of the cause of disease was analogous to that of the sanitarians of Europe, and he saw that the policy was for hygienic, not just aesthetic, purposes. Zhang suggested that government-funded garbage collection was a good basis for a Confucian "Kingly Way" of governance, but in
the end he did not discern the existence of a superior Western "sanitary
science."

A few in Tianjin would have been aware that foreign authorities in fully
colonial settings employed more invasive acts during outbreaks of epidemic
disease. Li Hongzhang received particularly unsettling reports about the
British handling of the 1894 plague epidemic in Hong Kong. These reports
described how Chinese who looked only slightly sick were given mixtures
of brandy and rhubarb by colony police. This noxious medicine made the
Chinese vomit, which was taken by the British sanitary police as a sign of
plague infection. The unfortunate victims were then whisked away to the
plague hospital where they were packed in ice, a treatment that resulted in
almost instant death. Li was most shocked to hear that dozens of Chinese
had been crowded into small huts by police and suffocated with sulfur gas.
An alarmed Li sought assurance from the British consul in Tianjin that
British Settlement police would not inflict such bizarre and frightening procedures upon Chinese residents in the event of a plague outbreak. The British
consul, Henry Buslow, tried his best to allay the viceroy's fears by patiently
informing him of the scientific basis for such procedures. "I explained to
His Excellency," the consul wrote, "that the fumigation was intended to dis-
infect the houses by killing the *germs* of the disease." Li reportedly inter-
jected with a laugh, "And it would suffocate the people *in* the houses, too, I
should think?" Buslow assured Li that the houses were not fumigated when
people were in them.[57]

It is possible that rumors of British interventions in the Hong Kong
plague were circulating in Tianjin by the end of the nineteenth century, but
they were not included under the rubric of *weisheng*. Readers of John Fryer's
translations might find that Western ways to health included wearing gas

masks, eating boiled meat, breathing oxygen, and renouncing wine. There was little sense, either in translated texts or in settlement administration, that elites in Europe had developed a powerful ideology linking the government, the police, the laboratory, and the people in one encompassing project of national health. If the late nineteenth century witnessed the emergence of a totalizing "hygienic modernity," there was little evidence of it in China, because no word existed to convey it.

5 Transforming *Eisei* in Meiji Japan

> When writing the draft of the National Medical Code [in 1875], I considered using words that were direct translations from original [Western] words—like *kenkô* [for "health"] or *hoken* [for "hygiene"]. But these words seemed too blunt and plain, and so I tried to think of other more appropriate terms. Then I recalled the word *eisei* [*weisheng*] from the "Kosôso hen" [Gengsang Chu pian] of Sôshi [*Zhuangzi*]. Of course the meaning of this term in the original text was slightly different [from Western concepts], but the characters appeared elegant and sounded tasteful, and so I chose them to signify the government administration of health protection.
>
> NAGAYO SENSAI, *Pine-Fragrance Memoirs*

In 1872, the Japanese government sent a thirty-four-year-old doctor named Nagayo Sensai (1838–1902) to serve as medical observer on an official embassy to the United States and Europe. Upon his return to Tokyo, he struggled to find a way to translate what he had witnessed abroad. In Europe and America, he perceived that state attention to health had become an essential cornerstone of governance. To varying degrees, each nation supported a web of engineering, education, policing, and laboratories that linked the health of the individual to the health of the nation. Each language had its own word to describe the system: in French, *santé; sanitary* in English; in German, *Gesundheitspflege, Sanitäts-wesen,* or *öffentliche Hygiene.* Nagayo hoped to find a Japanese word—conveyed in Chinese characters—that could adequately translate these meanings of expansive government provisioning for, and monitoring of, the health of its people. As he recalled in his memoirs a quarter of a century later, the word *eisei (weisheng)* from the Chinese Daoist classic Sôshi *(Zhuangzi)* struck him as a particularly appropriate translation. *Eisei's* characters for "guard" *(ei)* and "life" *(sei)* would give the new transplanted health system an "an elegant and tasteful" linguistic link to the past—albeit a link that reached back to the ancient past of Japan's neighbor, China.

Frederico Masini, in his meticulous scholarship on the formation of the modern Chinese lexicon, proposed that a radically new meaning for *weisheng* was "invented in Japan and imported to China at the end of the nineteenth century."[1] In the second half of the nineteenth century, Japanese scholars used Chinese characters to create a new terminology for words they encountered in European texts: *constitution, republic, science, rights, society.* Masini suggests that even though *eisei* was based on an existing Chinese term, the modern Chinese word *weisheng* should be considered as a pure neologism, a new word borrowed from Japanese since "the meaning that the word acquired in Japan was so different from its original meaning [to protect life]."[2]

Indeed, although John Fryer and others began to alter the content of *weisheng* in late-nineteenth-century Chinese treaty ports, the *eisei* that appears in writings of early Meiji medical elites is of a different order. For Nagayo Sensai and other builders of the Meiji state, *eisei* was a key link in the creation of a wealthy and powerful nation. Through the proper application of *eisei* in governance, an enlightened elite could lead the people to healthier lives. And where people's habits fell short of a hygienic ideal, the state had to intervene to impose health. *Eisei* linked the central government, the scientist, the physician, the police, the military, and the people in a joint effort to protect the national body. Through their linguistic imagination, *weisheng* had now become "hygienic modernity."

Hygienic modernity entered China in the twentieth century, but it was first translated and packaged as *eisei* in Meiji Japan. New scholarship examining translation as a process in Chinese has considered the "original" meanings of modern words such as *rights, liberty, machine,* and *society,* all of which were formed from classical sources. In tracing the development of these terms, scholars have hinted that these new words carried resonances from the past that significantly shaped their reception. Further investigation has highlighted how different individuals have deployed these words in different contexts, and how alternate translations competed for primacy.[3]

The role of Japanese translators as creator and mediator in this process is acknowledged, but seldom deeply pursued in scholarship on China. One can not consider the emergence of a word as powerful and complex as *weisheng* without considering the transformations it underwent in Japan. This is particularly important when one considers that "hygienic modernity" became a central strategy in the Japanese imperial expansion into Korea, Manchuria, Taiwan, and China. *Weisheng,* in its Japanese pronunciation *eisei,* was deployed over and over again in Meiji Japan, where it became an organizing principle in governance, a site of contestation over the relationship between the people and the state, and ultimately an indicator of the power of Japan vis-à-vis the rest of Asia. Certainly by the late nineteenth century, new valences of meaning emerged for *weisheng* in China, but these meanings had quite different resonances in comparison with what was emerging simultaneously in Japan. Japan was not the only birthplace of hygienic modernity, but Japan is where it assumed its recognizable shape and acquired its formidable power.

Several fine studies on the history of science, medicine, and public health in nineteenth-century Japan are already available in English. Within this literature a few scholars have begun exploring the ramifications of *eisei* in Japan in highly creative ways.[4] This chapter revisits this terrain and outlines the specific textual influences, the circulations between Japan and Europe, and the significant linguistic choices that went into the process of developing hygienic modernity in Japan. Threatened by Western imperialism, but not overcome by it, Japanese elites seized its tools and with them crafted their own apparatus to dominate Asia's future. This process was negotiated through languages that first invoked, and then attempted to sunder, Japan's connection to its Asian past.

NAGAYO SENSAI AND THE DISCOVERY OF EUROPEAN PUBLIC HEALTH

In his 1895 memoir, Nagayo Sensai used a Chinese-inspired idiom to convey his emotions on comprehending new meanings of health and hygiene during his first trip to the West in 1872. It was, he wrote, a bewildering but enlightening experience, like "seeing Mount Lu upon entering Mount Lu." Here one of the physicians who created Japan's modern public health system employed an allusion to a Chinese poem from the eleventh century:

> From one side, a whole range; from another side, a single peak,
> Far, near, high, low, no two parts alike.
> Why can't I tell the true shape of Mount Lu?
> Because I myself am in the mountain.

Composed by the Song dynasty literatus Su Shi upon visiting the scenic Mount Lu in Jiangxi province, this "Inscription Upon The Western Forest Wall" (Ti xi lin bi) had given rise to a Chinese idiom: "the true face of Mount Lu" *(Lu Shan zhen mian mu)*. In its use, this saying bypassed Su Shi's subtle Buddhist critique of earthly reality. Instead, "the true face of Mount Lu" meant to suddenly see the true nature of something that previously had been only partially comprehended. For Nagayo Sensai, going to Europe and seeing its administration of health was like "seeing Mount Lu from the inside": he was finally witnessing the full complexity of a system of medicine that he had previously glimpsed from afar.[5]

Nagayo Sensai was one of several physicians of Western medicine who were at the core of early Meiji state reforms. This immensely energetic and ambitious group, which included Ishiguro Tadanori, Matsumoto Ryôjun, and Gotô Shinpei, would ensure that health would be a central concern for the emerging Japanese nation. Nagayo Sensai was one among several, but his experiences are perhaps uniquely illustrative of the remarkable cultural and linguistic complexity of the early Meiji world. Nagayo's first glimpses of "Mount Lu" had come as early as the 1850s, when he began his study of Western medicine in Osaka. He gained other perspectives by reading translations of Western medical texts and working with Dutch physicians in Nagasaki. Finally, in 1871, Nagayo traveled to the United States and Europe as a medical observer on the Iwakura Embassy. Nagayo experienced medicine in a multilingual world of Dutch, German, Japanese, and English, yet he often framed his experience in terms of classical Chinese idioms. When he sought to name this new system of medical modernity—this "Mount Lu" that he had witnessed in Europe—Nagayo Sensai turned to a classic of Chinese philosophy.

Nagayo Sensai began his explorations of Western medicine at the age of sixteen, when he went to Osaka to study under the Dutch Learning *(rangaku)* scholar Ogata Kôan (1810–1863).[6] Dutch texts had become a window to the West after the Tokugawa shogunate excluded Europeans from Japan but allowed the Dutch to maintain a presence in Nagasaki. Medicine became one of the most attractive components of the language and science studies that made up Dutch Learning.[7] Since the early eighteenth century a small community of Japanese scholar-physicians had dedicated themselves to translating and learning from Dutch medical texts, in spite of government suppression and a general suspicion of the practice among the populace. Ogata Kôan was one of the nineteenth century's most active translators and practitioners of Dutch medicine. Ogata ardently sought to improve the status of his profession, and in 1838, he founded his own academy of medicine and translation, the Academy of Joy in Service (Tekitekisai juku, or Tekijuku).

At the academy, Nagayo Sensai learned about European approaches to anatomy, pharmacology, and medical ethics from his teacher's translated textbooks, particularly from Ogata's translation (from the Dutch) of the renown Berlin professor Christoff Wilhelm Hufeland's comprehensive medical textbook, *Enchiridium medicum* (Manual of medicine, 1836). In addition to using his translations, Ogata taught his students from Dutch texts, many of which were translations from the original German. In order to learn Western medicine, Sensai and his classmates had to struggle with Dutch-Japanese dictionaries and decipher the intricacies of Dutch grammar.[8]

After graduating from Ogata's academy in 1858, Nagayo Sensai journeyed to the western Kyushu port of Nagasaki, where he continued his study of Dutch medicine with a real Dutchman, the physician Johannes Pompe van Meerdervoort.[9] Under Pompe, Nagayo improved his spoken Dutch and learned how to run a hospital. He was also deeply impressed by Pompe's critique of Japanese public hygiene when cholera hit Kyushu in 1858.[10] The hospital founded by Pompe and the Tokugawa shogunate after the cholera epidemic went on to become Japan's first government-funded Western-style medical institution. In 1868, Nagayo Sensai became the director of the hospital and its affiliated medical school.[11]

Nagayo Sensai had immersed himself in European science texts, studied medicine in translation, and ran a small medical school: experiences that he later judged as mere fragments of Mount Lu. The opportunity for Nagayo to "enter Mount Lu" came in 1871, when he joined the Iwakura Embassy. Launched by Japan's new Meiji government, the Iwakura Embassy's original goal was to renegotiate the unequal treaties it had signed with Western powers. Ultimately the embassy's accomplishments as a fact-finding mission far outweighed its diplomatic achievements. Japan had witnessed the Qing empire's defeats at the hands of Great Britain and France, and the United States and other powers sought to "open" Japan to what appeared to be similarly devastating forces. The restoration of the Meiji emperor in 1868 gave legitimacy to a samurai-led program to strengthen the nation against incursions from the West. The Iwakura Embassy provided an opportunity for the new Meiji elite to scour the globe for ways to achieve national wealth and power. The embassy itinerary spread west to east across three continents, with ports of call including (but not limited to) San Francisco, Washington, New York, London, Paris, Amsterdam, Berlin, Rome, Vienna, and Moscow. For two years, the dozens of bureaucrats, nobles, and scholars who traveled with the embassy searched for the keys to modernity in the structure and function of the courts, elections, industries, legislatures, schools, prisons, and hospitals of every nation they passed through.

As the dean of Japan's first government-sponsored Western-style medical school, Nagayo Sensai focused on studying medical education in the West. The trip did not begin well for Nagayo. With the exception of being impressed by the presence of a sewer system and public hospital in a frontier city like Salt Lake City, he was generally bored and uninspired in the United States.[12] After he and his colleagues suffered racist slights from white professors at a medical school in Washington, D.C., Nagayo took his leave of the embassy and booked a passage to Europe.[13] He arrived in England months in advance of the embassy. After examining the sanitary works and public health organization of London, Nagayo moved on to Germany, which had recently gained a reputation as the new center for medical education in the West.[14]

In post-Chadwick England, public health had become "a kind of fundamental reform, an underpinning and sine qua non for all other reforms."[15] It is not clear if Nagayo realized that the primacy of public health had been accomplished in England only in fits and starts over the previous thirty years. After Chadwick's report, waves of cholera in 1848, 1853, and 1866 had added urgency to public health reforms, but concerns about the increasing power of government thwarted the sanitarians' vision of a state administered hygiene. London's Metropolitan Board of Works managed the engineering projects that would improve the health of the city, but the massive network of sewer pipes under the Thames was only authorized after the "Great Stink" of 1858 closed the houses of Parliament. During epidemic emergencies, numerous laws had been passed calling for the establishment of health officers in individual communities, but it was not until the Public Health Act of 1875 that a nationwide system of sanitary districts and health officers was formally established throughout Great Britain. In 1872 Nagayo would have witnessed the informal beginnings of such a system, where each district had a health officer and a sanitary committee responsible for the monitoring and reporting of epidemics and the guidance of health reforms. The participation of local councils in the hygienic needs of individual communities impressed Nagayo as particularly appropriate for Japan.

But it was in Germany that Nagayo felt he had finally "entered Mount Lu." Arriving in Berlin in 1872, Nagayo Sensai was not only poised to view impressive hospitals, shining laboratories, and the beginnings of a bourgeoning national public health bureaucracy; he also witnessed a society where physicians were major political actors and laboratory scientists shaped public debate. For the politically ambitious Nagayo, Germany offered a model for the central involvement of medicine—and medical experts— in the construction of a powerful and wealthy nation. In Berlin, Nagayo studied the organization and facilities of the Frederick Wilhelm University Medical School and its attached Charité Hospital. The first head of the faculty at the medical school had been C. W. Hufeland, the author of Ogata Kôan's translated comprehensive medical textbook. For Nagayo, traveling to Berlin was like making a pilgrimage to the source of his own medical knowledge. In his memoir, Nagayo remembered feeling conflicted emotions in Berlin. He deeply admired the university's traditions and laboratory facilities, but at the same time he felt deeply embarrassed about the comparatively meager facilities of his own medical school in Japan.[16]

While in Berlin, Nagayo Sensai noticed more than just the shining Bun-

Virchow

sen burners of the university medical school. A decade earlier, Rudolf Virchow, the social revolutionary and professor of cellular pathology, had been elected to Berlin's city council. As a politician who fervently believed in the power of vapors to cause disease and in the power of the state to create health, Virchow worked tirelessly to construct a miasma-free Berlin. Throughout the 1860s and 1870s, the councilman-professor pushed for the creation of a municipal sewer system so that miasma-causing wastes would not accumulate in the city's soil. Virchow also turned Berlin's hospitals, such as the massive Charité, into temples to light and ventilation. Through his political career and the publication of numerous essays on *öffliche Medezine*, Virchow the scientist shaped the politics of the city and made the municipal government responsible for the city's health.[17]

Pettenkofer

In the south of the newly unified German nation, another laboratory scientist, Max von Pettenkofer, was also influencing the architecture and politics of a city. As early as the 1840s, Pettenkofer held simultaneous positions as chemistry professor at the University of Munich and as medical advisor to the Bavarian Ministry of the Interior. Like Virchow, Pettenkofer was convinced that epidemics were caused by miasma-producing elements of filth lurking in the soil and relentlessly pushed the Munich government to construct sewer and water systems to purify the city. From his laboratory Pettenkofer quantified every aspect of hygiene—the composition of air, soil, water, and food; the value of ventilation; the quality of clothing; the function of cleanliness—and attempted to apply this data directly to the improvement of the environment. Pettenkofer's work was destined to be eclipsed twenty years later by Robert Koch's theory of germs. However, while in Germany, Nagayo learned of a triumphant Pettenkofer, a chemist-bureaucrat who was touted as the founder of Europe's new science of "experimental hygiene."[18]

In 1872, Germany under Otto von Bismarck was just beginning to weave together these regional public health phenomena into a nationwide system. But the outlines of a comprehensive, centralized state system to regulate the health of the nation already existed in German texts. Johann Peter Frank's *System einer vollstandigen medicinischen Polizey* (System for a comprehensive medical police), originally published between 1779 and 1817, described a totalizing plan for government responsibility for health. Frank postulated the development of a medical police force responsible for the removal of nuisances, the monitoring of epidemics, the execution of quarantine, and the enforcement of public and even domestic rules of hygiene.[19] While in Germany, Nagayo Sensai may have also encountered the works of Eduard Reich, whose magnum opus *System der Hygiene* (System of hy-

see Rosen article

giene) had just been published in 1871. In his *System*, Reich proposed four categories of health that were the concern of the state: moral hygiene, social hygiene, dietetic hygiene, and hygiene police. Nagayo would have immediately recognized the contemporary German thinking on health and the state embodied in the introduction to Reich's *System:*

> Hygiene is the totality of those principles, the application of which is intended to maintain individual and social health and morality, to destroy the cause of disease, and to ennoble man physically and morally. It deals with man in all his conditions and relations. Consequently, hygiene comprises the entire physical and moral world, and collaborates with all the sciences whose subject is the study of man and his environment. . . . It is the philosophy, the science, and the art of a healthy life for the individual, the family, the society, and the state.[20]

It was perhaps after reading such texts that Nagayo finally became aware of the significance and scope of the contemporary sanitarian movement in Europe:

> While investigating various medical systems as I was touring England and America, I often heard the words "sanitary" and "health," and when I came to Berlin I heard such terms as "Gesundheitsphlege" many times as I conducted interviews. At first I just took them at face value and did not think deeply about them, but as my investigations continued I realized that they did not simply mean preserving one's own health . . . I discovered that they referred to a special public administrative system that was responsible for the protection of the health of all of the citizens of the nation.[21]

Nagayo suggests that he had initially failed to grasp the comprehensive nature of the "hygiene" that he had heard spoken of so often in the United States and England. It took some time for him to comprehend a mode of preserving health that extended beyond individual responsibility to encompass the administration of a government and the construction of a society. For a national elite seeking to acquire modernity by quickly adopting complete systems of governance, the message contained in comprehensive works like Reich's *System der Hygiene* and Frank's *System einer vollstandigen medicinischen Polizey* proved exceedingly attractive. Indeed, after returning to Japan, Nagayo seemed to paraphrase Reich and Frank as he strove to define the way the Meiji government should administer health. Nagayo hoped to establish a new government entity that would

> form a single but comprehensive administrative department dedicated to removing dangers to life and ensuring the welfare of the nation. It would encompass all facets of life, whether great or small, that could

possibly endanger human existence, including prevalent diseases and epidemics; it would provide assistance to the impoverished and ensure the cleanliness of the land; it would control drinking water and sewage and regulate the construction of streets and houses as well as the manufacture of pharmaceuticals, dyes, and foodstuffs. . . . It would be an indispensable organization in the administration of the nation.[22]

With this rhapsody to comprehensive government administration and health, Nagayo outlined an ideal vision of hygienic modernity for Japan.

MOBILIZING ZHUANGZI IN THE SERVICE OF THE NATION

Upon his return to Japan, Nagayo Sensai's immediate goal was to establish an *öffentliche Medezine* system for the Meiji central government. For the Dutch Learning scholar turned state physician, finding an appropriate Japanese name for such a bureau was an essential first step. In his memoirs, Nagayo described the difficult process of translation. In his circumnavigation of the globe he had encountered terms such as *sanitary, hygiene,* and *Gesundheitspflege* (health care) used to connote both public and private approaches to disease prevention. Certain kanji combinations seemed to approximate these ideas: *kenkô* might be used to translate "health" and *hoken* (literally, preserving and strengthening) could translate "hygiene." However, it seemed to Nagayo that these terms conveyed a strictly private sense of individual actions to guard health. The German terms *Sanitäts-wesen* (sanitary system) or *öffentliche Hygiene* (official hygiene) described government structures, but Nagayo could not think of current Japanese equivalents for these terms. He hoped to somehow find a term that could incorporate the behavior of the individual but give priority to the role of the state.

In his memoirs, Nagayo suggested that in 1875 he finally turned to the Gengsang Chu chapter (Japanese, Kosôso hen) of the Daoist text *Zhuangzi* (Japanese, *Sôshi*) for the solution to his translation conundrum. In the Gengsang Chu chapter, Nanrong Chu asks Laozi to tell him the method of eluding death embodied in the "basic rules of guarding life." *Eisei* (*weisheng,* guarding life) struck Nagayo as the best term to capture the all-encompassing nature of his new government bureau for health. Describing his moment of linguistic triumph, Nagayo casually mentioned that the meaning of *eisei* in the original Daoist text differed considerably from the philosophy behind the state system he was trying to create. In this passage Zhuangzi proclaims that the best way to "guard life" is to become as spontaneous as a newborn baby, to "ripple along together" with all other things in the universe without a thought to purpose or destination—hardly the image that comes to mind when one thinks of Max von Pettenkofer or Otto von Bismarck. Moreover, Nagayo's crediting the *Sôshi* as the locus of his discovery seems a bit dishonest; as in China, the term *eisei* was commonly used to describe various dietary and exercise practices designed to strengthen the body's resistance to illness and age. If the word was in common use in Japan, why did Nagayo credit his choice to the hoary Chinese philosophy of Zhuangzi?

William Johnston has suggested that Nagayo consciously chose *eisei* because its first character, *ei* (Chinese, *wei*) conveyed the meaning of "policing or patrolling an area," and was thus related to the German concept of medical police that Nagayo wished to duplicate in Japan. In this interpretation, Nagayo, envisioning a highly centralized, interventionist state, had dubbed his organization the "bureau for policing life."[23] Nagayo was actually somewhat ambivalent about the suitability of hygiene police for Japan. In spite of his overall enthusiasm for the German model, Nagayo sought to conform with the regional variation of Japan and nurture the emergence of hygienically minded local elites; he actually supported placing the responsibility for local health with British-style citizens councils.[24] A more accurate appraisal of the meaning of *wei* would be akin to a military guard or fortress designed to protect something important or precious. Certainly Nagayo hoped that his new bureau would protect the life of the new Meiji state as it faced an uncertain future in a hostile world of armed Western imperialism. Nagayo's vision for *eisei* hoped to combine the best of the British and German systems. It was not only laboratories and quarantines: It also included education, welfare, and popular participation. The total sum of all these parts would create a healthy, strong populace that could both constitute and stand guard over the new nation. "Guarding life" was an appropriate term because in Nagayo's vision, the new bureau would protect the life of the citizen and the state.

Nagayo's explicit reference to the *Zhuangzi* was not just to display his erudition; it was also a way of honoring his mentor Ogata Kôan and his academy, the Tekijuku. The school's full name (Tekitekisai juku) could literally be translated as "The 'Delight Delight Studio' Academy," although to do so would be missing the point. The unusual doubling of the character *teki* (delight, joy) is an allusion to a passage in a chapter from *Zhuangzi* entitled "The Great Ancestral Venerable Teacher" (Da Shi Zong). This passage describes the attributes of Perfected Ones, the enlightened ancient sages whose profound character confounded those who tried to fathom it. They did not consider their own joy *(teki)*, but worked to fulfill the delight *(teki)* of others. At the same time, however, they did not compromise their principles in order to court fame or favor, even though such righteousness eventually cost them their lives.[25] With its complex allusions to exemplars of the Chinese past, the name Tekitekisai juku is only partially translatable into English as the Academy of Joy in Service. In nineteenth-century Japan, the doubling of *teki* in the school's name would invoke multiple associations of meaning for samurai educated in the writings of Chinese philosophy.

For many in the field of Dutch Learning, however, the use of *tekiteki* may have also been an allusion to an ideal of European medical ethics contained in Dutch texts. Ogata's founding of the Tekijuku coincided with the commencement of his work to translate C. W. Hufeland's *Enchiridion medicum*. In Japan, the most well-known section of the *Enchiridion medicum* was the final essay, "Die Verhältnisse des Arztes" (The relationships of the physician; Japanese, Fushi ikai), which had been translated separately and circulated widely among Dutch Learning scholars.[26] A brief treatise on professional ethics, this essay expressed Hufeland's wisdom on the profound responsibilities physicians had to serve their patients, their colleagues, and the public. The enthusiasm with which Hufeland's essay was translated and circulated in Japan suggests that its message appealed considerably to scholars of Dutch medicine who were struggling to establish and legitimize their profession. For early-nineteenth-century practitioners of Dutch medicine, the essay embodied the principled nature of an idealized European medical tradition, where *"der Arzt"* found joy in *"die Heilkunst"* of medicine and selflessly served his patients and his entire community.[27] As the first to translate the *Enchiridion medicum* in its entirety, Ogata Kôan was closely identified with Hufeland's work. The name of Ogata's school—the Academy of Joy in Service—quoted an ancient Chinese classic. At the same time, it paid tribute to a Berlin medical professor and conveyed the aspirations of a newly emerging hybrid healing profession in Japan. The very name of Ogata Kôan's medical academy highlights the abundance of East Asian and European cultural resources available to Japanese scholars of Dutch medicine—and the virtuoso manner in which scholars deployed those resources.

Thus for Nagayo Sensai, the choice of *weisheng* from the Daoist classic *Zhuangzi* was a tribute to his teacher and his school. It embodied multiple resonances that linked ideals of nationalism with the traditions of Dutch Learning and the prestige of ancient Chinese civilization. This moment embodied several significant aspects of Japan's situation in the early years of the Meiji regime. Nagayo Sensai and his medical community embraced European medicine within a world that valued Chinese culture. When translating Dutch they ranged freely through allusions to Chinese philosophers and poets. Nagayo Sensai originally operated in a world of intertexuality—and equivalence—that stretched from ancient China to nineteenth-century Berlin.

By the time Nagayo Sensai claimed to have invented a new *eisei*, however, the circumstances that had nurtured this rich creativity had begun to change. The teachers of Nagayo Sensai's generation had been drawn to European medicine before European imperialism loomed as a crisis for Japan. When Ogata Kôan established his academy, European medicine was not ascendant and powerful, the handmaiden of armies or colonizing authorities, but instead appeared as glimpses of anatomical diagrams and drug formulas in the pages of texts disassociated from their society of origin. Students of European medicine pursued Dutch Learning to further their own careers and satisfy their own curiosity, not to associate themselves with a dominant power or a symbol of Western-dictated modernity. This situation changed with the decline of the Tokugawa regime and the arrival of the Meiji Restoration. European medicine had become a key to wealth and power for the nation. A pilgrimage to Europe would reveal the proper path to medical modernity. Nagayo Sensai's reformulation of "guarding life" rested on old cultural allusions, but for Nagayo, *eisei* now meant "hygienic modernity," a way of radically transforming society, state, and the nation. Zhuangzi would lend his vocabulary to a concept that would become the key indicator of modernity for Japan, and ultimately a key rationalization for Japanese imperialism.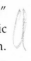

Nagayo Sensai had hoped to create a single meaning for *eisei*, one dictated by the state and by medical elites. But his choice of a "tasteful and elegant" word from a Chinese classic—one that also happened to be in common circulation in Japan, available for anyone to use—gave rise to numerous conflicting interpretations of the word in the early Meiji period. Old meanings for *eisei*, based on individual dietary regimes and practices, did not disappear when Nagayo named his government health bureau Eisei kyoka. Even among medical elites, there was no single, accepted mode of deploying vocabulary. Even as Nagayo Sensai built his bureau of hygiene, other scholars of Dutch medicine offered alternative approaches to "hygienic modernity" that were far removed from the state.

The First "New Hygiene": Eisei shinron (1872)

In spite of Nagayo's claim to originality, the first person to employ *eisei* in translating preventive health concepts from modern Europe was Ogata Kôan's son (and Nagayo's Tekijuku classmate) Ogata Koreyoshi. The younger

Ogata's work, *Eisei shinron* (A new treatise on hygiene), published in Osaka in 1872, predated Nagayo's post-Iwakura "invention" of hygienic modernity by three years.[28] Although the two had used the same word to convey their vision of hygienic modernity, the stark differences between Ogata's "new hygiene" and Nagayo's reformulated version demonstrates that no single definition for *eisei* existed in early Meiji Japan. In Ogata's treatise, the state is entirely absent. Instead the key to hygiene lies solely in the acquisition, by the individual, of a new and massively complicated set of vocabularies about the human body and the environment. In this regard, the message of Ogata's *eisei* is entirely comparable to that of John Fryer's Chinese *weisheng*. *Eisei shinron* renames the relationship between the natural world and the human body using the vocabularies of chemistry, physiology, and anatomy. Mastery of the language of the laboratory would guide the individual to achieve better health.

Eisei shinron is divided into two parts. The first part deals with the composition and metabolism of food and beverages. It presents the constituents of nutritious food (familiar from Fryer's *Huaxue weisheng lun*): gluten, protein, starch, sugars, minerals. It explains how the stomach digests nutrients, the blood circulates nutrients, and how the body excretes wastes. As in Fryer's *Weisheng bian* series, alcohol for Ogata rots the nerves and destroys the brain. The second section, entitled "Producing Progeny," details the anatomy and function of the human reproductive systems. Here Ogata describes the hidden reproductive organs of the female, measures and describes the inner anatomy of the male, and narrates the processes of conception and gestation. The proper regulation of sex and sexual organs, an essential aspect of *weisheng* in the East Asian context, is central to Ogata's definition of a modern *eisei*. The relationship between sex and health is something that the former missionary John Fryer, with his concerns about temperance and childhood education, excluded entirely from his reformulation of *weisheng*.

Another striking difference between Ogata's work and Fryer's translations lies in their use of language. Fryer's texts almost seem to hide the fact that they are translations of foreign works. Every attempt is made to naturalize foreign words by finding one, two, or three-character meaning-based "hypothetical equivalents" in Chinese. *Starch*, as a basic component of food, is translated as *xiaofen*, the powdery "starch" used to thicken sauces in Chinese cooking. *Albumin* is translated as *danbaizhi* (literally, egg white material). Transliterations of the sounds of foreign words are only occasionally used for chemical substances such as caffeine *(ka-fei-yin)*. In Ogata's work, however, the voice (and language) of the foreign expert, with his hundreds of new words defining the condition of hygienic modernity, is clearly preserved. Occasionally two-character kanji combinations suggest meanings in Japanese, whereas elsewhere combinations of multiple kanji convey the sounds of foreign words. Glosses written in phonetic kana in the margins provide Japanese pronunciations of the original Dutch words for each term. The appearance of Dutch in Ogata's work is not surprising. Ogata wrote *Eisei shinron* primarily as a text for medical students who would be expected to master foreign terminology. In contrast with Fryer's translation technique, *Eisei shinron* seems to embody a search for authenticity in the foreign. The result is a cacophony of new sounds and signifiers.

But these new vocabularies had not entirely succeeded in banishing other cosmologies: Foreign authenticity is not entirely complete. Ogata occasionally drew upon Chinese knowledge to fill in what he perceived to be gaps in Western knowledge. In the section on human reproduction, Ogata used a Daoist "anatomical fact"—the testicles are linked to the brain via the marrow of the spine—to explain why misuse of the sexual organs (through, for example, masturbation) led to more global disorders in the body. Since the scrotum is connected to the brain, Ogata reasoned, overuse of the sexual organs directly affected the functioning of the sense organs and nervous system. This Daoist anatomy allowed Ogata to provide a rational explanation for why sexual abandon led to blindness, deafness, bad breath, indigestion, acid stomach, baldness, and tooth decay.

Like John Fryer's *Huaxue weisheng lun*, *Eisei shinron* began to convey one of the first principles of hygienic modernity: the world was not composed of yin or yang manifestations of *qi*, but of various combinations of chemical elements. However, *Eisei shinron* highlights a specific moment in the process of constructing hygienic modernity in Japan. Shortly thereafter, in subsequent translations and publications, the use of alternate cosmologies and anatomies to fill in the gaps in European knowledge would disappear. For Nagayo Sensai and other early Meiji medical modernizers, the challenge to realizing hygienic modernity would become one of standardizing vocabularies and maintaining "authentic" representation of European knowledge. Japanese medical elites soon realized the diverse and rapidly changing nature of hygienic "truth" in the West. By the turn of the century, the pursuit of duplicating foreign authenticity would be discarded in favor of creating hygienic truth in Japan's own laboratories and clinics. But in the 1880s and 1890s, the continued pursuit of scientific authenticity compelled Japanese scientists to continue their pilgrimages to the centers of hygienic modernity in Europe. It also brought European experts to Japan to tutor eager students in the keys to modernity.

Modernity Kit: Eisei hanron *(1880)*

Eight years after the publication of *Eisei shinron*, another work on new hygiene emerged from the Tokyo Medical School. *Eisei hanron* (Comprehensive treatise on hygiene, 1880) was a compilation of the translated lectures of Ernst Tiegel, the Meiji government's first official professor of hygiene.[29] The book's title reflected the Meiji government's hope that one foreign expert could concisely, quickly, and accurately convey all of the principles of hygienic modernity directly to Japan's new medical elite. In many ways, *Eisei hanron* attempted to transplant in the minds of Japanese medical students a complete vision of the *öffenliche Hygiene* that had so thrilled Nagayo Sensai in Germany eight years before.[30] The official hygiene that Tiegel brought to Tokyo in 1880 was clearly the hygiene of Max von Pettenkofer, a vision entirely devoid of bacteria and obsessed with conquering miasma. In spite of the fact that this Munich approach to public health would soon be eclipsed by Berlin bacteriologists, *Eisei hanron* presented Meiji medical students with a comprehensive tool kit for the construction of an idealized European modernity.

Tiegel's lectures began with a very basic point: He sought to convey to his Japanese students the idea of "the masses," a collective of bodies that could be possessed of both health and disease. Tiegel encouraged the students to think of the population of the nation as one body, and the *eisei* official as both the policeman and the doctor to that body. Relying on a common late-nineteenth-century European trope equating illness with other forms of social disorder, Tiegel explained that disease killed citizens much in the same way that criminals and murderers threatened the population, and thus investigating and controlling disease was a basic responsibility of the state, just as investigating and controlling crime was one of the cornerstones of governance. First the state had to classify diseases as national, regional, or epidemic through the use of statistics. Then the state had to "diagnose" and eliminate the environmental factors that gave rise to public malaise.

In his discussion of the environmental causes of disease, Tiegel revealed himself to be a devotee of Pettenkofer's miasmal approach to disease causation. The environmental culprits of disease were the fouling airs that rose from the ground or from stagnant water. The stale air trapped inside the home and the smoky air of the factory could debilitate and kill. Bacteria lurked in water, but water also contained a large number of other harmful elements, including crystalline chemicals, dissolved gases, and microscopic insects.

To conquer the harms contained in air and water, Tiegel offered a complete kit of architectural, engineering, and administrative tools, all of which were to be orchestrated by the state. Government managed sewers, maintained water mains, policed building codes, and relocated unhealthy industries to the suburbs. In Tiegel's vision, the state should even design and construct sanitary toilets for public use. The sketches that illustrate this section of *Eisei hanron* project an idealized European version of a hygienic built environment, resplendent with cross-topped churches and gabled brick houses neatly arranged above orderly systems of underground pipes.

During his stay at Tokyo Medical School, Tiegel not only presented a template for German hygienic modernity: he also took time to scrutinize the hygienic quality of Japanese life. In these experiments, dubbed "Hygienic Investigations," Tiegel subjected Japanese objects to the laboratory scrutiny of Pettenkofer's scientific hygiene. He tested the ability of Japanese textiles to keep out harmful drafts, and examined Japanese straw sandals to see if they could prevent the harmful pollutants of the earth from reaching the Japanese foot.[31] In the bright new world portrayed by Tiegel in his lectures and reports, the combination of the laboratory and rational state administration was the key to the creation of a healthy, modern nation.

CONSTRUCTING THE CORPORAL NATION

In 1880 the world of hygienic modernity appeared tidy and complete in Tiegel's *Eisei hanron,* but for Meiji bureaucrats, the situation on the ground had proved far less orderly. Nagayo Sensai had drawn up plans for a bureau of health *(eisei kyoka),* which was established in the Home Ministry in 1875. The new bureau began its work by issuing regulations controlling medical licensing, burials, water supply, and waste removal. It also moved to establish a network of hospitals and medical schools throughout the country.[32] But devastating cholera epidemics swept over Japan from 1877 to 1879, resulting in the deaths of hundreds of thousands and demonstrating both the inadequacies of the new bureau and the huge gaps that lay between the state and popular conceptions of *eisei.*

In the cholera epidemic of 1877, health bureau intervention in the lives of Tokyo residents reached a degree previously only experienced by those suspected of serious crimes. Not surprisingly, the government met with stiff resistance. Sanitary police patrols inspected streets for cholera cases, concentrating their efforts on the poorer sections of the city. When cases were found, police posted public notices on victims' doors that announced *korera byô ari*—"Cholera Here"—and enforced in-house quarantine on the victims' families. Having a disease was no longer a private matter, but a public affair, publicized in the newspapers in dramatic accounts of police roundups of those who tried to escape quarantine. Cholera victims were forced from their homes and contained in isolation hospitals. Police disinfected homes with odd-smelling chemicals and burned the corpses of those who died from the disease.[33]

This unaccustomed intervention confused and angered people in Tokyo. Since so few of the sick who were put in quarantine returned alive, rumors about the isolation hospitals spread. In the popular imagination, hospital doctors were demons who drained patients of their life blood and plucked out their eyes. Patients, it was said, were put in coffins while still alive and hauled off to the incinerator. The renewed appearance of cholera in 1879 generated its own set of rumors, including the story that former U.S. president Ulysses S. Grant was visiting Tokyo in order to procure the liver of a Japanese cholera victim. Violent riots broke out against local authorities that were eventually quelled with military intervention.[34]

The cholera riots convinced administrators that a more effective public health bureaucracy was needed—together with a deeper indoctrination of society in the new principles of hygienic modernity. The appearance of a Central Sanitary Board, the evolution of a network of sanitary police (*eisei keisatsu*), the establishment of the Japan Hygiene Society, and the appearance of local neighborhood hygiene cooperatives (*eisei kumiai*) can all be linked to the subsequent waves of cholera that entered Japan throughout the 1870s and 1880s. In these crisis conditions, hygienic modernity could not be left to chance or to the gradual "enlightenment" of society, but had to be pursued vigorously by the state. In 1879, the first report of Japan's Central Sanitary Board stated, "Where hygiene is poor, it must be improved, where it is lacking, it must be imposed."[35]

Susan Burns has characterized this period as a time of intense debate between the state and society over the possession of the body. To what extent (and through what method) should the state intervene in the health of its citizens? To what extent was hygiene a private pursuit, and to what extent was it the prerogative of the state? To what extent could citizens maintain final control over their own bodies? These questions were complicated by the simultaneous bourgeoning in the 1880s of "domestic hygiene books," which emphasized "modern" techniques for the preservation of individual health and the health of families. An alarmed Nagayo Sensai claimed that

Japan had reached a "deadlock" *(tonza)* on hygiene, and felt compelled to publish an essay to correct mistaken understandings of *eisei*. Nagayo cautioned that hygiene was not about individual well-being, but about "disciplining the body" for the benefit of the health of society as a whole.[36]

As a multiplicity of popular understandings of health flourished and clashed with the state, new spokesmen for a centralized *eisei* emerged among the Meiji bureaucratic elite. The activities and writings of two men, Gotô Shinpei and Mori Ôgai , helped clarify and define *eisei* as a cornerstone of the modern Japanese state, and helped give *eisei* a central role in the formation of Japan's modern empire.

Gotô Shinpei (1857–1929) is synonymous with the idea of Japan's scientific imperial administration. He served as governor of Japan's first colony, Taiwan, and helped launch the Southern Manchurian Railway Company on the Chinese mainland before returning to Japan to end his career as the mayor of Tokyo. Significantly, Gotô began this long career of service to the empire in the field of *eisei*. His early essay, *Kokka eisei genri* (Principles of national hygiene, 1889), stands as one of the first major works on the philosophy of public health authored—and not simply compiled or translated—by a Japanese writer. In it, we find a biopolitical rationale for the modern state's intervention in matters of individual health.

Echoing themes found in the works of Herbert Spencer, Gotô first established that individual human lives were motivated by the struggle for survival and the desire to satisfy physical needs. When humans came together to form society, however, the struggle for survival between individuals ran counter to the interests of the whole. Therefore, the responsibility for the maintenance of health was transferred to the nation. The nation itself becomes a biological entity, a "national organism" *(yûkitaiteki kokkai)* or "corporal nation" *(jintaiteki kokka)* through which the satisfaction of the biological needs of the individual are realized.[37] In Gotô's vision, the state should not only intervene in epidemics, but should also provide a salubrious built environment, ensure basic welfare relief, and urge each citizen to develop an "enlightened" approach to personal habits. With a combination of biology and politics, *Kokka eisei genri* located the very survival of the nation, and the people within it, squarely in the central administration of hygienic modernity.[38]

Gotô's theory of the "corporal nation" reveals his early proclivities toward surveying, policing, and centralizing. As a twenty-one-year-old junior physician, Gotô initiated local surveys of the health situation in his native Aichi prefecture and established sanitary police in and around Nagoya. As an officer in the central government's bureau of health, Gotô not only continued his work setting up sanitary police, but also conducted numerous *eisei chôsa*, or hygiene surveys, of various prefectures. Gotô believed that in order to implement hygienic modernity, the state had to first understand local variation. Surveys could help the state diagnose and cure the benighted unhealthy habits of the masses, or help the state capitalize on any existing local customs that might profit from standardization and rationalization from above.[39]

Within months of publishing *Kokka eisei genri*, Gotô Shinpei was sent by the bureau of health to Munich, where he studied scientific hygiene under Max von Pettenkofer. In 1892, Gotô produced a doctoral thesis comparing various European systems of state medical administration, part of his goal to appropriate and shape techniques that would be suitable for Japan. After 1895, Gotô Shinpei would extended his unique methods of surveying, policing, and propagandizing the "corporal nation" to include the colonies of Japan.

The final contributor to shape the meaning of *eisei* in the late nineteenth century was the physician and novelist Mori Ôgai (1862–1922).[40] Mori Ôgai was one of the most prolific writers on hygiene in Meiji Japan. During his long career as a military officer, a medical professor, and (simultaneously) a novelist, Mori penned thousands of pages on *eisei*—essays on venereal disease, hospitals, women's hygiene, surgical techniques, nutrition, tuberculosis, malaria, public works, sanitary police, breast-feeding, and the hygienic value of *geta* (Japanese wooden clog-sandals). Mori made *eisei* into a science that encompassed everything: food, clothing, architecture, cities, police, armies, nation, and ultimately the Japanese "race." For Mori, a consciousness of hygiene was what made Japan modern, and more than any other writer in Japan, it was Mori Ôgai who created hygienic modernity.

Mori had studied German and medicine since the age of ten. After graduating from Tokyo Medical School (Tiegel taught his complete lectures on *eisei* during Mori's junior year), he became a ranking officer in the Japanese army medical service. In 1884, the Meiji government sent Mori to Germany to study military hygiene at the University of Berlin. The year after Mori arrived, the University of Berlin opened its Institut für Hygiene, with Robert Koch as its director. His diary from this period shows that during his time in Berlin, Mori was not confined to his laboratory bench: he frequented restaurants and cafés, networked with German and Japanese elites, wrote Chinese poetry in various Tang dynasty styles, and began a translation of Goethe's *Faust*.[41] But Mori did find the time to study the new bacteriological laboratory methods designed by Koch, who had just recently emerged as the triumphant discoverer of the tuberculosis bacillus and the cholera vibrio.

Mori's peripatetic mind was not content to focus solely on the microbe. He instead dedicated his medical career to thinking about the connections among organizations (especially the military), science, health, and culture (particularly Japan's). For Mori, Japan's acquisition of modern hygiene was what linked its destiny to that of the great nations of Europe—and clearly separated its identity from that of the ancient "Orient."[42] In *Eiseigaku tai-i* (An overview of hygienics, 1890) Mori explained the difference between *eisei* and older Sino-Japanese traditions.[43] On the surface *eisei* appeared similar to ancient forms of health preservation, but it was in fact a new science that had only been propagated in Japan in the past twenty years. Although ancient works such as "The Classics of Nurturing Life" or "The Precepts of Nurturing Life" focused on energies inside the body, the new science of *eisei* demonstrated how elements outside the body—air, water, food—influenced the health of the individual body and populations of people as a whole. *Eisei* was a science that taught how to manipulate environmental factors in order to decrease the incidence of disease. Utilizing a comparison with another science recently introduced into Japan, Mori suggested that the science of hygiene was perhaps best described as a sort of economics that facilitated rational planning for the improvement of health.

In tracing the history of hygienics, Mori praised the exhortations to domestic hygiene found in the ancient Chinese text *Zhou li*, but disowned the esoteric practices of Chinese Daoists that had influenced traditional Japanese health practices. According to Mori, Chinese Daoists were selfish hermits, eccentric aristocrats concerned only with their own longevity and well-being. Modern hygiene, on the other hand, was concerned with the well-being of society as a whole, and its work was situated squarely among the masses. If there was any clear historical precedent to modern hygiene in the global past, argued Mori, it was only to be found in European Christian charitable institutions such as hospitals and clinics, and, perhaps, in similar Buddhist enterprises in traditional Japan. Completing this historical sketch, Mori stated that the science of hygiene, by incorporating physics, chemistry, and other sciences, finally became established as a science in its own right in the modern world. Here it is clear that Mori's "modern world" is not limited to Europe, but also seamlessly includes Meiji Japan as well.

The rest of the work outlines the essential elements of hygienics around the world. Throughout these discussions, Mori Ôgai ranges back and forth between foreign and Japanese examples, seeking what is scientifically advantageous in different societies, regardless of origin. The urban planning of London, Berlin, Tokyo, and Vienna are all held to the same hygienic standard, yet at the same time Mori appreciates the varieties of customs and architectures produced by different natural environments. Japan fares no better or no worse than Europe on many counts. The stove and heating systems used in northern Germany and Russia are superior to the braziers of northern Japan, but Japanese architecture performs admirably well to ensure the circulation of air in Japan's hot humid summers. The narrow sleeves of European clothing protect the body from drafts and might be better for individuals of weak constitution, but Japanese women should not copy the European fashion of corset-wearing. Protein is an indispensable part of the modern hygienic diet, but Mori found that the Japanese diet could be sufficient in this regard, and cautioned his compatriots that they need not adopt the Western habit of eating large quantities of beef in order to be healthy. In *Eiseigaku tai-i*, Mori Ôgai demonstrates a confident hygienic cosmopolitanism. By grasping an international standard of science, he is able in the same breath to survey and critique the practices of both Europe and Japan. Through an understanding and implementation of the rules of hygiene, in Mori's imagination, Meiji Japan has indisputably entered the realm of the modern.

Mori's confidence in Japan's membership in the modern world was confirmed by the bacteriological discoveries of Kitasato Shibasuburô. Kitasato's contributions to *eisei* lay not in his writings for a general readership, but in the microbes he discovered and the institutions he founded.[44] He went to Berlin the same year as Mori and studied with Robert Koch in a far more intensive way than his more literary-minded classmate. He became master of his teacher's laboratory methods and soon emerged as an expert researcher in his own right. While still in Germany, he isolated the bacterium that causes tetanus in 1889, and the next year, Kitasato announced, with Emil von Behring, the discovery of diphtheria antitoxin. In 1893, he became the director of Japan's first Institute for Infectious Diseases, which began training Japan's own bacteriologists. By the last decade of the nineteenth century, Japanese youth were regularly going to German laboratories, then returning to find careers in the rapidly expanding civilian *eisei* bureau or the *eisei* section of the rapidly expanding Japanese military. He even replicated Robert Koch's accomplishments by discovering pathogens in far-flung colonial locales: in 1894, he and his mobile research team isolated *Pasteurella pestis* during an outbreak of the plague in Hong Kong. Mori Ôgai's vision of a Japan able to partake as equals in a global modernity was bolstered by Kitasato's 1894 discovery. But in that same year, Mori Ôgai's confidence in Japan's *eisei* was severely challenged as he faced death from disease on the battlefields of Manchuria.

EISEI IN THE WAR WITH THE QING

The Sino-Japanese War (1894–95) produced an unprecedented English-language document in the world history of military medicine: *The Surgical and Medical History of the Naval War Between Japan and China, 1894–1895*, written by the director of the medical department of the Imperial Japanese Navy, Baron Yasuzumi Saneyoshi.[45] Saneyoshi, who had studied medicine in Great Britain, noted in his introduction that no published medical history existed for any of the world's great naval battles, from ancient Greece to Trafalgar. Anxious to amend this situation during his administration, Saneyoshi in June of 1895 ordered the compilation of all ships' medical records into one major volume. Five years later this book was translated into English and presented as the world's first comprehensive account of all wounds received in all the naval engagements of a single war. The war between the Qing empire and Japan may have been fought over the control of Korea, but it also provided Japanese medical elites with the opportunity to demonstrate their mastery of modern medicine to the West.

The volume is a tour de force of medical observation. Schematic diagrams of battleships show the precise points of impact of Qing artillery shells and the position above and below decks of the casualties that resulted from each impact. Every wound received by every Japanese casualty in the Yellow Sea battles is catalogued, beginning with "Mutilation of Whole Body," followed by wounds to the skull, and proceeding down the body following a meticulous anatomical route: injuries of the eyes, injuries of the ear, upper extremity, upper limbs, lower extremity, and so on. The course and outcome of treatment for each of the 371 cases is recorded in elegant English prose, augmented by lavish photographs and color illustrations. The study proudly concludes that 70 percent of the wounded who were treated aboard ship or at the Sasebo Naval Hospital recovered from their wounds and were returned to active duty in the Japanese navy.[46]

If one compares this medical record of the Sino-Japanese War to the British medical debacle in the Crimea forty years earlier, it would seem that Japan had learned a perfect lesson in how to employ medical technologies and organization in the prosecution of war. The war itself had been a stunning success. The Qing forces who engaged with Japan's armies over con-

TABLE 1. Japanese Sick and Wounded in Sino-Japanese War

	Number of soldiers	Percent of (a)	Percent of (b)
Total on force (a)	178,292	100.00	
Total sick and wounded	171,164	96.00	
Battle-related wounds			
Gunshot, etc.	(approx.) 7,774	(approx.) 4.50	
Frostbite	7,226	4.05	
Nonbattle related	166,645	93.47	
Treated in field hospital (b)	115,419	64.74	
Beriberi	30,126	16.90	26.10
Dysentery	11,164	6.26	9.67
Malaria	10,511	5.90	9.11
Cholera	8,481	4.76	7.35
Total disease	60,282	33.82	52.23
Others	47,921	26.88	42.52
Sent back to Japan for treatment	67,600	37.92	

SOURCE: Date Kazuo, *Isei toshite no Mori Ôgai,* vol. 1, p. 365 (slightly modified).

trol of Korea had been decisively defeated. The Qing court, represented by Li Hongzhang, had been forced to pay a huge indemnity, open treaty ports to Japanese settlements, and even cede Taiwan and the Liaodong peninsula to Japan. To read the record of Baron Saneyoshi, the Japanese victory had been assured by the brilliant application of Western medical knowledge that had maximized the ability of citizens' bodies to serve the state.

What the naval officer did not mention, however, was that for Japan's forces, the greatest enemy had not been Qing artillery, but contagious disease. On fronts from Manchuria to Liaodong to Taiwan, many more Japanese soldiers succumbed to diseases than died of wounds in the entire war (see table 1). Wounds inflicted by Qing forces accounted for less than 5 percent of all casualties. Contagious disease (a category that in 1895 included the deficiency disease beriberi, whose cause had not been identified at the time) accounted for more than half of the cases treated in field hospitals during the war.[47] As head of the Japanese army's medical services in the Sino-Japanese War, Mori Ôgai saw the conflict over Korea as a "war with disease" that had been fought without much success. Behind the scenes, the war had been an extreme challenge to Japan's growing sense of hygienic modernity. Mori's reports from the field in Liaodong repeatedly emphasized the need for improved isolation of contagious disease, improved nutrition, more hygienic uniforms (that could, for example, prevent the thousands of cases of frostbite suffered by Japanese soldiers, or counter the chance of infection), improved management of the environment around military camps—in short, a redoubling of efforts in the field of *eisei*.[48]

When Mori returned from the war, he threw himself into the production of a comprehensive text on *eisei* for his students at the Imperial Military Medical Academy in Tokyo. In 1897, he published *Eisei shinron* (A new treatise on hygiene), later retitled *Eisei shinhen* (A new compilation on hygiene). To distinguish this work from Ogata Koreyoshi's earlier *Eisei shinron*, Mori's title might more accurately be translated as *A New Theory of Hygienic Modernity*. This work encompasses all the categories of knowledge on health and the prevention of disease that Mori had accumulated in his fifteen years as a student of *eisei*. In its modern reprint, it encompasses two volumes totaling more than thirteen hundred pages. Its table of contents alone presents the diverse realms encompassed and unified under hygienic modernity:[49]

General Theory
Gases
Reproduction
History
Climate
Hospitals
Life
Acclimatization
Prisons
Nutrition
Clothing
Vehicles
Food
Cities
Labor
Stimulants
Sanitation
Industry
Narcotics
Funerals
Epidemic Prevention
Race
Epidemic Diseases

Mori's summary of the science of hygiene was also enshrined in a new volley of post–Sino-Japanese War *eisei* regulations in the military, within Japan, and in Japan's colony, Taiwan, giving the government even greater power to inspect, enforce quarantine, and regulate the movement and lifestyles of people for hygienic reasons. Significantly, this strengthened capacity to administer hygienic modernity facilitated the formal acceptance of Japan's empire by the European powers—a new status reflected in Japan's port inspection regulations. Like the Qing empire, Japan's right to inspect foreign ships at its ports for contagious disease had been compromised by unequal treaties with Western powers. By 1899, with the end of the unequal treaties, Japan recovered all of its sovereign right to inspect and quarantine foreign ships at its own ports. That same year the Japanese colonial government in Taiwan established regulations for the Japanese control of port inspection in Taiwan. By the turn of the century, Japan demonstrated that it could, like the United States and European powers, be responsible for the *eisei* of Asia. The power to "touch the body" as a colonial administration marked Japan's arrival as an imperial power in its own right, and was one of the important modes through which Japan distinguished itself from its Asian neighbors.

Nagayo Sensai's moment of linguistic inspiration in 1875 points to an important conceptual and political shift in Japan that was to have radical implications for twentieth-century China. The word *eisei* once applied to a scattered variety of principles and practices related to personal health and sanctioned by Chinese cosmology. By the turn of the century in Japan, the meanings of *eisei* had coalesced around two new sites: the laboratory and the nation. All preventive practices advocated within this new *eisei*, from abstinence from alcohol to the burning of corpses, claimed to be based on universal truths emerging from laboratory experiments in chemistry, physiology, and the new science of bacteriology. At the same time, *eisei* implied that national survival was the ultimate purpose of disease prevention. The health of the individual was the business of the state, and the individual's preservation of his or her own health was for the greater good of the nation.

CONCLUSION

John Fryer and his Chinese colleagues produced texts on *weisheng* at the same time that the Meiji medical elite were producing a new *eisei* for Japan. Both groups produced texts designed to popularize new meanings about health and hygiene in their respective societies. Japanese translators produced numerous texts for an audience of medical and administrative specialists. By contrast, translations of *weisheng* in late-nineteenth-century China were not produced by physicians, nor were they produced by men centrally involved in Qing rule. The Qing did sponsor its own medical school—the Beiyang Navy Medical Academy, founded by British missionaries and taken over by the Qing in 1888—but the first Chinese graduates of that school did not leave any writings. Contemporary observers suggested that the graduates were not effectively employed by the Qing military until the early twentieth century. Certainly their impact on the operation of the Qing empire was not as great as that of Nagayo Sensai, Gotô Shinpei, Mori Ôgai and others on the operation of the Japanese empire. By the end of the nineteenth century, the extent to which new meanings of *eisei/weisheng* were constructed, embraced, and put into practice by national elites marked a distinct divergence between China and Japan. Although both had used the *Zhuangzi*'s term for translating new concepts of hygiene informed by laboratory science, the political and social content of the hygiene that they translated was not the same. Fryer's *weisheng* spoke to the amateur chemist and the general scholar about the chemical composition of the natural world. It warned Chinese youth about the dangers of alcohol and opium, and called upon each individual to make the right choice to ensure their individual health. By contrast, the *eisei* of Nagayo Sensai, Gotô Shinpei, and Mori Ôgai remained perpetually focused on public administration and presented a formula through which individuals could be subsumed under, guided by, and dedicated to the nation.

A dramatic example of the differences between Japanese *eisei* and Chinese *weisheng* can be found in discussions of the cholera epidemic of 1895 in Tianjin's first Chinese language newspaper, *Zhibao* (The Zhili gazette). Troop movements during the Sino-Japanese War unleashed cholera in East Asia in the summer of 1895. Its effects on the city of Tianjin became the focus of reporting in early issues of *Zhibao*, a newspaper owned by foreigners but written and edited by modernizing Chinese elites. The picture of *weisheng* that emerges from the *Zhibao* coverage of cholera demonstrates the persistence of Chinese approaches to health and disease at the turn of the century, and suggests that a public meaning for *weisheng* had yet to be devised in the minds of treaty-port Chinese.

The etiology of cholera in these newspaper accounts is diverse but rests primarily on Chinese terms. Relying on methods of conceptualizing disease first elaborated by the second-century physician Zhang Zhongjing, cholera as described in *Zhibao* is sometimes caused by damage entering the "three yins" of the body (the Mature yin of the Spleen, the Immature yin of the Kidney, and the Attenuated yin of the Liver).[50] Sometimes an external pathogen, identified as heteropathic *qi* or miasma *(xieqi, huiqi)*, gives rise to the disease. Other accounts hold that the improper eating of summer yin foods—cucumbers, watermelon, and Tianjin's beloved crabs—either cause the illness or trigger it after an external pathogen has entered the body. In all cases, however, cholera could be easily avoided through self-restraint. *Zhibao* published frequent warnings against the consumption of raw fruit and undercooked crabs, as their highly yin natures would be enough to trigger a bout of "sudden chaos." Most important, loss of *jing* would weaken the body's yin reserves. *Zhibao* frequently reminded individuals to "guard life through reducing desire."[51]

 Zhibao would not be unique in the turn-of-the-century world for maintaining conflicting views on the etiology of cholera. European scientists continued to disagree about cholera well into the 1890s. In Germany, the home of the germ theory, Max von Pettenkofer continued to subscribe to a multicausal view of cholera (miasma, impurities in the soil, improper eating) long after Robert Koch had announced the discovery of the organism that caused the disease. In 1892, Pettenkofer even consumed a beaker of cholera vibrio slurry in order to prove his point (he survived the encounter). Although one should acknowledge the diversity of approaches to cholera that existed across Europe at this time, it is highly significant that *Zhibao*'s coverage dwells primarily on sex and yin. Like Shanghai's first Chinese-language newspapers, *Zhibao* was owned by foreigners and produced by treat-port Chinese who were well-versed in "foreign affairs" *(yangwu)*: those who published in *Zhibao* included the famous reformer Yan Fu, whose essays on social Darwinism first appeared as lead editorials for the paper. *Zhibao* reported on events of the world, and occasionally contained dispatches from Hong Kong, Singapore, Japan, and Russia. But in their response to the epidemic of 1895, neither the *Zhibao* reporters nor the city they reported on seemed to have absorbed Western approaches to epidemic disease, or if they had, they subsumed them entirely within a Chinese idiom. Moreover, as portrayed in *Zhibao*, disease prevention in Tianjin in 1895 was entirely the responsibility of the individual. Local charities published in *Zhibao* the formulas for herbal medicines that could treat gastrointestinal disorders. By making otherwise specialized knowledge available to the public, Tianjin's elites demonstrated their concern for the public good. But nowhere within the pages of *Zhibao* did any of Tianjin's modernizing elites call for government intervention in the epidemic. The type of highly interventionist public response to cholera that took place in Meiji Japan did not occur in Tianjin, nor was it even imagined.

Instead, writers of *Zhibao* used individual-based concepts of guarding life both to criticize the Japanese invasion of Taiwan and to ridicule the idea that the Japanese possessed a superior kind of *weisheng*. *Zhibao* reports noted that cholera had taken a particularly heavy toll on Japanese forces during the first steps in the occupation of Taiwan. According to the paper, the reason the Japanese army lost so many soldiers was that they paid no heed to the rational rules of *weisheng*. It was common knowledge in China that the island of Taiwan was permeated by *zhangqi*, the endemic pestilent vapor that also lurked in the dense undergrowth of other southern provinces like Yunnan and Guangdong. The local Taiwanese people knew that in order to avoid *zhangqi*'s harmful effects, they had to practice sexual moderation, and as a result they were little troubled by cholera. But Japanese soldiers were of such lascivious habits, raping local women and frequenting brothels to excess, that they were immediately stricken with cholera.[52] With an ironic attention to detail, one article noted that the Japanese army's department of hygiene—in Chinese, the *weisheng bu*—had sent 1,759 medical personnel to Taiwan. These *weisheng* men "hurried back and forth, day and night, unable to rest" in their attempt to curb the epidemic, but their techniques (which remained a mystery in the article) had proved unsuccessful in Taiwan's environment. The true method of *weisheng* was possessed by the Chinese on Taiwan, not by Taiwan's new colonial masters.[53]

During the 1895 cholera epidemic, a multiplicity of activities were conducted by Japanese elites in the name of *eisei*. Mori Ôgai and Gotô Shinpei devised new methods to prevent disease by utilizing disinfectants, engineering, statistics, and police. Technicians at Kitasato Shibasuburô's Institute for Infectious Diseases applied Koch's postulates to isolate cholera vibrio from the feces of Japanese cholera victims. Tokyo sanitary police forcefully relocated suspected cholera cases to the city's isolation hospital, where victims feared they would be burned alive and referred to the physicians as "red and green devils."[54] One need not entirely agree with Warwick Anderson's assertion that Western medicine is, in all localities, essentially a colonizing force to see that from the perspective of medicine and public health, Japanese elites successfully avoided Western colonization in part by acquiring the ability to colonize themselves. By the turn of the century, the term *eisei*, as reconfigured by Meiji medical elites, embodied many of the elements associated with "colonial medicine": sanitary police, forced quarantine, mass microscopic examination of excreta, the suspicion and investigations of local sanitary habits. Yet Meiji medical elites were also convinced that the people of Japan could be tutored in civilization and enlightenment, and would willingly equate the goals of the state with their own. Thus *eisei* also included campaigns about diet, nutrition, and the habits of daily life in the hopes of transforming the people into the healthy constituents of the national body. At least in the minds of Meiji bureaucrats, physicians, and scientists, *eisei* by the turn of the century was hygienic modernity, a foundational element in the creation of a nation on par with the powers of Europe. In the twentieth century, *eisei* as hygienic modernity would become a foundational element in the creation of the Japanese empire. For certain parts of China, the introduction to this new vision of hygienic modernity would come suddenly and violently, with the arrival of the combined forces of the modern world's imperial powers.

6 Deficiency and Sovereignty

*Hygienic Modernity in the Occupation of Tianjin,
1900–1902*

Before us lies a great city, not only deserted, but sacked, looted, and
in ashes, by Christian armies. Only a few days before . . . this street
and the surrounding houses were a holocaust of human life. A day
later that long thoroughfare was a slow-moving line of homeless,
weeping human beings—their homes in ashes, without food, friend-
less, and, in many cases, their kindred left charred in the ruins of their
homes. This is not of the imagination; all that I mention I saw. . . .
This street was strewn with corpses; those of persons asphyxiated by
the fatal gases of the lyddite shells could easily be distinguished by
the yellow discoloration of the skin. Lily-feet, which were so expensive
at Shanghai, were here the appendages of mangled corpses that had
no more consideration than the carcasses of dogs, which also lined
the streets; but the camera cannot portray nor the pen describe those
heartrending scenes along this narrow street after the battle. Now
it is a pathetic scene of desolation.

JAMES RICALTON (1844–1929), photographer, on Tianjin in July 1900

La seule excuse de la colonisation, c'est la médecine.

HUBERT LYAUTEY (1854–1934), French military officer
and colonial administrator

In the summer of 1900, thousands of peasant practitioners of martial arts
began to attack foreigners and Christians in north China. Together with Qing
military forces, these "Boxers" lay siege to foreign outposts in Tianjin and
Beijing. In response, six Western nations, together with Russia and Japan,
dispatched a massive international relief force to rescue besieged foreigners, annihilate the Boxers, and chastise the Qing court.

The bloody suppression of the Boxer Uprising by imperial powers became a major turning point in the history of modern China. In James Hevia's
words, the aftermath of the Boxer Uprising "left a brand" on China, marking it in Western and Japanese discourse as a land boiling over with dangerous superstitions, a place in need of forceful redemption from a backward past. Paul Cohen has described how modernizing Chinese reformers
in the early twentieth century adopted this discourse, conceiving of the Box-

ers as "everything in Chinese society [they] wanted destroyed." The failure of the Boxer Uprising pushed the Qing court to enact destabilizing reforms, redoubled the political demands of local elites, spurred on the activities of anti-Qing forces, and led to the fall of the Qing in 1912. Even in
contemporary China, after a period of official praise of the Boxers as anti-
imperialist revolutionaries, the Boxers have returned, in the discourse of both
intellectuals and the state, as a specter haunting China's attempts at modernization. Myriad social phenomena, including the appearance of millions
of peasants streaming into China's cities (the "floating population"), the rise
of *qigong* sects such as Falun gong, and even the outbreak of riots at soccer
matches have caused exasperated intellectuals and nervous government
officials to invoke cautionary comparisons with the Boxer debacle. The Boxers have come to symbolize the deficiencies of China's culture, while the
humiliations China suffered at the hands of foreign armies in 1900 serve as
a reminder of what might happen if China's culture is not transformed.[1]

Although the Boxer debacle had a global effect on the polity and culture
of China as a whole, the direct impact of the events of 1900 fell dispropor-
tionately on a few locations in the empire. Tianjin was the Qing city most
devastated and most changed by the Boxer Uprising and its aftermath. Qing
forces, Boxers, and the international relief force fought a month-long siege
of artillery warfare over the most populous parts of the city. After weeks of
fighting, foreign troops finally blew open the south gate and stormed the
walled city. The ensuing combat, followed by the looting and destruction of
Chinese homes and yamens by foreign troops, left thousands dead, made
tens of thousands homeless, and stripped the city of its wealth. Many Western eyewitnesses to the violence, such as the photographer John Ricalton,
were shocked by the savagery that "Christian armies" had visited upon the
city. But the sack of Tianjin was not the end of the dramatic effects of the
foreign presence. For two years after the capture of Tianjin, the city was administered by a committee made up of representatives from the occupying
forces. This body, known as the Tianjin Provisional Government (TPG),
brought, in essence, an international colonial administration to one corner
of the Qing empire.

Preventing the outbreak of contagious disease was a central concern for
the TPG. The international relief force, as the military representative of all
the world's imperial powers, had brought along with it a full kit of hygienic
modernity to accomplish this task. The turn of the century had seen the triumph of the germ theory of disease and the establishment of tropical medicine in Europe, the United States, and Japan. By 1900, European powers had
established medical services in colonies stretching from Morocco to Viet-

nam. Relative latecomers to empire, the United States and Japan were now searching for microbes among the populations of their respective colonial possessions of the Philippines and Taiwan, even as they tutored populations back home in "the gospel of germs." To put this new knowledge into effect, the TPG formed a separate arm of the government expressly for the prevention of disease. The TPG, which used the language of international diplomacy (and the language of Pasteur) called this organization the *service de santé*. In Chinese, the *service de santé* was known as the *weisheng bu:* the department of *weisheng*. From the perspective of the Chinese in Tianjin, the most invasive procedures enacted by TPG administration—inspecting coffins, burning corpses, examining human feces, policing excratory behaviors, and spraying bodies with chemicals—were somehow done in the name of "guarding life."

Significantly, before the foreign powers would give Tianjin back to the Qing government, the Qing had to agree that it would establish its own *weisheng* bureau to continue the work of the TPG. *Weisheng* in China now had a new meaning: It encompassed government scientific control of sanitation, prevention of disease, cleanliness, policing, visual orderliness, and the detection and elimination of germs. Personal hygiene and public health administration had became markers of civilization and modernity in the context of high imperialism. *Weisheng* had became "hygienic modernity": a totalizing prerequisite for qualification as an autonomous nation. The Qing was forced to embrace and adopt this definition in order to regain its sovereignty.

The foreign suppression of the Boxers, and the dramatic impact it had on subalterns and elites alike in Tianjin, highlights the role of violence in the Chinese experience of modern technologies under the curious regime that some have called semicolonialism. Recent scholarship on semicolonialism has suggested that although violence was part of the legacy of imperialism, it did not permeate the day-to-day interactions between Chinese and foreigners in treaty-port settings. Because foreign powers were not able to "impose a colonial epistemology by force," the coming of the West did not result in a violent rupture with the past, and thus China's situation was marked by greater continuity, autonomy, and negotiation than colonialism elsewhere—that elsewhere being the model of colonialism, India.[2] Because of this lack of violence and total colonization, Chinese elites embraced the promises of modern technology with less ambiguity than their Indian counterparts, and also displayed less of a tendency to question the tenants of "Western civilization."

A close study of one particularly significant moment in China's semicolonial continuum, however, brings violence and rupture to the forefront. Through the suppression of the Boxer Uprising, foreign powers violently marked China, particularly China's peasants, with a stigma of backwardness. In Tianjin after 1900, hygiene was a cornerstone of a modernity imposed by occupying armies. At the same time, hygiene became the most basic constituent of an indelible rhetoric of Chinese deficiency. Those treaty-port elites who enthusiastically embraced hygienic modernity did so at the very moment when it was inextricably entwined with the violence of imperialism. In embracing hygienic modernity, they simultaneously escaped identification with Chinese peasants and evaded the violently imposed stigma of "lack" that the peasantry now bore.

The violence and rupture of 1900, although highly significant, was limited in time and place. Later the events of the Boxer Uprising and its suppression would be consciously fashioned as a memory of rupture and violence for the entire nation and the "Chinese people" as a whole. This constructed memory, and the backdrop it provided for interactions between Chinese and foreigners, varied in intensity, power, and immediacy within different parts of the terrain of "semicolonial" China.

INVASION AND CHAOS

There are no exact figures for the total foreign and native populations of Tianjin in the first half of 1900, before the arrival of the international relief force. By the turn of the century the total Chinese population of the walled city and its surrounding neighborhoods most likely numbered well over half a million, dwarfing the numbers of foreigners living in the concessions down river. The population of Tianjin had swelled in the last decades of the nineteenth century as country people sought relief in the city from increasingly harsh environmental conditions. The great famine of 1877–79 had been followed by more drought, alternating in places with the destruction of crops by flood and locust. The wealthy of Tianjin could ride out these lean times by diversifying their business interests in the south, or selling off valued possessions to curio-seeking foreigners. For most, however, life in Tianjin became increasingly crowded and dirty as the city absorbed the hardship of the countryside. Peasants were also drawn to the city by the promise of jobs. In spite of the increased trade brought about by the presence of foreign firms, unskilled laborers still found it difficult to make a living in the city. The vagaries of the international economy, combined with the vagaries of the increasingly silted-up Hai River, meant that there were not always great steamships to unload at Tianjin's docks, and newly arrived peasants competed with entrenched workers who had previously lost their jobs towing barges on the Grand Canal. Unemployed laborers were joined by Han soldiers demobilized after the defeat of the Qing in the Sino-Japanese War. Together they created a potentially violent underclass in Tianjin.[3]

By 1900, the cluster of foreign concessions clinging to the banks of the Hai had expanded; there were now a total of four foreign concessions in Tianjin. Japan gained a chunk of land along the Hai after their victory against the Qing in the Sino-Japanese War. Ironically, Germany asked for and received a part of Tianjin from the Qing government as a reward for its role in the Triple Intervention, an action that had prevented Japan from acquiring the Liaodong peninsula in its victory over the Qing.[4] The Japanese Concession was placed to the west of the French Concession, significantly positioned between the European zones and the Chinese city, whereas the German Concession lay to the east of the British Settlement, furthest down the river from the Chinese. By 1900, there had been very little activity in these two new settlements, and growth in the British and French areas had been slow. Early population statistics are sketchy, but in all likelihood there were fewer than two thousand foreigners living in the concessions before 1900.[5] For these foreign residents living in Western-style buildings two miles downriver from Tianjin's walls, the "real" Chinese city seemed a world away.

As early as January of 1900, while Tianjin's foreigners read in their newspapers about anti-Christian trouble stirring in Shandong, Boxing masters were already setting up altars in the fields outside of Tianjin's south gate and holding demonstrations of their techniques.[6] The Boxer movement (Yihetuan) had begun in impoverished regions of Shandong, a few hundred kilometers south of Tianjin. Angered that foreigners and Christians were bringing misfortune to the Qing, Boxers rose up against missionaries and Chinese Christian converts and moved north to spread their message of support for the Qing.[7] Recruits to the Boxer movement were quickly found among Tianjin's large underclass of demobilized soldiers, unemployed barge towers, and dockworkers. More bands of young peasant males straggled into Tianjin during the spring months of 1900, and by the arrival of the hot weather of June, tens of thousands of Boxers were said to be filling the walled city. On the night of June 15, watchmen in the British Settlement saw "men and boys approaching on many sides in the bright moonlight. They carried torches, shavings and oil, and tried to set fire to everything they could, indulging in hideous yelling when about 500 yards off."[8] The foreign chronicler ensures the reader that these attackers were "shot down like rabbits."

However, beginning the next day, Qing forces, who had thrown their lot in with the Boxers, began firing hundreds of shells at foreign buildings from cannons located atop the city walls and on the grounds of the Beiyang Military Academy. For almost a month, artillery shells from the north exploded over the French and British Concessions, while Boxer forces harassed the foreigners from positions in the south. The foreign legations in Beijing were similarly under siege by Boxer and Qing forces. Foreign powers responded swiftly and with deadly force.

In July of 1900, an international relief force of more than twenty thousand soldiers arrived in Tianjin. The force included units from eight different nations—Italy, Germany, France, Great Britain, Austria-Hungary, Russia, the United States, and Japan—hence it was known as the Eight Nation United Army *(baguo lianjun)* in Chinese. The majority of the troops were provided by nations (or nations with colonies) in the immediate vicinity: Japan (ten thousand soldiers), Russia (four thousand), Great Britain (three thousand, including Indians and Australians), the United States (two thousand soldiers, most deployed from the Philippines), and France (eight hundred).

Although united in their purpose against the Boxers and the Qing, there were intense rivalries between the armies that frequently broke out in hostilities. French and British troops (more specifically, Alsatian and Welsh) clashed, resulting in two dead and scores wounded. A Sikh soldier fighting for the British, incensed by racist insults from German soldiers, killed three of the kaiser's troops before he himself was shot. Such events did not appear in many Western accounts bent on praising the virtues of the force. As one chronicler put it, "These incidents do not, of course, belong to the glorious annals of warfare . . . and they may safely be omitted."[9] These conflicts highlighted the tensions of race, ethnicity, and nation inherent among the imperial powers themselves, tensions that contributed to the fractured character of foreign imperialism in China in the twentieth century.

In spite of these tensions, the international relief force was able to coordinate an assault on the walled city of Tianjin. Japanese troops led the attack, which involved using large amounts of explosives to blow a hole in the massive south gate. Once the city's walls were breached, chaos ensued.[10] Western troops robbed homes of silver, clocks, dishes, vases, and clothing, and also made off with the contents of the treasuries of Qing government offices.[11] Unable to distinguish Boxers from the rest of the population, foreign troops killed refugees as they tried to escape the city, arrested women who happened to be wearing red belts and executed men who had particularly long and thick queues.[12] As the fear and chaos spread, those of means left by boat to points west of Tianjin; the Grand Canal was said to be filled with boats of gentry, merchants, and officials escaping with their families and small armies of private guards.[13] Less fortunate refugees crowded into the northwestern part of the city, traditionally the Muslim quarter of Tianjin. There many Han underwent "instant conversions" and claimed to be followers of Islam, as it was rumored that the foreign troops believed that Muslims, due to their monotheistic religious beliefs, had not joined the Boxer movement.[14]

The residents of the city moved from one terror to another. Many had simply attempted to remain out of danger by lying low and complying with the demands of those in power at the moment. During the spring of 1900, while Boxers were marching at will through the streets, shopkeepers hid their imported goods and eliminated the character *yang* (literally, ocean, designating foreign origin) from their store signs. Many residents complied with Boxers when ordered to burn incense and light lanterns all night to show their support, and contributed rice, money, and food to the Boxer cause.[15] But when foreign troops overwhelmed the Boxers and occupied the city, many Tianjin residents posted white flags on their homes on which they had written in Chinese characters, *"Da riben diguo shunmin"* (Obedient subjects of the great Japanese empire).[16]

The symbolic surrender to the Japanese empire represented in these hundreds of white flags was not only due to the fact that the city's residents were more proficient in Chinese characters than they were in Roman or Cyrillic letters. To Tianjin residents accustomed since 1894 to the potential threat of Japanese armies in Manchuria during the Sino-Japanese War, the fall of the city seemed like the beginning of a long-expected Japanese invasion. The Japanese army now had a major share in the international occupation of the city. Almost half of the twenty-thousand-strong force was made up of Japanese troops, and almost one thousand of these troops stayed behind in Tianjin to maintain order.

Japan stood poised to act as an equal with the world's imperial powers as they enforced control over a corner of the Qing empire. As an Asian nation, Japan had to manage its position deftly between the nations of the West and the "Asiatic" world of China. It negotiated this position as a world-class imperial power in part through the deployment of a shared language of hygiene, sanitary policing, and bacteria—modern technologies encompassed by the Japanese term *eisei*.

THE TIANJIN PROVISIONAL GOVERNMENT
AND THE ENFORCEMENT OF HYGIENIC MODERNITY

The TPG was formed within days of the fall of the Chinese city. The central council was composed of one representative each from the Russian, British, Japanese, German, French, American, Austro-Hungarian, and Italian armies.[17] French was the official language of the TPG. It is not clear if French was used easily by all the members of the council, but French would have been no problem for the Japanese representative, Colonel Akiyama Yoshifuru. The cosmopolitan Akiyama had studied military science in France and was proud of his ability to communicate in the international language of diplomacy.[18]

The new government set out four immediate objectives: (1) To restore order to the city; (2) to improve sanitation and prevent the outbreak of contagious disease; (3) to ensure continued supplies for the united forces; and (4) to survey and secure the property left behind by the Qing government and Chinese citizens. Of these objectives, General Fukushima Yasumasa, the temporary commander of the Japanese forces, declared that sanitation and health were the most urgent tasks for the administration of the city.[19] Fukushima had been stationed in the Japanese embassy in Berlin in the 1890s and had witnessed Robert Koch hailed as a hero of the nation for his bacteriological discoveries. He was also a staunch supporter of Mori Ôgai's post–Sino-Japanese War push to reform the *eisei* of the Japanese military. In Tianjin, Fukushima came to the fore of all the occupying armies as a champion of *eisei*.[20]

The other members of the TPG were in agreement with Fukushima. Immediately after establishing a police bureau for the city, the TPG established Tianjin's first bureau of health, known in the official language of the TPG as the *service de santé (weisheng bu)*. It is unclear who decided to designate the bureau "*weisheng.*" It is quite likely, though unrecorded as such, that the name was put forth as the appropriate translation by the Japanese representatives, whose country already possessed a Chinese-character compound to name the government administration of health: *eisei*.

To head the bureau, the TPG appointed a Western physician familiar with the medical circumstances of the city: Dr. Renee Depasse, a personal physician to Li Hongzhang. Depasse had been one of the physician's attending Li when an assassination attempt felled the viceroy at Shimonseki in 1895. When not personally attending Li, Depasse served as a professor of medicine at Tianjin's Beiyang Navy Medical Academy, the medical school and hospital initially run by physicians of the London Missionary Society but then taken over by Li Hongzhang for the purposes of the Qing military. The TPG gave Depasse his own offices and command over a contingent of soldiers—mostly Japanese and Sikh—who helped to enforce sanitary regulations in the Chinese city.

The TPG had been formed at a significant moment in the history of medicine. By 1900, health administration was being altered by the growing hegemony of the germ theory of disease and the concomitant emergence of tropical medicine. Colonial rule throughout the world had allowed European (and Japanese) scientists to discover the microorganisms that caused many diseases, including diphtheria, tuberculosis, cholera, typhoid, leprosy, tetanus, and plague. The discovery of latent bacteria in the blood of healthy individuals, along with experiments in the process of acquired immunity, shifted the focus of disease prevention from a concern with the environment to a focus on humans as carriers. As Warick Anderson (following Bruno Latour) observed about the development of modern medicine in the colonial context, the concern about microbes "as social actors" made indigenous bodies and behaviors "the objects of ceaseless medical inspection and regulation."[21] Such inspections and regulations were to become commonplace in Tianjin under TPG rule.

The year 1900 also saw the emergence of a new science focused on non-human carriers of disease in the colonies. In 1899, former Qing Imperial Maritime Customs health officer Patrick Manson established the London School of Tropical Medicine, dedicated to the investigation of diseases in warm climates. The school's particular focus was on the newly discovered role that vectors played in the transmission of diseases such as malaria, sleeping sickness, and yellow fever.[22] Tropical medicine obliged the public health administrator to think about insects and insect breeding environments, but often the most immediate concerns focused on native populations as carriers of microbes that might affect whites. Although flying, creeping, and swimming vectors had been identified, colonial administrators versed in tropical medicine still sought ways to distance themselves from "unsanitary" natives.[23]

Knowledge of "microbes as social actors" did not radically alter the arsenal of public health management: administrations still cleaned streets, buried corpses, and drained sewers as they had in the past out of a fear of miasma. But the rationale for such actions had changed, and new invasive tactics were added to the administration of health, particularly the isolation, examination, and regulation of individual sufferers of disease and those suspected of harboring harmful germs. Even though well-established medical authorities in the colonies, particularly India, were slow to accept laboratory developments, military forces by the turn of the century had rapidly assimilated insights into bacteria and parasites, and these ideas were available to the physicians and medical officers involved in the occupation of Tianjin.[24] The TPG *weisheng bu* would not only intervene in the daily lives of Chinese in Tianjin in unprecedented ways, they would do so for reasons the city had not previously imagined.

Eliminating Filth

The first urgent task facing the occupying government was related to health and sanitation: it had to dispose of the numerous corpses left on the streets from the recent fighting. In Tianjin this was a particularly grueling task. The bodies of the battle dead were scattered around the city, and groups of dogs roamed about feeding on them. With summer temperatures reaching 100 degrees Fahrenheit, the corpses were rapidly decomposing. In order to avoid the outbreak of epidemics—particularly cholera—Depasse ordered Chinese laborers of the *weisheng bu* to dig large mass graves outside of the city wall. The bureau then unceremoniously dumped the bodies of the dead within them. This action repulsed rather than gratified Chinese observers, who were offended by the lack of ritual and respect entailed in these foreign-administered mass burials.[25]

After the initial disposal of casualties, the TPG continued its necromantic interventions by seeking to modernize the way that Tianjin buried its dead. Foreigners had long considered as highly unsanitary the northern Chinese custom of burying coffins in individual mound graves, which appeared as small conical projections that rose a few feet above the earth. Acre upon acre of fields to the south and west of Tianjin were bumpy with the graves of the city's dead. The TPG ordered laborers and soldiers of the *weisheng bu* to disinter hundreds of coffins outside of the city walls and move them to new "modern" native cemeteries. There the coffins were reburied "six feet under," according to the dictates of hygiene. The result was the visual transformation of Chinese cemeteries into smooth landscapes.[26] Chinese residents were also required to get TPG permits allowing the moving of coffins out of the city (there were no burial places inside the city walls). For the TPG, this was an ingenious method for gathering the basic stuff of public health: statistics on mortality rates. For the Chinese, it represented offensive government interference with private family ritual and an overly burdensome tax on death.[27]

In addition to corpse collection, the TPG embarked on a massive garbage disposal campaign. Regulations were promulgated specifying the sites where household garbage could be placed. The *weisheng bu* hired more than two hundred Chinese laborers to collect garbage, cart it outside of the city walls, and burn it. In two months, the bureau's "coolies" had moved an estimated two thousand metric tons of garbage.[28] The difficulty of providing wages for *weisheng* bureau workers was partially solved by using the labor of incarcerated persons who worked for no wage at all. One of the first actions of the TPG was to ban begging. Within five days after the prohibition on begging, the TPG had gathered five hundred men off the streets, washed and disinfected them, then put them to work as sanitation "coolies." These men kept the city clean and in return received food and shelter in a prison-like setting.[29]

Sanitation work also became a common punishment for transgressors of TPG laws. Upon arrest, the prisoner's queue was cut off and his head shaved. Punishment consisted first of wearing the cangue for a few days, followed by a sentence on a *weisheng* chain gang. At first elite Chinese observers noted approvingly that those assigned to sanitation duty were common hooligans *(tugun)*.[30] But as the number of TPG regulations increased and the effectiveness of the police force grew, people from many different strata of Tianjin society found themselves turned into sanitation coolies. In the words of one observer:

> I was walking outside the southern gate when I saw over twenty people who had been forced into labor. Their queues had been cut off, their heads shaved. They had peculiar uniforms on—half blue, half red—with the characters *wei sheng* embroidered on their chests. Their legs were chained together, and they were carrying heavy buckets of excrement and filthy water. Behind them, pushing them on, were several Sikh soldiers with guns. I stared at them for a long time, and I realized that among them there were two people who looked entirely out of place, one obviously a scholar, one a midlevel merchant. I have no idea what they had done to put them in this situation. Alas! The country is in such a precarious situation . . . and after the past few decades there are no Chinese left who are not coolies. What tragedy! What pain![31]

This scenario shows in stark terms the multiple hierarchies of class and race involved in the occupation of Tianjin, and how *weisheng* became associated with violence, punishment, and filth under the new regime. The remarkable sight of degree holders (even if of a low level), stripped of their robes, with queues shorn and legs shackled, symbolized for this observer the enslavement of the entire Chinese people. Men carrying buckets of excrement would not have seemed so out of place on the streets of Tianjin—collecting night soil was, after all, a common profession—but from the perspective of this Chinese observer, if a gentlemen did this work under a gun wielded by a "black" Sikh soldier, then Chinese had become the servants of the servants of the British empire. The observer distinctly notes the words *wei sheng* emblazoned on the laborers' uniforms, but it strikes him as two separate characters, devoid of any appropriate meaning in this context. This scenario demonstrates that reconfigurations of language take place not only in the texts penned by and read by intellectuals; the use of individual words on material objects, and their frequent replication and appearance on commodities, signs, office buildings, or even uniforms, can be a vehicle for the creation of new associations of meaning for many different sectors of society, including the barely literate. In the summer of 1902, Tianjin's residents were still puzzling through the strange and threatening content of the *wei sheng* that occupying armies had brought to the city.

Although the TPG *weisheng bu* sought to regulate the impurities of refuse and death, it also attempted to regulate another intimate physiological phenomenon—excretion. One of the earliest TPG regulations was a ban on public urination and defecation, a regulation that was, at times, enforced at gunpoint:

> A Chinese youth of fifteen was relieving himself in an open place when he was discovered and detained by a foreign soldier. The soldier ordered the youth to pick up his feces in his hands and move them to a remote spot. The youth did not want to obey the order, but the soldier threatened him with his bayonet, and so the youth had no choice but do as ordered. When the soldier saw the boy's hands made intolerably filthy, he just laughed and walked away.[32]

The proper placement of excretion and excreta has been the one element of personal hygiene and public health unequivocally embraced around the globe as a prerequisite of civilization.[33] At the same time, the inability to regulate excretion has been seen as the most basic marker of human deficiency. Even Gandhi criticized the Indian people for indiscriminate defecation, and proclaimed that the use of a spade to bury one's own feces was the absolute minimum requirement for a dignified human existence.[34] Colonizing powers and wealthier classes, as part of the creation of dramatic hierarchies, explicitly associated the colonized and the poor with excrement. Forgetting that all human beings share the same physiological processes, and forgetting that the ability to be excratoraly civilized is in part a function of economic well-being, the colonizer marked the colonized as "shitters."[35] In the above scenario the occupying soldier, under the pretense of enforcing hygienic regulations, forced the Chinese youth to perform a debased racial status by handling his own feces.

The TPG made public defecation a crime, but it took them two years to build public latrines in the Chinese city in order to facilitate excretory propriety. Called "government toilets" *(guance)*, these latrines were not exactly "public" as conceived of in present-day terms, but were run more like business franchises. The TPG *weisheng bu* granted toilet monopolies to private Chinese individuals, who collected usage fees for the government and maintained possession of the valuable night soil left behind by paying customers. The government toilets never totally solved the problem of public excretion in Tianjin: the usage fee of five *wen* for a visit that produced feces, one or two *wen* for a visit that produced urine, was beyond the means of Tianjin's poorest.[36]

Through these simultaneously public and intimate activities, the TPG began to demonstrate the new content of *weisheng* to Tianjin. *Weisheng* meant policing filth where it lurked in corpses, garbage, and feces. It involved the visual and olfactory reordering of public space, as bureau workers made Chinese cemeteries flat and smooth, removed rubbish outside the city walls, and concentrated smells around government toilets. It altered the human landscape of the city, transforming beggars into street sweepers and creating the appearance of sanitary chain gangs on the city's streets. *Weisheng* presented the power of the government to discipline, punish, and regulate the people. Scholars who committed infractions of the rules of *weisheng* might be stripped of their symbols of dignity (queues, scholars' robes) and be forced to labor in public wearing a uniform emblazoned with the characters *wei sheng*. Defecating in a field now brought with it the risk of death at the hands of an unpredictable armed foreign soldier. *Weisheng* as the policing of filth called for a standard set of public behaviors of all residents, no matter what their economic means or position in the community. It even meant giving the government a central role in the intimate family-based rituals surrounding death and burial. *Weisheng* now claimed to encompass and regulate life from the toilet to the grave.

Eliminating Germs

Much of the *weisheng bu*'s activities could have been performed without an understanding of bacteria. However, a discourse of germs added the weight of scientific authority to administrative decisions, a weight that was powerful enough to shatter walls. Foreigners had long noted the towering surrounding walls that were a distinct characteristic of Chinese cities well into the twentieth century.[37] As in Europe, city walls had been constructed for defensive purposes, and in China, they performed that task extraordinarily well. In 1900, Qing forces in Tianjin fired artillery at the foreign concessions from vantage points atop the city wall. Boxers hid behind the safety of the city walls for more than a month before foreign troops finally exploded the south gate. From the perspective of the occupying foreign powers, city walls represented an obvious threat to their security. They also stood as a major obstacle to the achievement of a desired transparent "governmentality" of the Chinese city.

Given the problems that Tianjin's walls had presented to foreigners, it was not surprising that the TPG wished to see them destroyed. What is surprising is that bacteria were cited as one of the major reasons for their demolition. According to the TPG, the city wall encouraged the proliferation of germs. The unsanitary poor built their reed and mud hovels against the walls, and pools of stagnant water collected on the ground around the walls. Both sites were breeding grounds for bacteria. To protect the health of the foreign community, the Chinese walls and the bacteria they fostered had to be eliminated. The Japanese representative to the TPG was particularly concerned that this obstacle to hygiene be removed, given its proximity to the border of the Japanese Concession.[38] The walls of other Chinese cities were removed because of the demands of modern transportation, especially the need for trains to have access to cities. Tianjin's walls came down because of the demands of hygienic modernity.

The TPG also made sex in Tianjin—at least sex for foreign soldiers—more transparent and more hygienic as well. Less than one month after the establishment of the TPG, the council discussed the question of opening supervised brothels for the troops.[39] The establishment of medically supervised brothels for military forces was a controversial but integral aspect of empire.[40] Although it had long been known that venereal disease was spread through sexual contact, the germ theory of disease bolstered the logic for the physical inspection and isolation of prostitutes. By the end of August 1900, a decision was made to establish one brothel each for Japanese, American, and British troops, and three brothels for the Russians.[41]

While the *weisheng bu* put hundreds of Chinese men to work providing sanitation services for the city, it also became the supervisor for perhaps an equal number of Chinese women who provided foreign troops with sanitary sex. It is unlikely that the women working in these brothels wore uniforms with *weisheng* embroidered on the chest pocket, and yet they would be aware that a government office regulated their work and government physicians examined their bodies—another remarkable manifestation of new meanings of *weisheng* in Tianjin. It is interesting to note that at the same time the TPG discussed opening "sanitary brothels," it debated closing down the numerous opium houses that existed in the city. This idea never came to fruition. Unlike the hopes expressed in John Fryer's *weisheng* texts, the *weisheng* envisioned by the TPG did not include the elimination of opium addiction.

A germ-centered vision of public health focused government attention on microbes lurking in and around things (like walls) and bodies (like those of prostitutes), but the bodies that harbored microbes were almost always seen as Chinese, and the bodies that labored under the threat of disease were foreign. Even though science had established that environments (dirty water) and vectors (flies, mosquitoes) were of utmost importance in the transmission of disease, the need to manage and to police "natives" was foremost in the TPG epidemic prevention measures.

Just as the TPG was to hand over control of the city to the Qing, its worst fears about natives as carriers of epidemic disease were realized. As cholera swept through the city in the summer of 1902, the foreign occupation attempted to impose highly invasive germ management techniques on the Chinese population of the city. In its attempts to do so, the occupation ran into the limits of hygienic modernity.

Policing Cholera, 1902

On June 2, 1902, cholera arrived in Tianjin aboard a steamship from Shanghai. In response, the TPG established a special "epidemic prevention police" who were empowered to enter homes to investigate suspected cholera cases. The routine followed by the epidemic prevention police would have been familiar to the hundreds of Japanese who were called upon to enforce TPG rules. Upon discovery of a person with suspicious symptoms, the epidemic prevention police summonned a doctor from the *weisheng bu* who determined whether or not the illness was true Asiatic cholera. If the diagnosis was positive, the epidemic prevention police forcibly escorted the victim to one of nine isolation hospitals around the city. Police also burned the patient's bed linens and clothes and placed the other residents of the home under quarantine for seven days. *Weisheng bu* workers disinfected the houses of cholera victims by covering all the surfaces with lime. Corpses of cholera victims and coffins were also covered with lime, as were all public toilets, sewers, and garbage heaps. Soon the city was blanketed with a layer of white as Russian troops brought in trains filled with lime for the mass disinfection.[42]

Chinese TPG cholera patrols gained a reputation for being less than scrupulous in enforcing hygienic regulations. It was said that some Chinese police extorted money from cholera victims' families, threatening that if they did not receive payment, they would notify the Japanese police officers, who would show no mercy to the victim or consideration for the family. The Chi-

TABLE 2. Cholera Cases in Tianjin, 1902

	Native City	Japanese Concession
Total population (approx.)	326,552	11,184
Chinese	326,552	10,064
Japanese	—	1,120
Total number of reported cholera cases	1,273	1,254
Chinese	1,273	1,223
Japanese	—	31
Total number of deaths	736	833
Total percentage of cholera cases to population	0.34%	11.21%
Chinese	0.34%	12.15%
Japanese	—	2.77%

SOURCE: Data from J. Tsuzuki, "Bericht über meine epidemiologischen Beobachtungen und Forschungen während der Choleraepidemie in Nordchina im Jahre 1902 und über die im Verlaufe derselben von mir durchgefürhrten prophylaktischen Massregeln mit besonderer Berücksightigung der Choleraschutzimpfung," in *Archiv für Schiffs und Tropen-Hygiene*, vol. 8 (Leipzig, 1904), 74.

nese police horrified families with stories of how foreigners would remove the patient from the family home, send him to the isolation hospital, pack the sick person in ice and force him to drink vile medicines. To avoid extortion at the hands of Chinese police or harsh punishment at the hands of the foreigners, many Chinese families concealed cholera deaths and tried to dispose of bodies in secret. This led inevitably to the tragic abandonment of corpses on streets or in the Hai River, without any burial rites at all.[43]

The Chinese city was not the only part of Tianjin hit by the 1902 outbreak. The newly created Japanese Concession, with its large number of Chinese residents, was particularly devastated by the epidemic (see table 2). The Japanese Concession suffered a 12.15 percent rate of incidence of cholera among Chinese residents, the highest rate in the city. Only a few Japanese succumbed to the disease, but the impact of this episode on the mentalities and memories of Japanese living in the concession went far beyond the scope suggested by the number of Japanese cases (see chapter 9).

GERMS, SEGREGATION, AND NATIONAL IDENTITY

As a result of the cholera of 1902, foreigners in Tianjin increasingly looked to separation and segregation from Chinese bodies as a strategy to preserve health—in spite of an understanding that cholera was transmitted through impure drinking water. British residents of Tianjin rethought the advantages of having Chinese servants. Editorials in the *Peking and Tientsin Times* assured foreigners that all would be well if they simply made their daily lives "conform to the simple directions of medical men." Foreigners would be all but immune to cholera if they boiled their water, cooked all vegetables thoroughly, and avoided raw fruits. This would all be more feasible, reported the paper, if foreigners would not rely so much on untrustworthy Chinese servants for their daily needs.[44] Europeans were assured that continued individual hygienic vigilance prevented the entrance of the microbe into their digestive organs, thus providing "an immunity which does not seem to extend to our native neighbors." Although the newspaper reminded readers that "the late M. Pasteur said the time would come when it would be looked upon as a communal disgrace if any one died of a zymotic or dirt disease," there was no sense of "communal disgrace" expressed at the deaths of Chinese in the native city. Recent European advancements in bacteriology had proved that the only way to ensure a community's safety from cholera was to provide a clean water supply for the entire population. Yet in Tianjin, most foreigners still held that individual hygienic vigilance saved them from the threat of cholera. In the minds of foreigners, Chinese were incapable of exercising such informed vigilance. They remained dangerous carriers, direct threats to well-being, and were best avoided, particularly in the intimate confines of the household.[45]

The Japanese physician and bacteriologist Tsuzuki Jinnosuke reached similar conclusions about the native population of Tianjin, although he did so through entirely different means. The Japanese Imperial War Board had sent Tsuzuki to Tianjin to conduct bacteriological and epidemiological observations during the 1902 epidemic. Educated in bacteriology at Germany's prestigious Marburg University, Tsuzuki arrived in Tianjin equipped with microscopes, petri dishes, agar, dyes, reagents, and a thorough knowledge of Koch's postulates.[46] He used this equipment and knowledge to scrutinize Tianjin's water, flies, and the excreta of Chinese cholera victims. Tsuzuki found the cholera vibrio in water samples from the Hai River, thus proving (for anyone who might have doubted it) that the river was the major source of infection. He was particularly proud of his careful experiments demonstrating that flies could transport cholera bacilli from human excreta on their tiny hairy legs and discharge them on unprotected food some distance away—a warning for anyone who ate food purchased at a Chinese market. He published his "Beobachtungen und Forschungen" (Observations and researches, 1904) in the premier German journal for tropical medicine, *Archiv für Schiffs und Tropen-Hygiene* (Archive for naval and tropical hygiene).[47]

Tsuzuki had a particularly dim view of Chinese sanitary habits. He bluntly concluded, "Der Prophylaxis sind die Chinesen unzugänglich" (the Chinese are incapable of enacting [sanitary] prevention). He also cautioned that the sanitary policing of the Chinese population would not be enough to guarantee the health of foreigners in the concessions. In terms of the public health of Tianjin, Tsuzuki warned that every colonial or military outpost had to act to protect itself. He advised the Japanese to stop relying on Chinese vendors for vegetables, meat, and, above all, water. Although he pinpointed water and flies as the vectors that transmitted cholera, he nonetheless sternly warned the Japanese residents of Tianjin to limit any unnecessary contact with individual Chinese if they wished to avoid contracting disease. For Tsuzuki, *eisei/hygiene* meant isolating bacteria, but at the same time it meant guarding the boundaries between the pure and the impure, the Japanese and the native of the Qing empire.

Tsuzuki's admonition against Sino-Japanese contact during the cholera epidemic reflected a general concern shared by many Japanese elites in Tianjin. Within the Japanese Concession, the Chinese population outnumbered the Japanese population ten to one. Unlike the European areas, the Japanese Concession shared a long border with some of the most densely populated (and poorest) areas of the native city. This proximity to the Chinese city, and the large number of Chinese within the concession, made Japanese elites particularly anxious about the threat of disease.

The Japanese Concession's location, literally wedged in between the Chinese and the Europeans, also symbolized another anxiety-provoking aspect of the Japanese experience in Tianjin. Japanese elites were determined to prove to Western observers that the Japanese were a superior form of Asian, far more capable than the Chinese of achieving modern civilization. Yet the location of the concession, and the poverty of the Japanese residents in 1900, made this distinction difficult to accomplish. Soon after the initial occupation of Tianjin, the Japanese commander, Colonel Akiyama, received a formal complaint from British military authorities that charged that the Japanese zone was unhygienic and posed a health threat to the European concessions. In his response, the French-educated cavalry officer conceded that some of the Japanese in the concession were of a deficient type and as a result did not entirely understand the importance of hygiene. However, he informed the British that it was wrong to suggest that *all* Japanese were dirty and ignorant, and assured them that the authorities would take proper precautions.[48] As was the case in many parts of Japan's "informal empire," the majority of Japanese who emigrated to Tianjin were poor adventurers seeking to improve their lot abroad. In the eyes of both European observers and Japanese authorities alike, these immigrants were of an inferior class, ignorant of both personal and public hygiene. The urgent task of distinguishing themselves from the Chinese in the eyes of foreigners inevitably helped make *eisei* an important part of the Japanese Concession administration (see chapter 9).

In the remarkable environment of early-twentieth-century Tianjin, foreign powers defined themselves not only in relation to the indigenous Chinese. Each concession constructed its identity and negotiated for status within a complex matrix of relationships among competing and cooperating colonizers. This situation was particularly acute for the Japanese as latecomers to the imperial scene, and more important, as "Asiatics" in search of an Asian empire. Victory over the Qing in 1895 (and soon, over Russia in 1905) helped raise European and American estimation of the Japanese, but reputations had to be constantly attended to, particularly when class distinctions among one's own compatriots threatened to confound distinctions between nationalities.[49] Adherence to the principles of hygienic modernity—at least on the part of the national elite—was a prerequisite to enter the ranks of advanced civilizations. Attention to germs, laboratory science, and medical police was part of what legitimized political authority. This would prove to be especially true for the Japanese, and ultimately true for the Qing as well.

DOMINANCE AND HEGEMONY IN OCCUPIED TIANJIN

It would be inaccurate to say that TPG rule was experienced by all Chinese in Tianjin as an unmitigated tyranny. Some of Tianjin's reform-minded elites learned to work within the new political order and even embraced its philosophy. Middle-men between the authorities and the Chinese population arose from various sectors of Tianjin society. Some members of the gentry functioned as the voice for Tianjin concerns, bringing military crimes and questions of refugee relief to the attention of the TPG. This role was especially vital since the TPG initially rejected all requests from Qing officials for any role in the administration of the city.[50] The TPG controlled locales primarily through its foreign-staffed neighborhood police bureaus, but it also worked in concert with neighborhood "directors" *(dong shi)*, local merchants or degree holders who were charged with making sure that TPG proclamations—the most frequent being those concerning public health and sanitation—were promulgated and understood.

For members of Tianjin's elite, it is quite likely that the occupation of Tianjin by foreigners was less onerous than the occupation of the city by Boxers. Some elites pointedly ignored the coercion behind TPG enforcement and even privately expressed genuine praise for the new regulations. The writings of Tianjin elites from the 1900–1902 occupation reveal that for some, life continued much the same during the occupation, in spite of the trauma, financial loss, and death that the initial military action had visited upon the city around them. Tianjin's elites were not personally affected by TPG regulations limiting public excretion or begging, and with their own private cemeteries and access to coffin-managing services through guilds or native place halls, they were most likely able to circumvent the offensive invasive modernization of family graves. Relatively buffered from direct experience of the coercive policies of the TPG, some of Tianjin's elite found that the occupation gave them the opportunity to have more contact with foreigners, particularly Japanese, whose language and knowledge they had been actively studying since the Qing's defeat in the Sino-Japanese War.

For example, the salt merchant turned educator Yan Xiu frequently entertained at least a dozen different Japanese acquaintances in his home during the occupation years. Some of these relationships had begun before the Boxer disturbance, others had been established only after 1900. Yan and his Japanese guests drank tea, discussed education and modernization, and exchanged works of calligraphy as gifts to solidify their friendship. Yan Xiu himself embarked on his first tour of Japan in the fall of 1902.[51] The journal of Hua Xuelan, a member of the prestigious Hua clan of Tianjin salt merchants, also shows that daily life seemed little changed except for an increase in contact with Japanese. Hua and his family were frequent hosts to Japanese army officers who would drop by to dine, drink, and chat. In more lighthearted moments, Hua's Japanese guests even staged sumo wrestling demonstrations in the courtyard. Taking advantage of the merchant's hospitality, Hua's circle of Chinese friends also exchanged calligraphy and other gifts with Japanese, and even sought advice from Japanese acquaintances on how to interpret directives from the TPG.[52]

Hua did note, with surprising indifference, the appearance of chain gangs being led through city streets by foreign soldiers. In contrast to the observers, he expressed approval of the improvements brought by TPG regulations, such as garbage collection, traffic control, and the remarkable phenomenon of a single-file ticket queue at the Tianjin train station, maintained by policemen who whipped anyone who stepped out of line. The preface to the 1936 edition of Hua's journal includes an apology for the camaraderie Hua demonstrated with the Japanese during the occupation. The Chinese editor, writing on the eve of the 1937 Japanese invasion of China, explained that it was not uncommon for gentry of the time to "lack race-consciousness." Given the tenor of the times, Hua and others were not entirely to blame if they "could not yet understand the real nature of imperialism."[53]

Hua likely understood the nature of imperialism quite well but reacted to it in a different manner than would be expected by a Chinese nationalist in 1936. In the aftermath of the violent suppression of the Boxer Uprising, many Chinese elites, particularly those in treaty-port cities, began to disassociate themselves from what they viewed as the backward superstitions of a peasant-centered Chinese culture. From the perspective of these elites, the violence of foreign armies in north China, although tragic, was nevertheless called down upon China by its own primitive culture and the irrational support given to the Boxers by a benighted Qing court. The critical stance of these elites with regard to Boxer practices such as spirit possession was not created by the arrival of a "scientific" West; many elites and government officials throughout the late imperial period looked upon such sectarian practices as tricks that could fool ignorant people and lead to social disorder.[54] However, the events surrounding the Boxers, combined with the presence of foreign models for thinking about the body and nature, contributed to an increased marking of Chinese cosmological models as "superstition" and an emerging construction of an unscientific Chinese "tradition." For many treaty-port elites, the Boxers and their violent suppression began a process of cultural bifurcation that would simmer throughout the New Policy reforms, fuel the republican revolution, and culminate in the iconoclasm of the May Fourth Movement.

Within this framework, Chinese elites comfortably entertained Japanese elites in their homes in the immediate aftermath of the Boxer suppression. In addition to a possible mutual appreciation of Chinese tradition, both were engaged in a similar project: distancing themselves from a perceived chaotic Other and obtaining for themselves, as fellow Asians, a position in the new order of "modern civilization." For both Chinese and the Japanese elites alike, this chaotic Other was primarily defined as a "superstitious," "backward," deficient China—although Japanese elites abroad might also seek to distinguish themselves, particularly for the benefit of Western observers, from their less sophisticated countrymen in the concessions. As Japanese participated in the occupation of Chinese cities, staffed police forces, and provided guidance for public health, they tutored the Chinese population in the means of "civilization and enlightenment." Chinese elites were desirous of performing this function in their own individual locales and would soon seek the opportunity to do so through newly established local assemblies and provincial parliaments. This occurred not under colonial rule, but within the framework of Qing sovereignty after the city reverted to Qing control. Even after reversion, a large number of Japanese advisors remained in Tianjin and helped shape the city's police, public health, and education systems. Chinese and Japanese elites, after having tea and staging mock sumo matches together during the TPG regime, would work together to construct a modern Tianjin in the beginning of the twentieth century.

The violence and coercion of the invasion and occupation of Tianjin created a rupture with the past, but for many Chinese elites it was not an unwelcome one. Foreigners dictated the conditions under which the Qing could regain sovereignty in the city, but this did not prevent Chinese and foreigners from working together closely to create modern administrations. To call this collaboration seems inaccurate, since the cooperation occurred under conditions of indigenous sovereignty, and yet one is struck by the remarkably close proximity between extreme violence and apparent hegemony, or the embrace by elites of the goals so violently forced upon the city in 1900. This "hegemony with dominance" was accomplished in part by Chinese elites' rapid move to distance themselves from a deficient China, combined with the experience of being temporarily colonized by a multinational force that included "fellow Asians."[55] A rapid and seemingly unambiguous embrace of the goals of the colonizer by Chinese elites was facilitated by the presence of Japanese, who appeared at once as foreign colonizers and as familiar cousins. Within this complex matrix of sovereignty, dominance, and modernity, *weisheng* would emerge as a central term of shared meaning and negotiation between Chinese elites and foreigners in early-twentieth-century Tianjin.

HYGIENIC MODERNITY, QING SOVEREIGNTY, AND THE JAPANESE MODEL

Foreigners were ultimately unable and unwilling to establish a total colonial government in Tianjin. Instead, they returned the native city back to Qing control, and each nation withdrew, with some anxiety, to the borders of its own settlement enclave. By 1902, Tianjin had become, in Gail Hershatter's term, a "fragmented city."[56] Austria-Hungary, Belgium, France, Germany, Great Britain, Italy, Japan, and Russia now all possessed concessions to the south, northeast, and east of the Chinese city, occupying vast stretches of land on both sides of the Hai River. None of these foreign powers showed any inclination to remain as colonial masters of Tianjin, yet all were wary that turning over the Chinese city of almost half a million souls to the Qing might be disastrous for their nearby settlements. For the foreigners, the Boxer Uprising and the cholera epidemic of 1902 demonstrated that Tianjin was infested not only with violent xenophobes, but with lethal germs as well.

The inability of the Qing government to maintain a foreign vision of sanitary order had been a persistent (but little-researched) rationale for continued foreign demands for additional territory and administrative jurisdiction in treaty-port settings.[57] Taking advantage of the foreign invasion after the Boxer Uprising, the British Settlement extended its territory several blocks inland from the Hai. This relieved the real estate crunch within its borders, but also brought the swampy "native" areas to the west of the original settlement under adequate sanitary administration. Epidemics could raise the specter of foreign expansion not only for treaty-port cities, but for the Qing empire as a whole.

The Qing's struggle for political autonomy after 1900 hinged upon its ability to recover Tianjin from foreign governments and reestablish Qing rule. In order to do this successfully, the Qing state had to demonstrate its determination to manage Tianjin in accordance with foreign expectations of municipal administration, expectations that had been embodied in the policies of the TPG. Foremost among these expectations was the establishment of a police force and a health department. Without the ability to administer hygienic modernity, the Qing would not be allowed to administer Tianjin, nor, potentially, the empire.

Tianjin finally reverted to the Qing on August 15, 1902. Yuan Shikai was placed at the head of a massive effort to remake the city to meet the dictates of the foreign powers. As described by Stephen MacKinnon, Tianjin was the site for experiments in Qing-administered modernity, including police, transportation, urban architecture, education, military, and government organization.[58] Central to these experiments was the creation of an infrastructure that would not only protect the health of Tianjin, but would also demonstrate to anxious foreign powers that the Qing could control disease without their intervention. Tianjin became home of the first government-administered municipal health department in China's modern history.

The establishment of a *weisheng* system was one of the most urgent, and most complex, aspects of the Qing's new autonomy. The presence of a health department assured foreigners that the Qing administration would use all the tools of science—from the microscope to the uniformed policeman—to check disease. It required a belief in germ theory, a determination to alter the environment for the sake of urban health, and a willingness to enter the homes and touch the bodies of all the men, women, and children of Tianjin. To view this entirely as a paradoxical form of colonial subjugation in the absence of the colonizer would be misleading. The Qing actively employed foreign advisors—particularly Japanese—to help oversee the creation of these new systems, yet at the same time Qing officials exerted considerable agency, consciously shaping the dictates of hygienic modernity to suit Chinese needs and Chinese bodies.

Yuan Shikai made Tianjin a center that generated multiple models of hygienic modernity for the empire. First, he created a regional contagious disease inspection system at major ports and along the rail lines of the northern coast. Second, he made military *weisheng* in Tianjin a crucial element in the modernization of the Qing New Armies. Finally, a municipal *weisheng* bureau in Tianjin began the important task of creating a hygienically modern citizenry while at the same time preventing the eight foreign concessions in the city from using bacteria as an excuse to expand their territory. In all three levels of these interlocking systems, hygienic modernity was consciously shaped to fit the Chinese people. At each level of the new system, Japanese advisors guided the Qing in the task of tailoring *eisei* to meet the needs of fellow "Asiatics."

The Beiyang Epidemic Prevention Office *(fangyi chu)* would make sure that foreigners would not have direct access to Chinese bodies at ports. Under the terms of treaty-port administrations, the health inspection of ship and train passengers was supposed to be a cooperative effort between Chinese and Westerners, but more often than not inspections were carried out by foreign personnel who "used Western methods to control Chinese people." At best foreigners carried out physical inspections with respect and with appropriate propriety shown to female passengers, but at their worst, their methods could be "extremely cruel." In particular, the medical treatments given to sick Chinese in the foreign isolation hospitals were seen as ill-suited to Chinese constitutions. Yuan Shikai sought to create a regional port inspection system that would put Chinese physicians in all positions so that "China could manage its own epidemic prevention vigorously and thoroughly" without outside interference.[59]

Like Li Hongzhang before him, Yuan Shikai used Tianjin as a center for building a new regional military force, and established a new military medical school for his New Army. Yuan Shikai's Beiyang Army Medical Academy *(junyi xuetang)*, founded in 1902, was based on a Japanese military model and employed instructors from the Japanese army.[60] The school's head instructor was Higara Seijirô, a high-ranking military medical officer who had come to Tianjin with the Japanese forces of the international relief expedition of 1900. Higara was instrumental in the founding of the Dôjinkai (Tongren hui, the Mutual Benevolence Society), a Japanese group that was dedicated to spreading a Japanese medical model in order to counter a perceived British and American medical hegemony in China.[61] Not surprisingly, *eisei* was a major part of instruction at the Tianjin school. The four year curriculum reflected the major categories of Mori Ôgai's *Eisei shinron:* It included courses in contagious diseases, bacteriology, general hygiene, military camp hygiene, military hygiene administration, school hygiene, and industrial hygiene. The army medical school created several generations of Chinese physicians who spoke Japanese and admired the medical modernity of the Japanese military. In addition, these physicians exposed thousands of New Army soldiers to the message of hygienic modernity by lecturing them in the importance of discipline, cleanliness, and germs. Japanese advisors were central in the creation of one of the first organizations in modern Chinese history that successfully realized the utility of employing modern biomedicine in the service of the state.

The Qing's first municipal health bureau, established in Tianjin in 1902, also showed the influence of Japanese (and German) models of hygienic modernity. The collected official regulations for Tianjin's *weisheng ju* reveal that the Qing's first modern health administration was designed to be as all-encompassing as any system envisioned by Peter Frank, Eduard Reich, or Nagayo Sensai. The overall mission of the *weisheng ju* was to do no less than "protect the lives of the people" *(baowei minsheng)*. This impressive goal included the varied tasks of providing "street cleaning, aid to the poor, medical care, and inspection and prevention of epidemic disease."[62] The new health bureau hoped to create an umbrella administration for all of the city's centers for poor relief, including those that had previously operated under the jurisdiction of different government yamens or merchant-gentry directors. This control of welfare had its practical side. As the TPG had done, the Qing-administered health bureau gathered indigents off the streets, cleaned their bodies, shaved their heads, doused them with disinfectant, and then put them to work cleaning the streets from whence they had come. Placing welfare under the direct administration of the *weisheng ju*, although part of the lofty ideals of "protecting the lives of the people," served to create an "in-house" pool of constant, cheap labor for the bureau's needs.[63]

Following a Japanese model, Tianjin's police also had many duties related to *weisheng*.[64] Tianjin's new five-thousand man force would have received instruction in sanitary policing at the Baoding Police Academy, a new provincial center for police training established by Qing officials under the guid-

ance of Kawashima Naniwa, the man famous for reforming Beijing's police.[65] *Weisheng* in Tianjin would only be invasive to the extent that Chinese police were capable of making it so. Police were to "encourage" residents to keep their houses tidy, to use public bathrooms, and to dump garbage
only in designated areas. They were to make sure that night-soil carriers
kept their lids firmly on their buckets. Police were to arrest "monks and old
women" who claimed to cure diseases with magical powers. Finally, police
were the first line of prevention against epidemic disease in the city. They
inspected markets for spoiled foodstuffs or meat that came from animals
that had died before being butchered. While walking their patrols, they were
to be on the lookout for individuals with symptoms of severe disease—a
child covered with sores, a laborer retching in the streets—and take any suspicious cases to the bureau's isolation hospital.

For the first decade of the twentieth century, the new Qing health bureau was surprisingly active in Tianjin. In the Chinese city, residents began
to sense the beginnings of a new *weisheng* as the sanitary police made their
rounds and as uniformed *weisheng* coolies swept the streets. Police could
always be bribed, and street sweepers might be less than successfully supervised, but inevitably the new health bureau began to make some changes
in daily life, even if only by altering where a laborer might relieve himself.
Restrictions on public defecation were no small matter, however. The disciplining of personal behaviors was a central element of *weisheng,* and
weisheng was a central prerequisite for Qing sovereignty. It was in the
aftermath of foreign occupation that *weisheng* fully appeared as hygienic
modernity for China's elites. By 1902 it was clear that *weisheng* not only
suggested a new way of thinking about individual health; it also was the
thing that linked the poorest individual to the very survival of the nation
within the new global order.

CONCLUSION

Weisheng as hygienic modernity may have been violently introduced by
foreign troops during the occupation of Tianjin, but Qing reformers moved
to make it as "indigenous" as possible: first, by adopting a model from a fellow Asian nation, and second, by attempting to place Chinese in positions
of authority. Tianjin's health bureau, like its army medical academy, was
based primarily on the Japanese *eisei* model, a system that had been reformed
and reshaped from European precedents by Nagayo Sensai, Gotô Shinpei,
and others. Qing reformers also took specific steps to create a *weisheng* with

"Chinese characteristics." Training Chinese physicians was an important priority, ensuring that foreigners would not be the only ones who would touch, examine, and treat Chinese bodies. Sovereignty—even sovereignty regained in the shadow of massive violence—allowed the Qing to choose among models and held forth the promise (though difficult to realize) that health might be administered entirely by Chinese.

In spite of these aspirations, Tianjin's new sovereignty could look remarkably like a case of colonial dominance. Between 1902 and 1911, Tianjin's various bureaus employed foreign experts from around the world. English was often used in communications between the German, Belgian, French, or Cantonese employees of the various bureaus. One might mistake Tianjin for a sort of "international city" were it not for the fact that foreign experts were there because the Qing had been forced to adopt modernity at gunpoint. There was nothing indirect or subtle about the initial violence of the international forces or the occupation of Tianjin, and yet there seems to have been a tremendous amount of consent about the new order among Tianjin's elites.

Just as the Boxer Uprising and its aftermath saw the consolidation of *weisheng* as hygienic modernity, a central gauge of civilizational superiority, the Boxer events saw the reconfiguration of *weisheng* as a marker of Chinese deficiency. Foreign troops attacked the Chinese city, destroyed its infrastructure, and disrupted society, then proclaimed the Chinese to be a chaotic and dirty race. Not only were the Chinese deficient in cleanliness, inherently disorderly, ignorant of germs, and incapable of preventing epidemics, the Boxers themselves had proved that Chinese ideas of the physical possibilities of the human body were absurd, superstitious, and unscientific. After the Boxer Uprising, *weisheng* became a science instructed by foreigners. Soon it was possible that the same young man who had once thought that his ability to manipulate *qi* could defeat foreign guns might be ordered by a gun-wielding foreigner to move his excrement to a more sanitary location for the sake of *weisheng*.

Weisheng as a discourse of deficiency allowed Chinese elites to distance themselves from the violence of the Boxer suppression. The foreign occupation may have brought about a violent rupture with the past, but at the same time it exacerbated a spatial rupture that existed between treaty-port elites and the denizens of the hinterland. These elites would not endure the burden of deficiency, hygienic or otherwise, and could best resist its onus by embracing modernity and its imperial agents. The Chinese peasantry (and urban underclass) were left to carry the label of hygienic deficiency, while Chinese elites worked at negotiating their status between the unwashed masses and the more "senior members" of the global hygienic order. Japanese military officers, after blowing up the city wall and beheading Chinese youth, served as a mediating link in this endeavor for Chinese elites.

Chinese elites certainly saw hygienic modernity as beneficial to the health of the city. *Weisheng* can not simply be reduced to discourses and violence when biomedicine and public health infrastructures ultimately bring longer lives and less suffering. Nevertheless, the arrival of hygienic modernity in China was closely linked to the arrival of devastating violence. Dipesh Chakrabarty has challenged scholars to "write into the history of modernity the ambivalences, the contradictions, the use of force, and the tragedies and ironies that attend it." He suggests that the ironies of modernity are nowhere more evident than in the history of public health, modern medicine, and personal hygiene. Chakrabarty points out that the triumph of an ultimately beneficial and benevolent modern health "has always been dependent on the mobilization, on its behalf, of effective means of physical coercion."[66] Although it is perhaps difficult to say that this has always been true of every case around the globe, certainly in Tianjin hygienic modernity arrived on the heels of destruction and was established at gunpoint. The ways in which this violence may have been experienced differently by different groups in treaty-port society illuminates China's fragmented, shifting, and sometimes paradoxical experience with imperialism in the twentieth century.

7 Seen and Unseen

The Urban Landscape and Boundaries of Weisheng

In the aftermath of the Boxer Uprising, hygienic modernity not only touched the body in Tianjin; it also touched the city and transformed it with its touch. Cities throughout China underwent dramatic changes in the first decades of the twentieth century. Towering defensive walls fell, trains looped in, and trams rumbled through streets. Single-story courtyard houses were demolished, multistory buildings with balustrades, portals, and domes rose in their place. While foreigners erected architecture that projected the power of capitalism and imperialism, Chinese reformers sought to display new values of progressiveness politics through construction of public spaces, public facades, and rational urban order.[1]

Frequently overlooked is the crucial role played by hygienic modernity, *weisheng*, in the transformation of Chinese urban space. Hygienic modernity called for the separation of functions in the urban landscape, the creation of things seen and unseen. For a city to be modern above ground required the construction of an alternate city under the ground, a city of pipes, drains, tanks, and gradients that would render wastes and water invisible.[2] Economic functions of the city were segregated so that potentially unhealthful activities would neither be seen nor smelled. Hygienic modernity even dictated the change of the human landscape: potentially diseased people had to be removed from the street, and potentially contaminating activities such as selling, buying, washing, defecating, and dumping were contained behind walls or within receptacles. The resultant *weisheng* environment would reflect a different visual aesthetic: linear, smooth, and ordered.

If nineteenth- and twentieth-century Europeans had difficulty making sense of the urban landscape in China, it was in great part because hygienic modernity had not emerged as an imperative in Chinese cities, an imperative that would spur government to override considerations of economics, individuality, and custom. In Tianjin, this imperative arrived with the international expeditionary force and proceeded to alter the city under foreign rule. Even after the return of the Chinese city to Qing administration, foreign concessions in Tianjin continued to exert an influence that went beyond their borders of sovereignty. Tianjin fostered no simple binary division between "colonizer" and "colonized," but instead gave rise to an unstable and contested hierarchy among many nations. Each concession attempted to mark its distinct identity—vis-à-vis China, and in relation to other foreign powers—through conscious manipulations of space and sanitary technology. In spite of sharing the same water-logged soil, the same polluted rivers, the same populations, and the same air, each sovereign area of Tianjin struggled to find its own solution to basic urban hygiene problems. Visual arrangements merged with sanitary arrangements to become vehicles for expressing national identity and national pride. Hygienic modernity became the means of creating hierarchical distinctions between the *weisheng* and the *bu* (not) *weisheng*, distinctions drawn not only between foreigners and Chinese, but among the imperial powers themselves.

Confounding this desire for architectural distinctness and sanitary separateness were the flows of the natural and human environment. Water, winds, people, disease, and excreta accumulated in and circulated through the city. On a daily basis the porousness of the city's enclaves was demonstrated by the presence of the human carriers of water and waste. Before the twentieth century, everyone in Tianjin (with the exception of the poorest) was supplied by the same "water system" and served by the same "sewer system," namely water carriers and night-soil carriers. These wiry, muscular men, with their wheelbarrows and burden poles, formed a ubiquitous presence on all city streets. Visions of a technologically mediated hygienic modernity had to negotiate with the tenacious need for livelihood represented by these men, whose eccentricities and violent proclivities earned them the moniker of "the Dark Drifters." These laborers, by circulating liquids of various degrees of purity throughout the city, served as the human link between the rich and the poor, foreign and Chinese, in pre-Boxer Tianjin. The twentieth-century desire to produce health and national identity through separation was at direct odds with one of the most basic arrangements of daily life in the city.

The tension and ambiguity in Tianjin's hygienic status, represented by the Dark Drifters, was preserved exactly because of the multiple political divisions of the city. In spite of reformists' claims to delineate civilized and uncivilized space through *weisheng*, neither Chinese nor foreigners could fully succeed in their desire to make the allegedly deficient "traditional" disappear from the urban terrain. Water carriers remained a fixture in Tianjin well into the 1950s and the first years of the People's Republic. Their profession's longevity was assured by their aggressive strategies of business and survival, but it was also guaranteed by the very political boundaries that made Tianjin the most complex treaty port in China. What was distinctively modern about twentieth-century *weisheng* was its association with the concept of a shared, public health. With so many divisions among municipal units, a true "public" administration could not emerge in treaty-port Tianjin. Hygienic modernity, a concept created by imperialism, was undermined by the fragmentations produced by imperialism itself.

THE MULTIPLE CITIES OF TIANJIN
City of Empires

Tianjin after 1900 became home to eight different empires, and each empire proclaimed its presence through distinctive arrangements of space and edifice. Great Britain, France, Japan, Germany, Russia, Austria-Hungary, Italy, and Belgium used their positions on the international relief force to establish new concessions in Tianjin or expand those already existing. Between 1900 and 1902, Russia, Italy, Belgium, and Austria-Hungary all claimed settlements on the north bank of the Hai River, while Great Britain, France, Germany, and Japan expanded their existing holdings on the south bank by more than 200 percent. By 1902, the total area of the foreign concessions was eight times the size of the (formerly) walled city (see fig. 4).[3]

The Boxer Uprising of 1900 transformed Tianjin into what I have termed a "hypercolony," a brash architectural, administrative, and cultural showcase of imperialism. Foreign powers existed in Tianjin not only in relation to Chinese administered space: they each stood, shoulder to shoulder, next to the representative spaces of other foreign powers. As foreigners expanded their control of land along the Hai River, a new type of urban environment arose in Tianjin, an urban environment akin to that which Timothy Mitchell has called "world-as-exhibition."[4] Mitchell used this term to describe the nineteenth-century European city, where a building was not simply an edifice, but a symbol of something beyond itself, and the city was "a place of discipline and visual arrangements . . . the organization of everything and everything organized to represent, to recall like an exhibition some larger meaning." In Tianjin, architecture was designed to

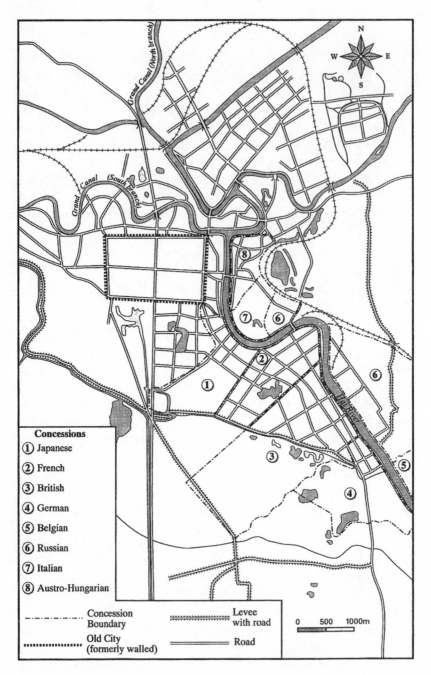

Concessions

① Japanese
② French
③ British
④ German
⑤ Belgian
⑥ Russian
⑦ Italian
⑧ Austro-Hungarian

—·—·— Concession Boundary
▪▪▪▪▪▪▪ Old City (formerly walled)
▬▬▬▬▬ Levee with road
▬▬▬▬▬ Road

0   500   1000m

Figure 4. Map of Tianjin, c. 1915, showing locations of the foreign concessions and an outline of the former walled city. From *Remaking the Chinese City: Modernity and National Identity, 1900–1950*, ed. Joseph W. Esherick (Honolulu: University of Hawaii Press, 200), 35.

exhibit a national essence, not just before a Chinese gaze, but also before an audience of multiple European and Asian empires. Tianjin became "world-as-exhibition," an exhibition of the world of turn-of-the-century high imperialism.

By the 1920s, Tianjin's multiple foreign settlements stood together as an array of quintessential European and Japanese architectures, all viewable in one day for the pedestrian willing to take an energetic six mile stroll up and down the banks of the Hai. Beginning a tour on the south bank, one would pass the Bavarian facade of the Club Concordia in the German Concession, the exaggerated parapets and massive towers of the British Settlement's Gordon Hall, the French Concession's pink-brick Hôtel du ville, and the imposing wooden *torii* arch of the Japanese Concession's Yamato Park. On the other side of the Hai, the fanciful turrets and steeply pitched roofs of Yuan Shikai's residence lent a Tyrolian atmosphere to the Austro-Hungarian Concession; in the circular piazza at the intersection of the Via Roma and the Via Marco Polo in the Italian Concession stood a fountain topped with a bronze angel commemorating the Italian casualties in the campaign against the Boxers. The Russian Concession boasted a few onion-domed churches and public buildings reminiscent of the architecture in the French Concession. The tour would end with the easternmost foreign outpost, the Belgian Concession. Since few Belgians had shown an interest in living in north China, the land here had been bought up by developers and turned into an industrial zone. As a result, the Belgian Concession boasted more smoke-stacks than residents, and our hypothetical pedestrian might be disappointed that the last concession on the tour bore no resemblance whatsoever to Brussels or Antwerp (see figs. 5–7).[5]

With the establishment of concessions and railroads, Tianjin became the boomtown of north China. In the first quarter of the twentieth century, waves of warlords, peasants, and foreign merchants came to the newly expanded city in search of fortune or simply a livelihood.[6] From 1902 to 1927, the city's population quadrupled from three hundred thousand to more than one million. The most impressive population growth during this time was in the foreign concessions, which grew from approximately fifty thousand in 1910 to almost a quarter of a million by 1927. Although the architecture that characterized the concessions was foreign, the majority of the residents were Chinese. By 1929, the British Settlement was home to approximately three thousand foreigners and thirty-six thousand Chinese. The smaller French and Japanese Concessions were the most densely populated, with fifty thousand and thirty-five thousand residents, respectively. The French Concession was home to only a thousand Frenchmen; the Japanese Concession

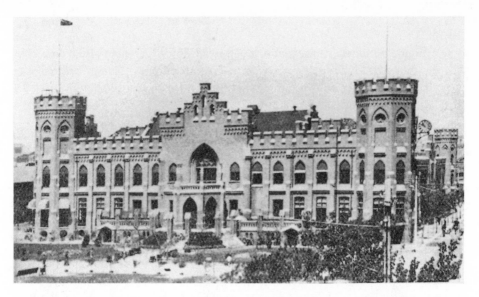

Figure 5. The British Settlement's Gordon Hall. Image courtesy of the Tianjin Academy of Social Sciences.

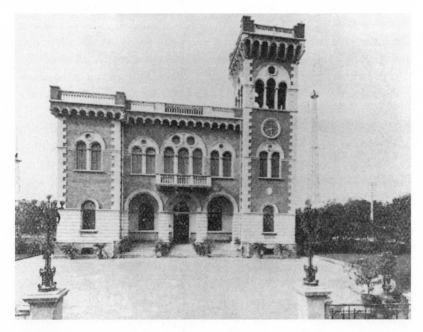

Figure 6. The Italian Concession's consulate building. Image courtesy of the Tianjin Academy of Social Sciences.

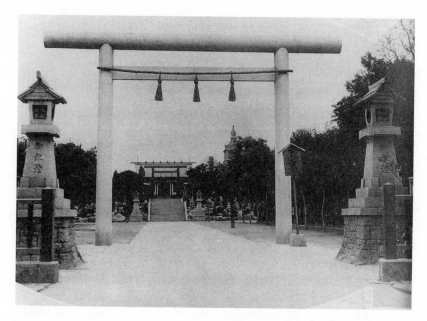

Figure 7. The *torii* at the entrance to the Japanese Concession's Yamato Park. Image courtesy of the Tianjin Academy of Social Sciences.

was home to between five and six thousand Japanese, constituting the largest foreign nationality in Tianjin.[7]

Different concessions became associated with different urban functions. The French Concession became the retail and business center of Tianjin, home to multistory modern department stores and office buildings. The British Settlement contained both the financial center of Tianjin and, in the suburban extramural extension, the stately homes of British and Chinese capitalists. The stylish architecture of the Italian Concession was a favorite for warlords (for example, Cao Kun) and intellectuals (Liang Qichao's "Ice Drinker's Studio" was actually a lovely Italianate villa). The Japanese Concession perhaps offered the greatest contrasts within its small area. It included the mansions that were home to deposed Manchu princes. It also included Tianjin's most popular red-light district, its narrow streets lined with brothels, gambling houses, and heroin shops.[8] The Austro-Hungarian, German, and Russian Concessions were relatively short-lived and were recovered by the Chinese administration after World War I and the Russian Revolution. Tianjin's concessions were jumbled places, where tiny minorities of French, Italians, British, Japanese, Russians, and Americans lived among a million Chinese, set to the backdrop of the architecture of imperialism.

The New Chinese City

After 1900, the modernizing Qing government abandoned the former walled city. When Yuan Shikai regained control of Tianjin from the TPG in the summer of 1902, Qing offices stood in ruin, looted and burned by foreign invaders. Rather than rebuild within the old city, Yuan chose a large tract of open land called "The Pit" (Yaowa), northeast of the old city, as the site for his new government district. Within six months of choosing the site, Yuan, like the British and French establishing their concessions forty years before, unceremoniously cleared the area of its numerous graves, and within two years the major roads and buildings of an entire new district had been completed.[9] The broad, straight avenues ran in a symmetrical grid, the ones running north-south named *jing* (warp) streets, the east-west roads named *wei* (weft) streets. Buildings that were a mélange of Chinese and foreign styles housed the Zhili provincial governor's office, the Tianjin Customs, the Changlu salt administration, the provincial and municipal courts, and other offices of Yuan's Beiyang administration. Throughout the 1910s and 1920s the establishment of new-style schools such as the Fisheries Institute and the Zhili Women's Normal School made this area the education center of Tianjin. A park, exhibition hall, and train station added a Western municipal atmosphere to Yuan's model town. A 1924 guidebook glowingly called this area the "gathering place of Tianjin's talent."[10]

But Yuan Shikai's "new Chinese city" lay far away from both the largest concentration of Chinese populations and the most commercially vibrant sectors of the city. Modern bureaucrats, young students, and professors of fisheries technology populated this rationally ordered area, and yet their projects of modernity took place out of the sight of the vast majority of Tianjin's residents. The municipal garden's exhibition hall might host educational displays of art, industry, and hygiene, but the people who benefited from the exhibits were a minority of "Tianjin's talent." Unlike the infamously restricted parks of the British Settlement, the municipal park of the new city was a place where Chinese were free to enter. However, its distance from Tianjin's metal workers, pig-bristle sorters, and flour mill workers ensured that its impressive grounds and modern buildings remained quiet, refined, and empty.[11]

The Old Chinese City

After 1902, the walls of the Chinese city were gone, but their location was marked by a tramline that circled the city where the walls once stood. Western-style buildings lined the outer streets, but within the old city, architecture and space remained much the same as before. By the 1920s, government and commerce had shifted to identifiably "modern" sections of Tianjin. With the opening of modern department stores and office buildings in the French Concession, the once prosperous North Gate neighborhoods became marked as the abode of the working class. Transport workers, shop clerks, rickshaw drivers, tanners, prostitutes, and doctors of Chinese medicine all struggled to make a living in the area that had once contained some of the most flourishing commercial streets of the city. Commerce had not entirely abandoned the neighborhood: the native place associations of sojourning businessmen were still located here, including the Fujian-Guangdong Hall and the Shanxi Hall. The Tianjin Chamber of Commerce also established its headquarters in this area. But in comparison with the multistory department stores and cafés of the French Concession, the old city commercial districts began to represent the "traditional economy" of the city.

To the west of these commercial streets lay an area where religious activity had once flourished but was now in dramatic decline. The exotic architecture of Tianjin's major mosque still dominated the landscape in the Northwest Corner neighborhood and served as the center of worship for the area's thousands of Muslims. But many of the city's Daoist temples, including the City God Temple, the Dragon King Temple, the Temple to the Immortal Lu Dongbin, the Temple of the Two Loyalists (dedicated to Guan Di and Yue Fei, also called Double Temple), and the Great Medicine King Temple had either been destroyed or converted into schools or police stations.[12] The Great Medicine King Temple was defunct, but hundreds of doctors of Chinese medicine and sellers of herbal medicines still lived on or near the street that bore its name. In the 1920s and 1930s, the doctors of Medicine King Street faced increasing challenges to their business. Not only were foreign-educated doctors draining off some of their clientele, but the wealthier customers who were dedicated to Chinese medicine preferred to visit traditional doctors who had offices in the foreign concessions.[13]

Part of the allure of the foreign concessions and the visibly more Westernized areas of the Chinese city was the perception that these neighborhoods were cleaner, more healthful, more orderly—more possessed of hygienic modernity than the neighborhoods north of the old city wall. By the 1920s, the Northwest Corner neighborhood bore the stigma of being *bu weisheng*. Using the new rhetoric of hygienic modernity, Chinese guidebooks to the city state that the poor Han and Muslim residents of the neighborhood were "unsanitary in their habits," and urged Chinese tourists to stay away from this district.[14] Only two decades after the occupation of Tianjin, sophisticated Chinese travelers were being urged to guard their health by separating themselves from their "unsanitary" countrymen.

It is ironic that this way of marking bodies and populations occurred at the same time that hygienic modernity was being created through massive private and government investment: in architecture, sewers, water pipes, and paved streets. *Weisheng* was not a property inherent within the bodies of the middle class—it required constant regulation and vigilant policing. Natural flows of people, disease, smells, and water drifted through the city. The maintenance of hygienic modernity was a perpetual attempt at regulating those flows, fueled by the anxiety of maintaining boundaries within a borderless hypercolony.

REGULATING FLOWS OF PEOPLE: CONSTRUCTED HYGIENE IN THE BRITISH SETTLEMENT

The roads of the British Settlement recalled the empire and its heroes. Elgin Avenue intersected with Gordon Road not far from London Road. The marble portals of banks and businesses lined Victoria Road, sometimes known as the "Wall Street of North China." Beyond the Weitze Creek, in the area that the settlement took over after the Boxer Uprising, broad commercial buildings gave way to the trees, spacious yards, and mansions of Edinburgh Road and Singapore Road. In spite of the paeans to Britannia emblazoned on the road signs, the population of the British Settlement was more than 90 percent Chinese. By the 1920s, more than thirty thousand Chinese lived and worked in an environment that attempted to mirror the image of the British metropole.

Daniel Headrick has observed that in colonial Dakar, segregation was justified on types of buildings and hygienic habits. All Africans in Dakar were proclaimed French citizens, but there were two types: Africans who could "be subject to the sanitary regulations applicable to Europeans," and those who could not.[15] By contrast, Chinese within the boundaries of the British Settlement were not able to vote for officers on the municipal council until 1928, but all residents were subject to the same regulations that dictated the size, construction, and uses of their homes. Unable to exclude on the basis of race, the regulators of the British Settlement sought to legislate segregation through the hygienic standards of buildings.

A vast majority of the British Settlement's municipal by-laws of 1919 dealt with the interconnected concerns of sanitation, hygiene, and visual arrangement of the built environment. Within the by-laws' capitalized passages and margin headings one can detect the anxieties of British business-men attempting to plan a bourgeois urban space against the backdrop of per-ceived Chinese characteristics. DANGEROUS STRUCTURES built along native lines fall into neighbor's yards. CHINESE-OWNED BOILERS and machinery explode if not operated by foreign engineers. STAGNANT POOLS of water emanating from Chinese privies flood streets. Pig-offal and other OFFENSIVE MATTER accumulates, or alternately OFFENSIVE MATTER is sloshed about on the streets in the buckets of Chinese night-soil carriers. Traditional medical practitioners are unversed and unlicensed, and "gaming houses" and "bawdy houses" lurk behind edifice walls. Above all, there is a fear of OVERCROWDING, along with a fear of CHOLERA, DIPHTHERIA, MEASLES, SCARLET FEVER, SMALLPOX, TYPHUS FEVER, BUBONIC AND PNEUMONIC PLAGUE, ERYSIPELAS, AND MENINGITIS. The image that arises in the 1910s is one of a British minor-ity anxiously surrounded by a dirty population prone to accidents, crowd-ing, gambling, whoring, and epidemic disease.[16]

The first two decades of the twentieth century had been relatively healthy for the British Settlement, but epidemics surrounded this island of salubrity, adding to fears of Chinese as carriers of contagion. Cholera struck the city in 1895, 1902, 1907, and 1909. In 1911 plague killed tens of thou-sands of people in Manchuria and several hundred in Tianjin. In 1917 mas-sive flooding of the Yongding ("Forever Stable") River inundated the en-tire city, bringing cholera, dysentery, and the plague in its wake. Although foreigners in the British Settlement were relatively immune from the ef-fects of these outbreaks (in part because they enjoyed a steady supply of treated water), children's diseases such as scarlet fever and diphtheria were still a problem. And even though many Chinese residents of Tianjin had been vaccinated against smallpox, the sight of smallpox-infected rural poor who sought refuge in the city during the floods of 1917 helped to convince foreign observers that they were threatened by a plague- and parasite-ridden Chinese population.

By the late 1920s, the world of the British Settlement had become in-creasingly complex, in need of more ordering and more boundaries, but seemingly with fewer attendant fears of racially specific hygienic lack. Dur-ing the 1920s, the British Settlement witnessed increased trade, a building boom, and the influx of prosperous Chinese. The quiet and refined south-eastern section of the British Settlement had become a favorite site for the homes of tremendously wealthy retired warlords, former Qing officials, re-publican-era governors, and their many relatives. The defeated warlord Sun Chuanfang's massive mansion (which, from the exterior, resembled a fantastical European equestrian academy) was a stone's throw away from the sleek lines of warlord Wang Zhanyuan's modernist residence. The former Qing diplomat Zhou Xuexi's Italianate villa competed for Mediterranean splendor with Sun Songyi's Spanish-style mansion two blocks down on Singapore Road. Within these ostentatious dwellings, Chinese lived far more regally than the vast majority of the settlement's European and American residents. Tianjin's growing population of middle-class professionals lived in comfortable multiroom apartments in large, architecturally distinctive apartment buildings, or in attached row houses that gave some of the settlement's streets the feel of a Brooklyn brownstone neighborhood.[17]

The growing wealth in the settlement (for both Chinese and foreigners) and the growing technological complexity of hygienic modernity are reflected in the sanitary regulations section of the settlement's building codes. A series of specialized pipes of specific diameters was required to link water closets, sinks, and drains to an underground sewer system. Gradients were carefully measured, access vents were mandated at regular intervals, and smoke was forced through pipes to test their soundness.[18] The world of John Fryer's *Juzhai weisheng lun* (The hygiene of residences), with its multiple pipes and blueprints of household containments and circulations, had finally arrived in Tianjin. Indoor plumbing was not mandated by law, but municipal by-laws no longer specifically mention night-soil carriers, indicating that increased wealth had slowly made the night-soil carrier a rare sight in the British Settlement.

Overall, by the 1920s, the British Settlement seemed to have erased many of the explicit signs of racial distinction from their regulations. Regulations were no longer specifically aimed at an inherently dangerous and dirty Chinese population. Chinese residents of the settlement would not gain a voice on the ratepayers association until 1928; even before then, a Chinese middle and merchant class was enjoying residency in the shady lanes and neat brownstones of the British Settlement. The Municipal Council seemed content to dictate the dimension of pipes and chimneys without invoking the specter of an inferior horde. Racial hierarchies were eliminated through the seemingly neutral architectural demands of hygienic modernity. Life in the British Settlement was expensive. Intent on being the most hygienically advanced of the foreign areas, the British Municipal Council made standard a middle-class British-built environment that few Chinese would be able to afford. Through building codes, the British Settlement legislated out the Chinese poor and preserved its British facade. Most of the thirty-six thousand Chinese who lived in this environment were economically far better off than most of their one million compatriots living in the Chinese city. Hygienic modernity provided two services for Europeans and Chinese residents of the settlement: It helped maintain the distinctive visibility of British borders in a Chinese world, and it allowed Chinese elites to distinguish themselves through the markers of architecture and cleanliness.

Hygienic modernity was not a natural characteristic of the settlement, but was maintained through vigilant policing. Influxes of refugees were still a problem during the warlord years; control over Chinese-administered Tianjin switched hands several times between 1922 and 1928, and each warlord battle brought with it a fresh influx of refugees into the concessions. Refugees were packed away into missionary relief camps, and any lingerers might be among the several hundred arrested each year by settlement police for "breach of sanitary regulations" *(bu zun weisheng guiding)*.[19] The Municipal Council also reserved the right to close down any "candle-house, melting house, melting-place, soap-house, slaughter-house, place for boiling offal or blood, or for boiling or crushing bones, or any pig-sty, necessary house, dunghill, manure pile, hide-yard, or wool cleaning factory," a regulation that indicated the need for constant vigilance against creeping incursions of Chinese economic life.[20] Hygienic modernity in the British Settlement mandated the setting of boundaries in stone and concrete. At the same time, it attempted to prevent the indiscriminate flow of noxious gases, liquids, and people through its portion of Tianjin, even though these circulations resulted from, or were the basis for, the livelihood of the city.

REGULATING FLOWS OF GASES AND SMELLS:
THE CHINESE CITY BUREAU OF HEALTH

The British Settlement was not the only locale in Tianjin that sought to regulate the built environment and stop promiscuous circulations for the sake of health and appearance. In the Chinese-administered city, these tasks fell to the newly created *weisheng ju* (health bureau), the inheritor of the TPG's *service de santé*. From the 1907 regulations of the health bureau it is obvious that *weisheng* had grown to encompass everything from the visual order of the city to the control of bacteria. Through its force of health inspectors, sanitary police, and street sweepers, the health bureau eliminated untidy walls, organized garbage, rounded up beggars, and monitored food vendors.

The health bureau also sought to control the smells of the Chinese city. In pursuit of that goal, it spread lime and creosote on the city's public toilets, but it was quite another matter to control the production of gases by small industries in the Chinese city. Taking a page straight from a sanitarian's handbook—or from John Fryer's *Huaxue weisheng lun* (Chemistry and hygiene)—the *weisheng ju* regulations identified the gases emitted by factories and workshops as prime disease-causing agents. Unfortunately these gases were also the very products of Tianjin's main economic activities. Unlike Shanghai, Tianjin in the 1920s had few large factories. Its economy was smaller, smellier, and more closely linked to the hinterland. Workshops received the pig-bristles, goat hides, camel hair, and wool bundles that came into the city from Inner Mongolia and Manchuria and processed them so they could be shipped abroad. The hooves and bones from the numerous cows, sheep, and goats herded outside the city were boiled down into glue in huge vats owned by individual entrepreneurs. The chemical dyes used for homespun fabrics came from urban backyard factories.[21] Regulating the gases emitted by these myriad tiny industries pitted the health bureau against the livelihood of the population. Hygienic modernity could only be approached through a combined strategy of negotiating with city business interests, employing the modern rhetoric of sanitary science and "the public," and the levying of the coercive force of the state.

In the first decade of the twentieth century, the Chinese city health bureau began an all-out campaign to move dye manufacturers from locations within the city, arguing that the smoke they produced was bad for the city's *weisheng* and could cause lung disease. In response, the companies petitioned the bureau through the Tianjin Chamber of Commerce, arguing that it was economically unfeasible for them to move operations away from their potential customers in the center of the city. The health bureau persevered, portraying itself as the champion of the public interest against commercial desires for self-enrichment, invoking the importance of a new phenomenon—the *weisheng* of a city: "This bureau is responsible for protecting the city's health [*weisheng*]. Therefore we must vigorously attempt to eliminate all things that harm health. If we acted only in accordance with individual merchants' private [*si*] convenience and did not consider the great inconvenience to the people of the city, then we would be violating our bureau's original mission."[22]

In a last-ditch effort, the dye manufacturers offered to erect tall chimneys to take the smoke high into the air where it would be "dispersed by the winds." The health bureau replied that it had been proven "by chemists in scientific experiments" that the smoke produced by the dye-manufacturing process did not rise in the air, therefore the chimneys would be useless. The bureau successfully insisted that the Chamber of Commerce require these businesses to move their operations beyond the Weitze Creek, away from the populated areas of the city.[23] The government had prevailed over commercial interests to defended the *weisheng* of the city.

The health bureau could also come down with surprising force on smaller violators of *weisheng* regulations. Men attending smoky vats of boiling pig skin were sentenced to wear the cangue in public for ten days.[24] Slaughter-house operators were fined and their businesses moved out of neighborhoods where elite residents complained about "pestilent vapors" *(yiqi).*[25] The health bureau acted as a de facto enforcer of zoning regulations, removing cottage industries from the streets and alleys of Tianjin's more affluent neighborhoods in the native city. While such activity reduced the presence of noxious smells and unsightly messes from some of Tianjin's streets, it also served to remove the presence of the workers who labored in such in-dustries: the night-soil dealers, the tenders of cauldrons, the haulers of car-casses. Although the residents of Tianjin's more elite neighborhoods could continue to use the products of these industries, the manufacturing process itself, and the laborers who participated in it, would be rendered invisible in these neighborhoods by the dictates of hygienic modernity. Resident elites and government officials sought the same goals for different reasons: the health inspector pursued bacteria, the neighborhood spokesmen feared pestilent *qi*. Their combined common interest removed workers to the pe-ripheries of the city: the Three Stone Slabs neighborhood north of the Grand Canal, the South Market section, the southern and eastern suburbs outside of the Weitze Creek, and the areas to the north and west of the former city wall. As poor laborers and noxious industries became more concentrated in these neighborhoods, the label *"bu weisheng"* was increasingly attached to them. Protecting the *weisheng* of some Chinese meant further stigmatiz-ing the lives of others.

REGULATING FLOWS OF WATER AND WASTE

Although gases threatened if they circulated too freely through the city, so too did water. Water was a prime carrier of disease and inspired vigilant mon-itoring and control. At the same time, massive amounts of freely flowing water— needed for drinking, cooking, washing things and bodies, and most of all, for flushing away impurities—was the cornerstone of hygienic modernity. Each concession sought its own solutions to the problem of water and waste management, but the modern impulse to create distinct bound-aries in the name of hygiene was constantly thwarted by human and or-ganic elements that resisted containment.

Water determined which areas were *weisheng* and which areas were *bu weisheng*. Removing water and waste from sight while eliminating human intermediaries became the ultimate hallmark of hygienic modernity. Areas that managed to acquire underground pipes to bring clean water into homes and take waste water away not only eliminated unsavory waste-water vats and cesspools from their neighborhoods, but also removed the presence of unsightly laborers from their streets. However, the political divisions and economic realities of treaty-port cities ensured a heterogeneous hygienic state in spite of this hygienic ideal. Constructed and managed by different private companies and concession governments, sewer pipes and water pipes were unevenly distributed and began and ended abruptly. Some areas in the city had water pipes but no sewers: here tap water might spring from a gleaming brass faucet, but no pipes existed to drain away the effluvia of toilets and sinks. In other neighborhoods, the municipal government might provide water and sewer pipes, but residents could not afford the expensive porcelain and tile fixtures of an indoor modern bathroom, known as the *weisheng jian* (literally, a hygienically modern space). Water was the one element of *weisheng* that was most intimately tied to variations in income level and government efficiency. The complete circle of hygienic modernity—indoor sanitary facilities forming an unbroken chain with purified running water on one end and underground sewers on the other—became a virtual monopoly of only a small portion of the foreign concessions. But this exclusive monopoly was accomplished only through a fierce struggle with Tianjin's powerful water carrier and night-soil carrier guilds.

THE DARK DRIFTERS

Many men in Tianjin made their living by carrying things.[26] Tianjin was a merchants' city, and merchandise had to be moved. Barges that came up the Hai or the Grand Canal had to be unloaded and their goods delivered to warehouses. Bulk bundles from warehouses needed to be distributed to retail shops. Foreign trade meant even more goods were moved along the city streets by human power: bales of cotton, bundles of pig-bristles, sacks of dried herbs, and loads of coal traveled between the docks and the shops of the city. Borne on backs, slung from burden poles, or pushed along on wooden wheelbarrows, goods circulated through the city through the muscle power of thousands of individual men.

Water was no exception to this transportation logic. Like cotton, grain, or coal, drinking water was a commodity moved by men with wheelbarrows. Tianjin's particular geography produced this situation. Lying close to the sea in a major salt-producing region, Tianjin's wells produced a brackish, saline brew. The city was surrounded by rivers, but most of them served as the dumping ground for the region's millions. Water from the southern branch of the Grand Canal had not yet flowed past the city and its drains, so it was deemed more suited for drinking than water from the Hai River. Throughout the city there was a demand for Grand Canal water, and yet for most neighborhoods, the Grand Canal was miles away. Water carriers collected water from specific sites along the banks of the Grand Canal, loaded it into buckets and wheelbarrows, and traveled along preassigned routes to the households of the walled city and beyond. Hundreds of thousands of customers paid for the convenience of having water regularly delivered to their door.

Waste was also a valuable commodity that traveled around the city in the buckets and wheelbarrows of workers. The link between the alimentary canal and the farmer's field began early every morning when a good man or woman of Tianjin dumped the nightly accumulations of the family chamber pot into the bucket of the neighborhood night-soil carrier. Night-soil carriers went from house to house, crying out their arrival to awaken sleeping residents, consolidating each family's product into their larger buckets. They would pour the unwanted liquid element into nearby canals or rivers, and take the reserved drier matter to spots where it could be spread out to dry. Night soil guild managers then sold the valuable fertilizer to farmers, who used the feces to bring forth the food that would in turn produce more excrement. The night-soil trade flourished as a vital economic and ecological link between any Chinese city and its surrounding countryside.[27]

On any given street in Tianjin, one could find carriers of water and carriers of waste passing in a constant stream, moving from suburb to city center and back again with their wheelbarrows or burden poles and buckets (see fig. 8).[28] The majority of these men belonged to guilds that regulated transport routes and set fees. Different guilds staked out specific territories along the banks of the Grand Canal and claimed exclusive right to retrieve water at those spots. Guilds lay claim to delivery routes and customer bases in different neighborhoods throughout the city. Although these territories were often negotiated by representatives from the upper echelon of the guild structure, territorial disputes sometimes broke out into violent battles among the laborers themselves.[29] In the popular imagination, fights between water transport guilds were always the doing of the legendary Dark Drifters.

Tianjin was known throughout north China as the home to street toughs

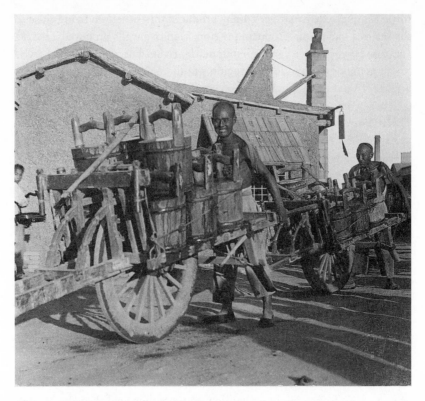

Figure 8. Tianjin water carriers, early twentieth century. Image courtesy of Library of Congress.

known as *hunhunr,* an odd Chinese phrase of obscure origin which Gail Hershatter has translated as "Dark Drifters."[30] The *hunhunr* (pronounced something like "hwr-hwr") were loosely organized groups of day laborers, swindlers, and gamblers who inhabited the streets and alleys of nineteenth-century Tianjin, distinguished by their swaggering walk and flamboyant dress. Although not exclusively associated with water and night-soil carrier guilds, there was considerable overlap between the two. The presence of Dark Drifters imparted a violent edge to Tianjin's neighborhoods. When not engaged in street brawls, they maintained their reputation as fearless fighters by swaggering about, dressing in accessories such as scarves and open shirts, and publicly demonstrating their indifference to pain. Stories of Dark Drifters proving their mettle by cutting off pieces of their own flesh, jumping into vats of boiling oil, or baring their chests to welcome oncoming knives may or may not have been exaggerations. What is more certain is that conflicts between rival Dark Drifters groups were frequently resolved by staging violent rumbles in the streets of Tianjin. The influence of Dark Drifter gangs reached from the level of night-soil carriers through the upper echelons of Tianjin merchants, ensuring them a ubiquitous and powerful presence on the streets of the city.[31]

In the minds of many of Tianjin's foreign residents, these brawny, proud water carriers fell far short of the ideals of hygienic modernity—and colonial servility. Although in most foreign households a chain of Chinese servants mediated between the Dark Drifters and the genteel cup of afternoon tea, the source of the water and its means of conveyance to the home provided a cause for considerable anxiety. Attempts to find water in the concession areas proved a failure—well water was sulfurous and far too salty to drink. Beginning in the late nineteenth century, various foreign settlement authorities searched for means to sunder the common human bond of Tianjin's watery environment, but not all could break entirely free.

THE BRITISH SETTLEMENT: LIQUID INDEPENDENCE

Residents in the British Settlement shared anxiety about water and the Chinese who delivered it, but there was much debate about the proper role of the government in solving the problem. The issue of a public water supply had been discussed in the British Municipal Council in Tianjin since the 1880s, but it was only after the cholera epidemic of 1895 that serious debate began about the virtues of government intervention in the water supply. Although many in the British Settlement accepted the explanation that cholera was caused by the presence of bacteria in drinking water, there was still no consensus that the government should be the entity responsible for removing bacteria and other contaminants from water. An 1889 editorial in the *Chinese Times* urged "municipal interference" in the British Settlement's water supply, noting that in outposts of the British empire such as Hong Kong, Bombay, Shanghai, and Sydney, the "expatriated Englishmen can . . . now drink without the fear of death in the pot." The editorial conceded that some British residents held that the filtration and cleansing of water was an individual responsibility and duty, but it called this "a flimsy objection" when in England the home government was already involved in such "socialistic" enterprises as poor houses, free schools, and "even free breakfasts." To further the point, the editorial then raised the specter of British reliance upon Chinese water carriers and domestic servants to supply, precipitate, and boil water. It was the "notorious inefficiency of Chinese servants" that provided the most convincing counterargument to those who counseled against a municipal water supply.[32]

After the cholera epidemic of 1895, the question was no longer whether or not the municipal council would be responsible for water supply, but rather from what source the water supply would be drawn. Some optimistic residents (and gardening enthusiasts) held that the Hai River could provide a healthy supply of water for drinking with enough left over to "turn our sparsely covered grass patches into bright green lawns, and our sickly floral display into brilliant flower gardens."[33] Others called the Hai "a mere drain of the filth and refuse of half a million natives from Tientsin city," a source that "no civilized community" should consider.[34] Convinced of the ability of sanitary technology to render the Hai water drinkable, the plan to use water from the river was approved. By January 1899, the British Municipal Waterworks had completed its plant along the river, including water tower, pump house, filters, and settling tanks. Treated water was pumped through a ten-inch main laid under the main roads, and four-inch branch pipes that ran to all the side streets in the settlement.[35] Property owners rapidly converted their buildings to include indoor water pipes, and by the turn of the century most British Settlement residents were using water from indoor taps.

Soon the residents of the British Settlement discovered that having their own municipal water supply did not produce the desired effect of freeing them from interaction with and dependence upon Chinese. Although municipal water was filtered multiple times, it still needed to be boiled, a task that in most households was the responsibility of Chinese servants. British residents were therefore warned that the provision of municipal water did not entirely free them from vigilance over their Chinese domestics: "Since the water is very well clarified by the Water Works, an excellent opportunity may be thereby afforded for the Chinese to neglect the measures for purification . . . and this will prove a menace to the public health instead of a blessing."[36]

British residents also discovered that although the waterworks supplied them with water through impersonal pipes, the lack of a sewer system in the settlement meant that they still had to deal with Chinese intermediaries to get rid of water once it was used. Before the advent of the waterworks, the Chinese water carriers who brought in fresh water also contracted with foreign households to remove dirty water. These men now refused to carry dirty water out of houses that no longer used their fresh water services, or else asked exorbitant fees to do so.[37] The British Municipal Council made the completion of its sewer system a priority. By the 1930s, advancements in water treatment technology also allowed the British to draw water almost exclusively from settlement wells and use the Hai water solely as an emergency supplement.[38] Ironically, almost as soon as the settlement had finally acquired its liquid independence, it relinquished its independent existence as an outpost of the British empire, first to Japan, and then to the Nationalist government of China.

THE JAPANESE CONCESSION:
NEGOTIATIONS AND COMPROMISES

The Japanese Concession provides an instructive comparison with the British Settlement. From the beginning of the Japanese Concession in 1896, the Chinese always outnumbered the Japanese, with the exception of the years of the Japanese occupation (1937–45). Association, negotiation, and cooperation between certain segments of Chinese society and Japanese Concession authorities was the inevitable mode of operation. Dr. Tsuzuki's *eisei* advice from the 1902 cholera epidemic—to separate and segregate from the Chinese—was a practical impossibility.

The environment of cooperation in the Japanese Concession was manifested in the composition of its Residents' Association *(kyoryûmindan)*. Any resident of the concession who paid a minimum level of taxes to the municipal government could vote for a representative, and taxpaying residents, regardless of nationality, could run for a seat. By 1914, the number of Chinese representatives to the Japanese Concession Residents' Association outnumbered Japanese representatives. By 1925, the Japanese consulate, which retained decision-making authority in the concession, cut the number of representatives to sixty and mandated that at least half must be Japanese citizens.[39] In some ways, the Japanese Concession stood as a unique locus of "East Asian cooperation" within the treaty-port environment of Tianjin. However, all positions of authority were held by Japanese citizens. Residents' Association records are filled with the enumerated names of Japanese businessmen, diplomats, and physicians, but below the level of leadership, other subpositions are filled by anonymous *shina jin* (Chinese). The "East Asian cooperation" of the Japanese Concession appeared to be more a system of "East Asian tutelage," with Japanese in positions of authority.

From the first year of its establishment in 1907, the *eisei bu* (health department) of the Japanese Concession Residents' Association began maintaining careful statistics on contagious disease within the concession. It became immediately apparent that intestinal disorders were the most frequent complaint, including typhus, dysentery, and infant diarrhea. Second to intestinal disease were "nervous disorders," including "neurasthenia" *(shinkei suijaku)* and hysteria *(hisuteri)*, which were associated with the "special conditions" of living abroad. Authorities pointed out a number of causes for the unhealthfulness of the concession. They blamed Tianjin's climate, tracing outbreaks in disease to the disruptive changes in weather that occurred during the fall and spring. Health officers also emphasized the importance of household hygiene in overcoming these diseases, and encouraged Japanese residents to alter their private habits in order to better adapt to Tianjin's climate. Japanese would have to get used to living in "foreign-style" houses with indoor heating, and avoid using coal braziers for inside their houses. But hearkening to the experience of cholera in 1902 and the warnings of Dr. Tsuzuki, medical authorities placed the primary blame for the predominance of gastrointestinal diseases in the Japanese Concession on impure water supplies and the improper disposal of excrement.[40]

The central public health concern for the concession became the management of waste water and excreta. During the first few years of the settlement, Japanese residents, like Chinese residents in the old city, contracted with private Chinese carriers who hauled away human waste to be used as fertilizer. In the eyes of the concession authorities, however, the men who did this did not pay attention to hygiene, and frequently let buckets spill on the streets. Moreover, they were "the lowest sort of characters" who used foul language, worked at an extremely slow pace, and extorted extra money from households. Throughout the 1910s there was considerable debate among concession authorities about the most efficient and economical waste disposal plan. A feasible strategy would not only work within the concession's budget, but would also have to take into account the power of the Chinese night-soil carriers' guild.[41]

Finally in the 1920s, the Residents' Association founded the Cleanliness-Preserving Section (Japanese, *hojôka;* Chinese, *baojing ke*), a compromise between the interests of the Chinese night-soil carriers and the interests of hygienic modernity. The concession Residents' Association provided a monopoly contract for the night-soil carriers, who agreed to work under Japanese supervision. Every morning the *hojôka* workers would collect the contents of the concession's privies and chamber pots and remove them to a designated station at the end of Fukushima Street, near the southwestern edge of the concession, bordering Qing-administered lands. There the solid waste was separated from the liquid waste, and the solid waste was carted away by peasants. The liquid waste was then dumped into the drainage pipes beneath the streets into the concession's incomplete sewer system.[42]

Building a sewer in the Japanese Concession proved to be an engineering challenge that would require the finest resources in the Japanese empire. *Weisheng* in Tianjin demanded constant effort in part because the natural environment itself resisted boundaries and separations. Set on a flat plain that drained nine rivers into the sea, Tianjin was a city of *keng*, a word that means any depression in the earth where water gathers: a pool, a swamp, or a cesspool. Water lived in intimate connection with land, and Tianjiners lived in intimate connection with their *keng*. The *keng* of Tianjin had names; the *keng* at the four corners of the walled city were even eulogized in poetry. In some places, *keng* were part of the drainage system of the city: they held water that might otherwise collect in the homes of the people and kept it there until summer rains flushed it into the city moat and on into the Hai River. In other places, they were simply the product of neglect. But the cost of draining water from land could be high. Common experience held that one could never truly eliminate the water from the land—eliminating a *keng* in one area usually meant the birth of a new *keng* nearby. Early maps of the Japanese Concession clearly show that this was the environment awaiting Japanese developers. The concession appears as a small orderly grid of streets suspended between two bodies of water: the Hai River on one side, and a series of interconnected *keng* on the other. Any expansion would require parting the water from the land.

The Japanese began installing sewer pipes under the main streets near the Hai River—Yamaguchi Street, Asahi Street, and Fukushima Street—as early as 1908.[43] But municipal sewer installation within the Japanese Concession was affected by the expansion of private buildings on the other side of the border in the Chinese-administered area. This area, originally a marshy no-man's land, became known as the "Sanbuguan"—the "Three No-Cares"—because neither the Chinese, the Japanese, nor the Western authorities showed any desire to govern it. Private landfill projects on this land in the 1910s altered the drainage of the area, and soon the main thoroughfare of the Japanese Concession, Asahi Street, was being flooded with the backwash from the Sanbuguan area. Finally with the help of engineers from the South Manchurian Railway, a comprehensive drainage plan was drawn for the concession. By 1929, the concession Residents' Association had laid a pipe network of over ten kilometers under all the of the concession's streets. It had been a tremendous struggle. In spite of the self-congratulatory mode of the concession history on its *eisei* accomplishments, it had taken, from the formal founding of the concession in 1896, a total of thirty-three years for the Japanese Concession to provide sewers for a mere eight-by-ten block area.[44]

This long-awaited sewer system still did not eliminate the need for the *hojôka* service, since the majority of households in the concession did not have indoor plumbing. The expense of purchasing and installing such equipment, as well as the additional expense of water fees and maintenance, limited the number of households who could flush directly into the underground drainage system. As late as 1928, only eight hundred households and businesses had indoor flush facilities. As a result, more than three thousand homes in the concession used the *hojôka* service, a number that represented about 70 percent of all households. Of the eight hundred households that had flush toilets, one hundred still used the *hojôka* night-soil service because, as the Residents' Association explained, "Many Chinese women still had the habit of using chamber pots."[45] The concession authorities still received numerous complaints against the Chinese night-soil carriers, who reportedly continued to use crude language and violent resistance against their Japanese supervisors. But because of the economics of the concession and the strength of the Chinese laborers' organization, the *hojôka* system continued. Japanese bacteriologists ran the health bureau of the Japanese Concession, but ultimately their vision of hygienic modernity was compromised through the process of living life in China.

NAVIGATING THE WATERS OF IMPERIALISM: THE NATIVE CITY WATERWORKS

The inability of individual concessions to solve their water problems provided Chinese and foreign entrepreneurs in Tianjin with an excellent business opportunity. Founded in 1903, the Tientsin Native City Waterworks Company (Ji'an zilaishui gongsi) eventually supplied water to the Chinese-administered districts of Tianjin and all the concessions of the city—with the exception of the British, who preferred their own water. The Tientsin Native City Waterworks was an independent company that provided water for profit to any part of the city that was willing to pay its rates. Throughout its forty-year history, the company deftly negotiated the complicated political boundaries of the city, signing contracts, laying water pipes, and building sewers through land administered by Chinese, French, Germans, Italians, Japanese, Belgians, Russians, and Austro-Hungarians. In its role of provider of potable water to almost every district in the city, the Native City Waterworks came closer to being a true municipal health institution than any other organization in republican-period Tianjin. In the absence of a unified municipal government for the city, a private company was perhaps the only entity that could bridge troublesome political barriers with a water network.

Like any other purveyor of liquids in the city, the Native City Water-works had to contend with the economic interests of human water carriers. The laying of pipes throughout the city not only failed to eliminate the traditional water bearers of Tianjin, but even generated a new group of Chinese entrepreneurial intermediaries involved in the management and maintenance of water shops and water hydrants. In a city where livelihoods were hard-won and staunchly defended, the waterworks' business of providing water was constantly negotiated not only with government bureaus and concession governments, but also with individual Chinese competing for a role in the business.

The Tientsin Native City Waterworks Company was founded by a combination of Chinese and Western investors. The Chinese investors included Ma Yuqing, a comprador for a foreign match company, and Chen Jiyi, one of the original founders of the Shanghai Waterworks. Western investors included the American Charles Denby, the secretary of the TPG; Wilhelm Pappe, a German businessman; and J. Holmsburg, a Danish engineer. The company was established in November 1901, while the city was still under foreign occupation. Two and a half years later, in March 1903, the company began providing filtered water to the native city.[46]

Rather than use water from the heavily trafficked Hai River, the company drew water from the smaller southern branch of the Grand Canal, just as Tianjiners had done for generations. The company established its pumping station on the Grand Canal at a location upriver of the more populated part of the city. This location, called Mustard Garden, or Jie Yuan, had been the site of a large private garden established by the salt merchant Zha Riqian during the early eighteenth century. By the late nineteenth century the estate had fallen into disrepair and suffered the indignity of serving as a barracks for occupation armies in 1900.[47] Finally the once-magnificent compound that had hosted the Qianlong emperor was razed and replaced by a modern water plant that included a sixty-thousand-gallon capacity coal-fueled steam pump, three huge settling ponds, and two slow-filtration tanks.[48] The company established its headquarters in the northwest corner of the old city, across the street from the City God Temple. Photographs of the City God Temple from the early twentieth century show the water company's 110-foot high water tower dwarfing the former center of ritual life in imperial Tianjin.[49]

With the blessing of Tianjin's Columbia University–educated Customs superintendant, Tang Shaoyi, the company began laying water pipes through the most populous parts of the Chinese city. From 1904 to 1910, Tianjin's streets were in a constant state of construction. First waterworks company employees dug up earth and laid pipes, then the government public works bureau covered them over and paved the streets. The tram company then laid down trolley tracks on the newly paved streets, while the telephone company and electric company installed wires above.[50]

Such a rapid, extensive modernizing project, undertaken by several independent entities at the same time, proved extremely difficult to coordinate. Frequent conflicts arose between the waterworks company and government bureaus concerning responsibility and payment for construction work. Cooperation between bureaus and companies was complicated by the multitude of nationalities and languages represented—management of the tram company was Belgian, the electric company was French, and the water company predominantly British and Danish. The Chinese municipal bureaus themselves in the early twentieth century still employed many foreign managers and technical consultants from Germany, France, and Japan. Many of the Chinese engineers and clerks in the employ of the various bureaus and companies were southerners from Guangdong, Fujian, or Shanghai. English was the lingua franca of this Babel-like assemblage and remained the language of many official communications until after the 1911 Revolution. Communications between the various departments and the water company reveal clerks and managers valiantly struggling with English while at the same time struggling over contested payments and responsibilities.[51] The establishment of a water system in the 1910s revealed the strange combination of hypercolonialism (Danes, Russians, French, and Americans suspended in mutual suspicion and cooperation), sojourner economies (many of Tianjin's early "modernizers" were southern Chinese), and Qing sovereignty that characterized turn-of-the-century Tianjin. This multiplicity of modernizing elites, however, never operated in an environment solely comprised of other elites. The cooperations and conflicts between elites in treaty-port Tianjin were perpetually conducted within the context of Tianjin's workers, water carriers, and Dark Drifters.

THE HUMAN FACTOR OF MODERN WATER

The Native City Waterworks maintained a constant vigilance over the one factor that, from the perspective of management, stood as both the most serious threat to water quality and the most challenging competition to their business—the numerous Chinese laborers, shopkeepers, and "entrepreneurs," both within the employ of the company and without, who sought to profit from the supply of water in Tianjin. To understand the magnitude of this "threat" to the company, one must first examine how water was actually delivered to the majority of consumers in the city. Unlike the contemporary conception of water flowing upon command into private sinks and tubs, water in Tianjin was handled by as many as three levels of human intermediaries before it reached the teacups and cooking pots of the city's Chinese residents.

Unlike the newer, Western-style buildings of the concession areas, few of the residences and shops of the Chinese city had indoor plumbing. By the 1910s the network of Native City Waterworks pipes ran under most of the major streets of the old city and surrounding commercial districts. The pipes came above ground not in private residences, but on street corners through open hydrants and taps. If individuals wished to use the company water, they had to purchase "water tickets," which could then be exchanged at the tap for water at the rate of ten gallons for one cent *(wen)*.[52] Initially these hydrants were manned by laborers from the water company who collected water tickets and operated the tap. As metering technology improved, the water company shifted from direct management of taps to renting out to entrepreneurs who established "water shops" *(shuidian)* around the taps. The company left the collection of water tickets and the distribution of water up to the shop owner. The company simply sent meter readers around to each shop to determine how much water had been sold and billed the owner for that amount. The growth of the water shop business far outpaced the growth of indoor plumbing in the Chinese sections of the city. By 1929, there were 558 water shops in the Chinese city, accounting for 78 percent of the water company's business.[53]

While some sections of the city had water shops on every other corner, water carriers still provided the service of delivering water to many individual households. The water company did not seem to concern itself with any disputes, territorial or otherwise, among the water carriers themselves, but they were deeply concerned about the potential for adulteration of their product at this stage in delivery. Once the water left the tap in the water shop, it was essentially out of the company's control. The waterworks could only request that the municipal authorities of the native city and the concessions punish those water carriers who made a practice of filling only half their cart with the company's water, then filling the rest with water drawn directly from the Hai River.[54] Less threatening to the public health, but equally threatening to the company's profits, were those water shops and water carriers who mixed company water with water obtained from artesian wells. Water from artesian wells was as clear as the company's filtered water but tasted considerably saltier, and the mixed product, if masqueraded as the company's water, raised complaints from consumers. Most onerous to the company was that artesian well water sold for an average of thirty cents per one thousand gallons, much lower than the company's rate of one yuan per one thousand gallons, yet water carriers sold it at company water prices and thus cleared higher profit margins for themselves at the cost of lower sales to the company. Unable to control the actions of water carriers, the company decided to "wage war" against the artesian wells by temporarily undercutting their prices in an attempt to drive them out of business. The tactic was only partially successful.[55]

PRIVATE WATER VERSUS PUBLIC INTEREST

Conflicts between the water company and water carriers typified the tension between Chinese and foreign elites on one hand, and the Chinese workers of the city on the other. Another line of fracture within the treaty-port environment lay between the private water company and the forces of Qing/Chinese sovereignty. Beginning with the years just before the 1911 Revolution and continuing into the Nationalist era, the water company frequently clashed with municipal authorities. The presence of a foreign-managed private water company violated many Chinese administrators' sense of what "the public" should be in their city. With the rise of Chinese nationalism through the first three decades of the twentieth century, clashes between the water company and the government became more intense.

During epidemics, the waterworks cooperated with municipal authorities to alter its price structures. During the cholera outbreak of 1907, the company cut its rates in the poorer, more populous sections of the city by two-thirds, and informed the health bureau that they were actually willing to sell the water at a loss in order to aid the public health. At the same time, the company was quite pleased that the bureau advised the people of Tianjin to use the company's water as a way of avoiding disease.[56]

The company was less amenable when the Tianjin police director Yang Yide demanded that the company supply more fire hydrants for use in the native city. This demand, written soon after the founding of the republic, was among the first communications to the company from the Chinese government that was written in Chinese, not English. The company was obliged to have a Chinese clerk translate it into English for the benefit of the foreigners on its board of directors. In the letter, police director Yang Yide, a disciple of Yuan Shikai, held forward the case of Japanese urban modernization as an example the company ought to follow:

> The more houses there are in a place the more fire hydrants should
> be erected and the more pipes laid in the ground, such that they may
> become of service in case of a fire and against other misfortune. During
> the 32nd year of Ming Chue [Meiji], at Tokio Japan, the natives of this
> country began to improve their water-supply and they erected 50–60
> fire hydrants to be used free of expenses in case of fire. . . . There is up
> to now erected [sic] 2,500 of these fire hydrants in the said town. . . .
> Now the Tientsin Native City Water-Works Co. has only laid pipes
> in such places where there is a chance of making a profit by sale of water,
> but in populous and important places there are none. The waterworks
> company ought to make the water easily accessible everywhere for the
> public, and should assist the public in its precautions against fires, and
> not only think on [sic] making a profit.[57]

The original text of the company's response is particularly telling of its latent worries as a private, foreign-managed service in a Chinese city. It begins by stating that the company had the public good in mind when it provided fire hydrants free of charge, and blamed any loss due to fire on the "old fashioned fireguilds" that "turn up at the fires with their gong-banging crowd of useless people, who are only in the way for the proper fire brigade." The letter continues:

> You further write that at Tokyo in Japan, there are 2,500 fire-hydrants.
> Now we must tell you, that Tokyo is many times larger than Tientsin,
> *and besides, the water works is a Municipal water works and estab-*
> *lished by the Government of Japan.*[58]

The last phrase referring to the Tokyo waterworks as a government-controlled entity has been crossed out in the original draft and was most likely deleted in the version sent on to the Tianjin police. The company did not wish to remind Yang of what he was already highly aware—that most of the modernizing projects in Meiji Japan so admired by the Chinese were conceived and managed directly by the Japanese government. A company such as the Tientsin Native City Waterworks possessed the capital and equipment to undertake modernization schemes that the Qing and the republican state were unable to accomplish—a situation that left a bad taste in the mouth of many Chinese administrators. It is quite telling of the condition of Chinese treaty ports that the Native City Waterworks Company was able to maintain control of its business until 1941, in spite of long-running battles between it and the Nationalist government health bureau through the late 1920s and 1930s. The waterworks were finally taken over by the Nationalist government in 1945, but only after the company had been seized from foreign managers by the Japanese in 1941. In the political environment of treaty-port Tianjin, many of the nationalizing dreams of Chinese patriots were only realized when "Japanese" companies were handed over to them by victorious Americans as part of the spoils of World War II.

CONCLUSION

In mid-nineteenth-century Europe, a few voices expressed admiration for an "Oriental" approach to the circulation and recycling of human waste. Victor Hugo called the sewers of Paris a wasteful system that left "the land barren and the water tainted." The famous chemist Justus von Liebig admired the civilizations of China and Japan for sustaining high agricultural production for thousands of years through the application of human waste to the soil. In contrast, Liebig portrayed the British international search for fertilizer made from bones or guano as the workings of "a vampire . . . on the breast of Europe, and even the world, sucking its lifeblood without any real necessity or permanent gain for itself."[59] But such sentiments were not to last in an era when the invisibility of waste and water was becoming a definitive marker of "Western civilization."

Water and waste reveal the complexity of the strange colonial politics of a Chinese treaty port. Multiple imperialisms created fragmented municipalities in Tianjin. A company formed by British and Chinese investors bridged the divisions between the city's "little empires." Hundreds of thousands of Chinese residents in the city received treated water, but economic disparities made sure they received it in ways quite different from their wealthier Chinese compatriots. Under conditions of "hypercolonialism" in Tianjin, the health of "the public" lay almost entirely within the realm of "the private"—a private company provided clean water to those who could pay, and indoor sanitary facilities were only available to those who could afford them. These disparities and differences mapped imperfectly over the division between foreigner and Chinese. In the 1930s, a Japanese resident in the Japanese Concession might still have to turn his excreta over to a Chinese night-soil carrier; the British had devised a closed water system that eliminated the night-soil carrier from the streets. Water that poured from pipes and faucets distinguished wealthier Chinese from their compatriots who received their water in buckets from Dark Drifters. Chinese administrators' dreams of creating a public water supply were unlikely to be realized in an environment where Chinese were also co-owners of the private water concern, and coercive power was in the hands of the nations behind the concessions. If post-Boxer *weisheng* was new, it was because it added a public dimension to conceptions of health. Imperialism had brought *weisheng* as public health to Tianjin, but then it worked against the creation of a comprehensive public administration that could make a difference to the health of the city.

After 1900, as the territory and influence of foreign concessions grew, reformers in Tianjin began to create multiple internal divisions within the city: between humans and water, between foul and fragrant, between public and private, and between rich and poor. Before the early twentieth century, neighborhoods in Tianjin, although generally known as relatively wealthy or poor, exhibited a fairly large degree of intermingling of classes and functions. The house of the wealthy merchant might be in the vicinity of the house of the peddler or the servant, or in the same neighborhood as the slaughterhouse or the glue maker. Some homes were far grander than others, but all shared the same general structure and function. After the Boxer Uprising, zoning laws and health bureaus separated residential and industrial functions, and hygienic modernity dictated the shape, appearance, and use of buildings in specific areas. Although never able to stop the flow of humans or the flow of rivers through the city, some concessions labored mightily to eliminate from their streets any signs of wastes, waters, or the men who carried them. Through the application of hygienic modernity to urban space, some areas of the city made the functions of daily living invisible. Slaughterhouses, dye makers, and pigskin boilers moved out. Water and waste ran silently under the streets. Hygienic modernity dictated what was seen and unseen.

Post-1900 Tianjin became a showcase for European and Japanese imperial ambitions in East Asia. The built environment of the new concessions displayed these ambitions not only for the Chinese, but before an assembled audience of foreign powers. The thing that unified this patchwork of national styles was a commitment to hygienic modernity, expressed through the maintenance of boundaries between the sanitary and the unsanitary. The regime of invisibility gave rise to hygienic hierarchies. Those areas where the products of daily life could be clearly seen were proclaimed *bu weisheng*, a marker of deficiency vis-à-vis the hygienic ideal. In spite of rhetorical tendencies to proclaim hygiene a product of inherent characteristics, the borders between *weisheng* and *bu weisheng* required constant patrolling, constant effort, a constant influx of capital and labor. Only a few enclaves in

Tianjin, most notably the British Settlement, were able to achieve a state of virtual hygienic modernity by establishing a separate water and sewer network. By embracing foreign architecture and foreign bathroom fixtures, Chinese elites could continue their project of separating themselves from their "deficient" compatriots through strategies of *weisheng*. But for most, such separations were incomplete or impossible. Human ties created by waste and water would link rich and poor, Chinese and foreign in Tianjin well into the 1950s.

8 *Weisheng* and the Desire for Modernity

Health had fled to a remote place.
LIU NA'OU (1900–1939),
"Etiquette and Hygiene"
(Liyi he weisheng)

In the 1930 short story "Etiquette and Hygiene" (Liyi he weisheng), the writer Liu Na'ou created a vision of modern Shanghai embodied in a sexually liberated Chinese woman, Keqing, and her sophisticated lawyer husband, Qiming. Toward the end of the story, Qiming takes a walk from the gleaming International Settlement to the Chinese city. Once Qiming enters the Chinese neighborhood, he has entered a "danger zone." His nostrils are assailed by "ghastly stenches." Prostitutes solicit customers in alleys smelling of urine. Liu Na'ou observes that in the Chinese city, "health had fled to a remote place," and all that was left was a world of noise and smells. Shumei Shih, in her analysis of "Etiquette and Hygiene," notes that Qiming "willfully alienates himself from the Chinese throng" in order to revel in his own cultural superiority, but in the end his own hygienic habits are also brought into question: The reader learns that Qiming frequents Shanghai's brothels and may himself harbor the germs of disease.[1]

The modern life of Shanghai, represented by the buildings on the Bund, is marked by its desirable state of *weisheng*. Liu Na'ou's protagonist demonstrates, through his refined hygienic sensibilities, his ability to separate himself from the impoverished Chinese Other. But by ironically illuminating Qiming's penchant for frequenting potentially diseased prostitutes, Liu Na'ou seems to question the feasibility of Chinese elites breaking away into a state of hygienic modernity. For both the Chinese city and for the modern Chinese elite, "health had fled to a remote place." Desire for a hygienic modernity might be thwarted at any turn, by the intractable presence of the poor, or even by the invisible germs of disease inherent within the body of the modern Chinese.

Liu Na'ou's short story, with its fortuitous inclusion of *weisheng* in the title, provides an illustrative framework for consideration of the discursive uses of *weisheng* in republican-era Tianjin. During the 1920s and 1930s, Tianjin's popular media were permeated with similarly paradoxical and complex representations of *weisheng*. *Weisheng* resonated through advertisements, lecture halls, movie theaters, wall posters, newspapers, magazine articles, and government propaganda as a wide variety of actors used the word to help them imagine the condition of modernity. The meaning of *weisheng* was not fixed, nor was the field of power in which circulation took place dominated by any one element. Ultimately, however, *weisheng* was intertwined with desire, a desire for a modernity—often marked as foreign—that existed just out of reach. How far away this desired hygienic modernity resided depended on the situation. For the sophisticated middle-class individual, it might be easily obtained through the purchase of a commodity. For elites contemplating the masses of Chinese people, hygienic modernity lay far away, obtainable only through a medical revolution or a moral revolution that could bring the absolute standards of the West to China. *Weisheng* was even used to decry biological deficiencies hidden within the very genetic material of the Chinese people. By the 1930s, some believed that "health had fled to a remote place," a hidden, microscopic realm, and could only be obtained by altering the genetic material of the "race" or by conquering the germs that lurked on the skin and in the blood. The standard for this imagined hygienic modernity was always a distant and idealized West/Japan, where all was robust and free of germs.

This chapter considers four "cases" of *weisheng* from Tianjin of the 1920s and 1930s. The first case explores evidence of *weisheng* in the advertisements from Tianjin's major republican-era newspaper, *Da gong bao* (L'Impartial). Here the term *weisheng* was frequently used to conjure up desire for a wide range of commodities, objects that promised to propel the consumer into the robust and/or sexy but always germ-free condition of modernity. The ambitious plans of the Guomindang (GMD) and the critiques launched by Tianjin's new medical elite form the center of the second case. The arrival of the GMD in 1928 fueled hopes for the advent of a modern state *weisheng* regime, but those hopes became more modest as the Nanjing decade (1927–37) wore on. By the 1930s, a small but diverse group of foreign-educated doctors in Tianjin used *weisheng* to express their disappointment in both the Nationalist government and in the Chinese people. The third case begins with a lecture on *minzu weisheng*, or racial hygiene, given in Tianjin in 1935 by the "father of Chinese eugenics," Pan Guangdan. Educated in Ivy League schools in the early 1920s, Pan returned to China convinced that GMD-style reform could never offer China a "way out" from its predicament of deficiency. For Pan, the key lay not in educating the mind, but in altering the bodies of the Chinese "race" through eugenics. The last case considers the physician of Chinese medicine, Ding Zilang, who critiqued the underlying premises of modern *weisheng* and put forth a revitalized Chinese medicine as the way to achieve health and to resist imperialism. Ding rejected the idea, clearly expressed in the other three cases, that health was an entity that was "always already" in the sole possession of a desirable, modern West/Japan. Significantly, Ding also rejected the germ theory of disease, an idea that by the 1930s had become a centerpiece in Chinese elite's understandings of the deficiencies of their "race."

CASE I. THE CONSUMER

In the 1920s and 1930s, *weisheng* could easily be purchased in many stores throughout Tianjin. For one and a half yuan, one could obtain *weisheng* in a pill. A few *yuan* more would buy *weisheng yi* (underwear; literally, hygienically modern clothing) to wear under a Western suit. A substantially larger investment was necessary to make one's home *weisheng* through the purchase of *weisheng qiju* (hygienically modern appliances for the bathroom) such as a flush toilet and porcelain sink. Once one's bathroom had been transformed into a hygienically modern space *(weisheng jian)*, a variety of *weisheng* chemicals could keep the body in hygienically modern shape. Advertisements for *weisheng* products abounded in Tianjin's major newspaper, the *Da gong bao* (L'Impartial). Ideals of health promoted by these products varied with time and with the gender of the target audience for the commodity. Significantly, all of the products that claimed to provide hygienic modernity for the consumer were imports. British underwear, Japanese toothpaste, and American pills promised to make the consumer as comfortable, as fragrant, and as strong as a foreigner. This message of desire for the foreign Other was not always explicit in advertisements for *weisheng* commodities, and yet the foreign nature of *weisheng* was never ambiguous.

Gendered images of suffering and health contained in advertisements reveal the imagined structure of a hygienically modern consumer world. Manufactured in Canada by an enterprising pharmacist and marketed through extensive advertising networks throughout English-speaking countries and the British empire, Dr. William's Pink Pills for Pale People promised better health for men and women from St. Louis to Singapore.[2] In the early 1920s, Dr. William's Pink Pills for Pale People (in Chinese, *Wei lian shi da yisheng hong se bu wan*, which sounded something like "The famous doctor Great-and-Honest-Scholar's red supplement pills") was one of the "foreign goods" most frequently advertised in Tianjin's newspapers, or, for that matter, in any newspaper around the world. Dr. William's Pink Pills offered Chinese customers a *weisheng zhi dao:* illustrated literally as a path upon which Chinese sufferers walked toward a bright, healthy future.[3] Dr. William's pills employed the same testimonial advertising technique in China as it did in England and America. The descriptions of ill-health in the testimonials paint a revealing portrait of the physical complaints that Chinese advertisers imagined the consumer to suffer, and present the characteristics of the happy, healthy lives that male and female consumers of this foreign medicine might have desired.[4]

In advertisements from the early 1920s, the ideal consumer is portrayed as the male head of a traditional multigenerational family. He is possessed of a foreign education and modern ideals of political progressivism, but socially he is still the master of his household, one who makes judicious decisions that will improve the health of the women, youth, and elderly in his care. Often a male head of household is the assumed reader, but the health of the women and children in the family is at issue: "Is your esteemed wife thin and sickly? Are your Excellency's children weak and lethargic?"[5] A closer reading of Pink Pills advertisements reveals that women are the predominant target audience. Women experience headaches, a loss of appetite, a ringing in the ears, irregular menstruation, and a wan complexion. New mothers experience a lack of energy and a paucity of breast milk. Children are thin, weak, colicky, and in danger. With such compromised health, women can not fulfill their filial duties as mother, wife, and caretaker for the family's elderly.[6]

The underlying problem for all of these discomforts is a weakness of what is called *xue,* which could be translated literally as "blood," but could also be perceived by Chinese readers as something else. Charlotte Furth has demonstrated that the concept of *xue* in Chinese medicine differs from the biomedical idea of a red liquid that regularly circulates in vessels from the heart throughout the body.[7] Instead, *xue* is a yin form of *qi,* a basic quality of the energy material that ebbs through, collects in, and makes up all human beings, but it is particularly crucial in the health problems of women. Pink Pills claim to *bu xue,* a commonly found phrase in Chinese medicine, meaning "to Nourish Blood." In spite of using this familiar phrase from Chinese medicine, the *xue* of Dr. William's pills, is, however, a decidedly red-colored, circulating liquid, an entity that needs to be "thick and fresh" if men are to have strong bones and muscles and if women are to be vibrant and energetically filial.[8] True to its patent medicine character, Pink Pills can cure everything from insomnia to intestinal worms, but the product's overall virtue lies in its ability to strengthen the inherent weaknesses in the blood of Chinese men and women.

To attribute the symptoms of deficiency encountered in Dr. William's Pink Pills advertisements solely to the stresses of an increasingly modern treaty-port lifestyle would not be entirely accurate. In his comparison of the foundations of Western and Chinese medical thought, Shigehisa Kuriyama has pointed out that Chinese pathology consistently emphasized the condition of emptiness, *xu*. Unlike Greek medicine, which feared plethora and overabundance within the body, Chinese medicine emphasized lack as the primary cause of imbalance.[9] The traditional Chinese pharmacopoeia abounded with recipes to *bu xue:* Nurture Blood. The bodily complaints portrayed in Pink Pills advertisements are familiar from Chinese medicine, but they simultaneously echo the infirmities described in American and British advertisements from the same period. Pink Pills for Pale People represents a belief that bodies around the world are essentially the same—and that Western medicines do the best job for all bodies.

In the early 1920s, Japanese medicine also promised to deliver a state of *weisheng* to Chinese consumers by boosting the spirits and alleviating bodily weakness. Jintan (in Chinese, Rendan; literally, benevolent elixir) was one of the earliest and most ubiquitous Japanese products on the East Asian market.[10] Jintan styled itself as essential to health *(weisheng zhi yao)*, an efficacious medicine to use against stomach complaints, headaches, faintness, colds, and general malaise. A vague promise of a robust Japanese modernity was conveyed through Jintan's distinctive trademark, which pictures the upper torso of a Japanese naval officer, resplendent in epaulets, commodore's hat, and waxed mustache. Significantly, Jintan was developed following the Japanese victory in the Russo-Japanese War, and its military trademark projects a manly picture of a triumphant Asian health. "The time has come!" proclaimed one advertisement, and Jintan was the sign of the times. Overworked Chinese scholars and slender Chinese beauties could use a medicine represented by a modern Japanese general to boost their flagging vitalities.[11]

Although both men and women suffered from tired blood, digestive disorders, and general malaise in these advertisements, the ideal state of health for each sex differed considerably. Women who had achieved a state of health were good wives and virtuous mothers, but their happily healthy men were successful businessmen, polo players, and above all, officers in the military. A dashing, mustachioed precursor to the Hathaway shirt man appears in advertisements for "hygienic" Western clothing in Tianjin in the 1920s. What was hygienic was not the Western suit or shirt modeled by this professional-class Western figure, but the particular type of underwear he wore beneath them. The Chinese man could achieve the same warmth, comfort, and hygiene that lent confidence to the Western businessman if he purchased this medically approved underwear, imported from "England and America," for three yuan a pair. Elsewhere Chinese men could be confidently masculine as long as they took Western medicine to keep their bowels regular. Dr. William's Clearing and Leading Pill (Qing Dao Wan) was a "secret tactic for *weisheng*" that countered "the greatest enemy of hygiene and physiology": constipation. A Chinese military officer with epaulets, waxed mustache, and formal hat accompanied Qing Dao Wan advertisements, along with the testimonial of a military man who had suffered from constipation for more than ten years until he began taking Dr. William's pills. In this era of warlord armies, the desired state of health for a modern male consumer in treaty-port China was a robust and fearless modern soldier with regular bowels.

Male sufferers in the 1920s were often portrayed as thin, stooped-over Chinese scholars, cradling their throbbing heads or clutching their aching backs within the cramped surroundings of their indoor studies. Their somatic deficiencies often stem from weaknesses of morality or habit. Opium addiction makes men so weak they faint as they walk down the street. Teachers spend so much time in the classroom or hunched over their writing that they neglect physical exercise, and as a result suffer from headaches, backaches (which may have also indicated sexual deficiencies), and constipation.[12] In advertisements selling *weisheng* in the early 1920s, The Sick Man of Asia was decidedly an intellectual, whereas the desired state of being was the opposite: a man of decisiveness, virility, and power.

By the 1930s, an interesting shift had taken place in the gendered images used to sell *weisheng* products and in the nature of *weisheng* itself. Although *weisheng* in the 1920s was associated with virtuous, kind mothers, a decade later *weisheng* had become an attribute of single young women who were clean, healthy, and sexy at the same time. *Weisheng* had become less a question of internal health and moral integrity, and was now associated with surface appearance, physical allure, and, significantly, the elimination of germs and odors from the skin. By the 1930s, seductive Shanghai movie stars endorsed Lux soap for its ability to keep their skin attractive and *weisheng*. Alluring Chinese models praised Lever's hygienic medicated soap (Lihua weisheng yaozao) for performing the dual function of keeping the skin supple and removing body odor.[13] Occasionally there is the suggestion that body odor is produced by bacteria, but thankfully, eliminating bacteria could be sexy. In one advertisement from 1937, a few drops of the "German antibacterial medicated liquid" Lysol, poured in the modern porcelain bathtub, helps preserve the *geren weisheng* (personal hygiene) of a nude bathing beauty (see fig. 9). Lysol makes this woman beautiful by exterminating *(shamie)* all the bacteria on her skin. It is also particularly effective in disinfecting and deodorizing her vagina *(yin dao)*. At the bottom of the advertisement, an anthropomorphized bottle of Lysol waves its fists and kicks its legs at a group of devilish germs that flee before it. The germs of disease lurk on the external and internal surfaces of a woman, but an erotic hygienic modernity can be achieved through the application of German disinfectants, applied while privately luxuriating in the American Standard tub of a modern bathroom *(weisheng jian).*[14]

By the 1930s, advertisements of *weisheng* products were often associated with sex, and not with domesticity. Nancy Tomes, in her work on the popular reception of germ theory in the United States, has demonstrated how health, hygiene, and "the gospel of germs" became the central domain of the American housewife in the first half of the twentieth century.[15] Charged with keeping her house clean and her family safe, the female homemaker needed to acquire a knowledge of germs. It seems that a similar middle-class domestic phenomena was occurring in treaty-port China. Advertisements designed to appeal to homemakers touted the healthful benefits of American Standard toilets and the clean manufacturing processes of Nestle's chocolate, Borden's milk, and Asahi beer. However, in newspaper advertisements aimed at a general elite and middle-class audience in China's treaty ports, *weisheng* by the 1930s seemed to be associated less with domesticity and more with sexuality. The desire for health in the service of one's public and domestic duties gave way to a health that could facilitate desire. In Tianjin, Lysol was advertised to clean vaginas, not kitchen counters.

The bathing beauty in the 1937 Lysol advertisement disinfects herself in order to distinguish herself from the unhygienic sexuality of the prostitute. Frank Dikötter has shown how an anxiety-tinged discourse emerged among Chinese health modernizers in the 1920s and 1930s as they explored the parameters of a newly biologized female sexuality.[16] Gail Hershatter has shown that at the same time, the prostitute emerged as a symbol of the intersection of sexual allure with contagion and disease. The prostitute became, in Hershatter's words, at once "a deadly conduit of disease" and a symbol of the anxieties created when modernity allowed "women to cut loose from the respectable social controls imposed by the family."[17] Liu Na'ou's protagonists in the story "Etiquette and Hygiene"—the prostitute-visiting husband and the sexually liberated wife—capture perfectly these seemingly inescapable paradoxical relationships among modernity, desire, and disease.

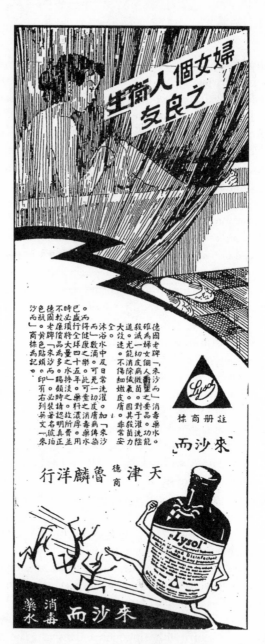

Figure 9. "A Good Friend for Women's Personal Hygiene." Advertisement for Lysol from Tianjin's major daily newspaper, *Da gong bao* (L'Impartial), 26 July 1937.

The young, apparently virtuous woman depicted in the *Da gong bao* advertisement soaking in a tub full of Lysol is attempting to extricate herself from these unpleasant paradoxes through the use of an imported German disinfectant. Commodities for medicines and personal products hint at the anxieties of modernity in 1930s treaty ports, but by conveying the benefits of foreign science and sanitary engineering, these products promise an ambivalence-free path to hygienic modernity.

CASE II. THE GUOMINDANG PHYSICIAN

Imported objects may have fulfilled the desire for *weisheng* for a small percentage of middle-class consumers in Tianjin, but many professionals and patriots longed for a strong government that could bring hygienic modernity to the city as a whole. Tianjin's vigorous health bureau of the Yuan Shikai era had faded after the 1911 Revolution, leaving the job of monitoring Tianjin's health to the city's police and the increasingly understaffed and underfunded Northern Epidemic Prevention Service (Beiyang fangyi chu). Increasing desires and hopes for *weisheng* in Tianjin were spurred by the arrival in 1928 of a consciously modernizing Nationalist regime to the Chinese city.

Christian Henriot, Frederic Wakeman, Gail Hershatter, William Kirby, and others have shown how Chiang Kai-shek's government attempted to bring forth a modern China in southern cities during the Nanjing decade of 1927 to 1937.[18] In Shanghai, Nanjing, and other cities in the lower Yangtze region, GMD-controlled municipal governments built modern offices, improved urban infrastructures, polled and registered populations, expanded police forces, established government-directed social organizations, and created an extensive propaganda network. Medicine and public health were among the professed keystones of the Nationalist vision of Chinese modernity. Numerous physicians educated in modern biomedicine—what was commonly called "Western medicine"—supported the Nationalist regime and sought an active role in bringing about a medical revolution in China. From the perspective of medical modernizers in Nanjing, such a medical revolution would entail the establishment of modern hospitals, the creation of a strong medical education system, the suppression of "old style" Chinese medicine, and the promotion of state public health policy predicated on the germ theory of disease.[19] Knowledge of bacteria would not only promote healthier habits among the general population, but would also facilitate government intervention in the event of an epidemic, and thus help promote the new nation's sovereignty.

The idealistic vision of Nanjing's central Health Ministry physicians was shared by many physicians of Western medicine in Tianjin, but Tianjin's unstable political situation in the 1920s and 1930s did not offer ideal conditions for the development of a medical revolution. Tianjin was not under the direct control of the Nanjing government, but was in the region where competing warlords were held in tenuous allegiance to Chiang Kai-shek. In 1928, the Nationalist Party registered eight hundred members in the city and began forming a municipal government, but beneath the surface of unity lurked various factions aligned with Yan Xishan, Feng Yuxiang, or relatives of Chiang.[20] Public health institutions begun in 1928 suffered discontinuity of government support, changes in medical personnel, and insufficient budget. Dreams of medical modernity in Tianjin were victim to the same instabilities that plagued many cities in China during the Nanjing decade. The idealistic officers of the Nationalist-era municipal health department did put in place the organizational infrastructure for Tianjin's public health that served as the basis for the *weisheng* system that remains in Tianjin to this day. Unfortunately, reformers ran out of time and money, and given their meager resources, it was sometimes more possible to talk about *weisheng* than to provide it.

Providing Weisheng

The Nationalists who arrived in Tianjin in 1928 revived the ideals of hygienic modernity of the turn of the century New Reforms period. In significant contrast with Yuan Shikai's "semicolonial" health department, however, the Nationalist health offices in Tianjin were staffed entirely by Chinese physicians, some of whom had been educated in the West's most prestigious medical schools. The background of the department's most active health reformers illustrates the creation of a new medical world in Tianjin. The first head of Tianjin's Nationalist government municipal health department was Quan Shaoqing. He had begun his medical education at Li Hongzhang's Beiyang Navy Medical Academy, and later went on to serve as instructor and dean of Yuan Shikai's Army Medical School. In the 1920s he did graduate work at the Harvard School of Public Health. According to Chinese accounts, Quan had even served as a health inspector with the municipal government in Boston. The official health department photograph portrays Quan as an extremely neat and disciplined-looking man, clad in a crisp Western suit with vest and watch fob. With his round horn-rimmed glasses, close-cropped hair, and neatly trimmed mustache, Quan might easily have been mistaken for a Japanese bureaucrat.[21] The first director of the Nationalist regime's public hospital, Li Yunke, studied medicine at Berlin University from 1926 to 1929, and was one of the most visible members of what had grown to be known as the "German-Japanese" faction of medicine in Tianjin.[22] Quan and Li were joined by a handful of men who had studied abroad and returned to their country with ambitious goals for the transformation of Chinese *weisheng*.

In the first two years of the GMD government in Tianjin, the health department established two public hospitals, created "health stations" to monitor the outbreak of disease in each district of the city, carried out free vaccination campaigns, registered physicians and drug manufacturers, inspected factories, established a medical contract system for state employees, and developed health services for the poor. On the planning board, these blueprints for Tianjin's hygienic modernity looked exceedingly thorough, but their implementation was often limited. Significant steps were made in planning an infrastructure, but political instabilities in north China and lack of funding frustrated the progressive ideologies of Nationalist-era health officers. The health department made a difference for many in Tianjin, but it had neither the time nor the resources to transform the health of the city.

The Tianjin Municipal Hospital (the Number One Municipal Hospital) was symbolic of the ambitious vision of hygienic modernity that Nationalist reformers entered Tianjin with, and the limits that those visions faced. In 1928, Tianjin's poor could receive treatment at a number of small missionary hospitals around the city. As part of its program of asserting a revitalized national sovereignty, the GMD hoped to establish a hospital that would serve as the basis for a new government-funded medical system. Originally planned in 1928 to encompass several new buildings and a government-funded budget of two hundred thousand yuan, by 1930 the hospital's budget had dropped to thirty thousand yuan, only half of which was funded directly by the government. The municipal hospital had to content itself with a few buildings on the grounds of the Italian Concession mansion of the deceased warlord Cao Kun.[23] With a small staff of thirty (including doctors, nurses, and medical technicians), the municipal hospital clinic treated an average of two hundred patients a day. Most sufferers came to the hospital for treatment of broken bones, tumors, skin infections, and eye disorders— illnesses that Chinese felt Western medicine could successfully treat. Patients included rickshaw drivers who had been hit by cars, injured flour-mill workers, men and women wounded in episodes of domestic violence or in street brawls, victims of botched abortions, and the occasional tubercular office clerk.[24] On the average, more than 90 percent of all patients were *gong fei:*

treated for free upon presentation of proof of their residence and poverty from their district government committee.

Seeing as many as ten thousand patients a month on a shoestring budget was difficult and exhausting business. During epidemics, such as the cholera outbreak of 1932, the clinic handled as many as twenty-five hundred patients in a week. The hospital frequently ran out of vaccines and had to conserve supplies. Contracts to provide medical care and inspection for the city's largest textile and flour mills further taxed the resources of the hospital. Administration fought over requests to refund fees as small as ten cents.[25] Municipal hospital employees were dedicated health workers, but for those educated abroad, the conditions of serving thousands of the city's poor with minimal government support was a particularly grueling experience.

Talking Weisheng

While the municipal hospital attempted to make dents in the suffering of the city, other Nationalist-era health workers spread a "gospel of germs" in public lectures in Tianjin's public schools and exhibition halls. Such talks were by no means the first time that Tianjin residents had been lectured about contagious diseases and hygiene. Western missionaries and Chinese Christians had been preaching the importance of a healthy body for the past thirty years. The Tianjin YMCA, established in 1895, was a center for the spread of information on a particular type of modern hygiene, one that included washing hands, wearing Western-style clothing, and playing basketball.[26] Hygiene and physical education were central to the curricula of the city's new schools, like the Nankai Middle School, where such famous political figures as Zhou Enlai began their progressive education.[27] The activities of these education institutions had given rise to Tianjin's hygienically aware middle class. It also helped produce Tianjin's handful of physicians of modern biomedicine, men who had studied in foreign and foreign-staffed institutions in Beijing, Shanghai, Tianjin, or, in a few limited cases, Berlin or Boston. During the years of the Nationalist era, these men represented a thin stratum of healers in Tianjin. By 1931, the city's population of one and a half million supported only 115 registered doctors of Western medicine. In the late 1920s and 1930s, a few members of this tiny community attempted to spread the word of hygienic modernity to the city's masses.

Nationalist-era health department lectures were a form of triage aimed at defusing the administrative crises of epidemic disease.[28] Rather than focus on the chronic, endemic diseases that were the main problems in the city—disorders like tuberculosis or malnutrition—lectures dealt with cholera, smallpox, and plague. Lecturers sought to convince audiences that bacteria caused disease, with the hope that once this principle was understood, the populace would cooperate rather than resist government inspection, vaccination, and quarantine measures. The first step was to convince audiences that their "traditional" understandings of disease were mistaken and dangerous. Health department lecturers warned city residents that *huoluan* was a very serious, anomalous disease, and not just a common summer stomach complaint that one should expect to catch every year. New residents from the countryside had to abandon all of their colloquial names for serious gastrointestinal illness: "sudden attack" *(fa sha)*, "gut-wrenching attack" *(jiaochang sha)*, "camel attack" *(luotuo sha)*, or "dangling foot attack" *(diaojiao sha)*. There was only one disease, cholera, that was caused by one type of "comma-shaped bacteria," and nothing else.

Department physicians would then go on to explain the connection between bacteria and government epidemic prevention techniques. Lecturers called upon Tianjiners to be receptive to the isolation of neighborhoods, quarantine for individual sick people, or the burning of cholera victims' clothes and possessions. Citizens had to abandon their "selfish feelings," think about the good of their fellow citizens, and allow the health department to do their work. Lectures put a positive spin on government interventions: even quarantine was to be viewed in a positive light. Physicians and nurses were as caring as family members, and quarantine was always temporary. Once people recovered, they could rejoin their family permanently. Placing so much value on seeing each other during the short duration of an epidemic was foolish and harmful to the city's *weisheng*. Health department physicians warned Tianjiners that commercially marketed "Emergency Relief Water" (*jiuji shui*, oral rehydration solution) was unreliable, and Chinese treatments such as acupuncture or scraping *(guafa)* were sure to result in death. They pleaded with Tianjiners to trust Western medicine and the wisdom of the government during times of crisis.

Unable to provide clean water and sewer services to everyone in the city, overburdened health department workers attempted to reduce epidemic disasters in Tianjin by talking about *weisheng*. Such public education programs were important and could save lives: by submitting to the definitive "Western" treatment of having liquid injected into the skin through a needle, victims of severe cholera could avoid death from dehydration. Imparting such knowledge to Tianjin's people could ease the stress of government interventions once epidemics had already erupted, but this sort of "talking cure" was only part of the most effective approach to epidemic prevention, the ultimate goal of the health department. True prevention would require more funds, more personnel, and more investment in infrastructure than was forthcoming from the Nationalist regime.

Talking about *weisheng* reached its height during the Nationalist government's New Life Movement (Xin shenghuo yundong). Launched in 1934 by Chiang Kai-shek and his wife Soong Mei-ling, the New Life Movement sought to revitalize the Chinese nation by reforming the bodily habits of the Chinese people.[29] Chiang's movement was, in many ways, an attempt at improving the "etiquette and hygiene" of a nation. Faced with the threat of Communism and the increasing threat of war with Japan, Chiang and his wife combined the doctrines of Christian missionaries with organizational insights from Japan, the Soviet Union, and Germany to form a program for national revitalization. Reforming the way Chinese looked and acted in public was, for Chiang, the key to maintaining China's sovereignty.

Although New Life claimed to be a mass movement, it primarily reached individuals who were already encompassed by state-affiliated organizations such as GMD youth groups, government offices, hospitals, and schools. The centerpieces of the New Life Movement were long lists of hygienic do's and don'ts. Prohibited behaviors included public spitting, loud talking, public scratching, slouching, and other such violations of modern decorum. Other directives were positive statements for personal and domestic cleanliness, including guidelines for showering, haircutting, and fingernail trimming. Some regulations sought to dictate the smallest aspects of personal appearance, mandating the buttoning of top buttons on shirts and the frequent shining of shoes.[30] Although some aspects of the New Life Movement were related to the improvement of health, most were aimed at creating a disciplined population whose most intimate habits were monitored by the state.

There is little indication that the New Life Movement had much impact at all in Tianjin. It was propagated most energetically in state offices and in institutions that dealt with middle-class youth, zones of society where Nationalist Party organization—and the message of hygienic modernity—had already penetrated. For example, during the New Life Movement at Nankai University, students who had been indoctrinated in hygiene for years at missionary schools or modern Chinese academies were now urged to remember to use "public chopsticks" *(gonggong kuaizi)* when removing food from serving plates at the cafeteria. Monitors levied fines against anyone who spit in public. Once a week, students aired out their bedding, while rooms were sanitized with carbolic acid spray to kill germs and bedbugs. In the summer, students participated in mandatory fly-catching exercises. Regular exercise and regular showers, always a part of school policy, were now a government mandate.[31] Even the municipal hospital received New Life dicta for improving hygienic appearances. For the physicians who had been laboring so mightily to improve the health of Tianjin's masses in the face of budget cuts and tremendous suffering, the New Life dicta to comb hair and shine shoes must have appeared particularly petty. There was no increase in public hospital funding or staffing as a result of the New Life Movement. Instead, doctors were ordered to keep the collars of their shirts and jackets buttoned up at all times, while orderlies and janitorial staff received stern lectures from New Life activists about the evils of spitting.[32]

Some of Tianjin's reform-minded physicians found government propaganda hollow and ineffectual, and criticized the Nationalist regime for not doing enough for the city's health. In the eyes of some, the government was placing its energies in cure for a few while it let the city's environmental hygiene languish. Public latrines in Tianjin were rarely cleaned or disinfected, water was distributed unequally, and the Chinese city still lacked a sewer system. Critics blasted the Nationalist administration for concentrating on high-profile medical projects like public hospitals instead of simply building adequate sewers: "Now the government's call to 'build a new Tianjin' fills our ears. I think what today's Tianjin needs the most are sewers to drain the open cesspools and eliminate the dirty water accumulated inside the city. . . . These are far more important steps toward improving Tianjin's hygiene than establishing public hospitals or doing *weisheng* propaganda work."[33]

The harshest criticisms of the Nationalist government came from a small group of Tianjin physicians who had been trained abroad. In 1930 they established the journal *Weisheng zazhi* (Hygienic modernity magazine) to convey their opinions about the health of the city and its inhabitants. The back of each issue featured prominently the names of each contributor and, most important, the foreign country where he had received his medical degree. With Western standards constantly in mind, these doctors from France, England, the United States, and Japan constructed a harsh critique of the Nationalists around an unfulfilled promise of hygienic modernity.

The writers of *Weisheng zazhi* constantly contrasted the successes of industrialized foreign countries where they had achieved their medical degrees with the deficiencies of China. Mortality rates for China were never compared with other developing nations, but were compared instead with those of the United States and Europe. In these nations, superior public health infrastructures and knowledge of bacteria (and not economic development) made mortality rates less than half of that of China. Articles on contagious disease were frequently embellished with English terminology, but given the inaccuracy and superciliousness of many of the glosses, their addition served to invoke foreign authority rather than effect any actual technical clarification.[34] Monetary figures—such as the expense of running a modern public health bureau, or the economic value of a human life—are expressed first in U.S. dollars, and then in Chinese yuan, indicating that the standards of what was appropriate or expected in health and medicine were set in the world's wealthiest nations.[35]

The foreign-trained physicians of *Weisheng zazhi* did not criticize the government alone: Many articles lambasted the deficiencies of the Chinese people as well. The "average Tianjin resident" exhibited a profound ignorance of *weisheng*. In their ignorance, they attributed outbreaks of disease to the weather, left their chamber pots on top of the *kang* (heated sleeping platform), drank water out of Tianjin's polluted rivers, and worst of all, ate unhygienic (and uncivilized) objects such as deep-fried locust.[36] But if the Chinese people were ignorant and diseased, it was the government that was to blame for not properly providing modern infrastructures through which they could improve their lives.

Foreign-trained physicians in Tianjin seemed to live in perpetual frustration at the deficiencies of the Chinese people and the shortcomings of the new, "modern" Chinese national government. From their perspective, health in China had indeed "fled to a remote place." Between the standard of an imagined West and their perspective on Chinese realities lay a gap that propelled their desire for an ever-receding hygienic modernity.

CASE III. THE EUGENICIST

In 1935, Tianjin was host to a lecture by the famous "Father of Chinese Eugenics," Qinghua University professor Pan Guangdan. Those in attendance probably noticed that Pan took to the podium with a jerky gait; the slender, bookish professor had suffered a severe injury when he was young and walked with the aid of a prosthetic leg. Once behind the podium, Pan spoke with a straightforward clarity, even bluntness, about his topic for the evening: the impossibility of using social reform to improve the deficient health of the Chinese. For Pan, eugenics alone was the only effective form of hygiene for the race *(minzu weisheng)*.[37]

"Just what is racial health *[minzu jiankang]*?" Pan asked his audience. Everyone talks about health, Pan went on to explain, but no one really understands what it is. "When we compare ourselves to the various peoples of the West, or even to the Japanese people, most of us think that our physiques are quite deficient and not as good as theirs."[38] Pan felt no need to elaborate on the obvious truth of this statement. He then argued that the definition of health should not end with the individual physique, but should include the mental and moral capacities of the entire race. Even there the Chinese fell short. Pan considered the ambition, spirit, intelligence, ability to think scientifically, leadership quality, and organizational talent of the Chinese, and found that the race as a whole was insufficiently endowed *(bu zu)* or lacking *(qian que)* in every category.

In a brief recounting of the Chinese people's history, Pan suggested that natural selection had already produced a type of human specimen that was well adapted to China's harsh climate. This inheritance, however, had not prepared the Chinese to face the challenges of the twentieth century, when Chinese people had to compete with different human types from around the globe. Pan allowed that a few areas in China had produced relatively healthy populations. These genetically superior areas seemed to coincide with the more economically developed zones of the nation, including the area around Lake Tai, the provinces of Guangdong and Hunan, and Manchuria.[39] The north China plain (with its major cities of Beijing and Tianjin) was pointedly absent from Pan's list. One wonders how the Tianjin audience might have reacted to this appraisal of their genetic fitness. But any regional specificity in Pan's lecture was overshadowed by the constant repetition of a handful of key words describing the Chinese race as a whole: deficient, lacking, incomplete.

Pan spoke with a direct simplicity that belied his elite intellectual background. Pan's father was a holder of the highest level of Confucian degree who had served as a scholar in the Qing court's Hanlin Academy. Pan himself had a bachelor's degree from Dartmouth (class of 1924) and a master's from Columbia.[40] Even though his background in eugenics stemmed from his American education, Pan was able to tailor his eugenics message to make it compelling to a Chinese audience. Pan's dire words of warning about the overwhelming challenges of the twentieth-century world would have resonated strongly with audiences in Tianjin in 1935. A few years earlier, Japan's military occupied the northeast provinces and established the puppet state of Manchukuo. The creeping encroachment of the Japanese military into north China had increased the profile of Japanese soldiers and police in Tianjin's Japanese Concession. Japanese and Koreans were increasingly involved in the city's now-massive drug trafficking business.[41] Increasing acts of violent agitation against the Japanese presence by Chinese nationalists resulted in an undeclared underground war between Japanese secret police (and their Chinese collaborators) and Communist and Nationalist operatives, a war that was waged in the streets of the Japanese Concession and the nearby Chinese-administered city.[42] With great fanfare, the Nationalist government had announced many reform and reconstruction projects from its capital in Nanjing, but it seemed unwilling, if not incapable, of mounting any serious resistance to the Japanese in the north. Although he never mentioned Japanese imperialism specifically in his lecture, all who listened would automatically understand what Pan meant by the inability of the Chinese to face the "challenges" of the era.

Pan's lecture continued with an ironic criticism of charitable and government attempts at improving the health of the Chinese people through public health *(weisheng)* programs. The basis for Pan's critique was far removed from that of the Western-educated physicians who criticized the Nationalist government's *weisheng* administration. Pan did not accuse the Nationalists of having a lack of commitment to health, but rather he argued that their very intentions were wrong. Those who believed that improved environment and improved education could uplift the race were simply being naive. In fact, in Pan's view, improvements in medical services and sanitation represented a misallocation of resources. The reconstruction programs so popular in Nationalist China would only weaken the health of the race as a whole by increasing the chances of survival for the weak, thereby altering the process of natural selection. Charities and government programs only wasted money by saving the genetically unfit.

After Pan reminded the audience of their deepest anxieties and scorned the *weisheng* efforts of idealistic reformers, he then presented his vision of eugenics *(yousheng)* as the only viable means of *weisheng* for the Chinese people. The best way to improve the health of the people was to improve the genetic stock of the population by increasing the numbers of those who were genetically superior. For Pan, health was based first and foremost in heredity, not behavior. Successful hygienic modernity, therefore, was not a question of promoting healthy practices or a healthy environment, but was instead a question of breeding an inherently healthy race.[43]

Pan's vision was for the most part a positive eugenics program, one that encouraged early marriage and high fertility rates among those deemed genetically superior. In his 1935 Tianjin lecture, Pan did not explicitly discuss the sorts of negative eugenic interventions that were becoming more common in Western countries, such as the sterilization of the "genetically unfit." Pan seems to have been content to let China's high rates of infant mortality, famine, and epidemic disease act as agents of "natural selection," weeding out the weakest genetic specimens among the peasant masses. But Malthusian mechanism alone was not enough to provide the dramatic boost in quality needed by the Chinese race in the twentieth century. Instead it had given rise to the very species that his eugenics plan hoped to eliminate: the selfish, unscientific, passive, face-loving, noncommittal Chinese Everyman.

The characteristics of this Chinese Everyman were much on Pan Guangdan's mind as he prepared his Tianjin lecture, for the work that had engrossed him from 1933 to 1935 was a translation of the American missionary Arthur Smith's classic text, *Chinese Characteristics* (1894). Earlier Pan had translated excerpts from Yale professor Ellsworth Huntington's 1924 work, *The Character of Races,* which included several chapters on natural selection and the evolution of the Chinese people.[44] Huntington's book inspired Pan to turn to Smith's work. Pan translated and edited fifteen out of Smith's original twenty-seven chapters, including those describing the Chinese "Absence of Nerves" (Meiyou "shenjing" de zhongguo ren), "Disregard of Accuracy" (Bu qiu biaojun de zhongguo ren), and "Absence of Public Spirit" (You si wu gong de zhongguo ren). In 1937, Pan published his translations of Smith and Huntington, together with the texts of his own essays, in a volume that epitomized his philosophy: *Minzu texing yu minzu weisheng* (Racial characteristics and racial hygiene).[45]

Pan Guangdan was not the only modern Chinese thinker who was influenced by Arthur Smith. Lydia Liu has shown that Lu Xun, China's most modern literary figure, encountered Smith's works in Japanese translation and was profoundly impressed by what he read.[46] The fictional characters in Lu Xun's short stories were veritable walking catalogues of Smith's *Chinese Characteristics.* Lu Xun's best-known creation, Ah Q, is a rural simpleton who is easily angered, easily contented, insensitive to the suffering of others, and insensitive even to his own suffering. The difference between Lu Xun and Pan Guangdan, however, lay in their approach to the solutions to China's predicament. Lu Xun had abandoned his medical studies because he saw China's maladies arising from diseased souls, not diseased bodies. Literature and social criticism were for Lu Xun the best foundation for change. Pan and other advocates of eugenics had instead embraced the body as the vehicle through which China would find its "way out" *(chu lu).* While others spoke passionately of improving China's education, health, and environment, Pan proclaimed racial hygiene as the ultimate solution for China.

Pan's *Minzu texing yu minzu weisheng* ends with a clarion call for eugenics, entitled "Minzu weisheng de chulu" (Racial hygiene: The way out).[47] The presentation of racial hygiene as a "way out," or "escape route" echoes the first paragraph of Pan's *Racial Characteristics and Racial Hygiene,* from a guest preface written by the sociologist Li Jinghan:

China has always been an isolated, self-contained country. If it weren't for contact with the Western races, then we would still be a world unto ourselves, and we would have no way of seeing our own weaknesses and strengths. Ever since the Opium War, our doors have been flung wide open. We have been defeated time and time again and suffered every kind of oppression from outside forces. Now we suddenly realize that our race is a sick race. We are all looking for a medicine that will cure us. We are all searching for the path to salvation: we are all searching for a way out [*chu lu*].[48]

In Li's logic, China suffered horribly at the hands of imperialism, and yet without imperialism, the Chinese people would not have an awareness of their own nature, their limitations and good points, or, as Li figures it, their "shorts and longs" *(duanchang)*. After China's "opening" to the rest of the world, the shortness and longness of things is determined by the standard of the West. Although Li criticizes the viciousness of imperialism, he does not criticize the adoption of Western standards. For both Pan and Li, this new "universal" standard is an inescapable reality. What must be escaped, then, is not the Western standard itself, but the Chinese people's inability to meet that standard.

Pan's biological approach to Chinese deficiencies dictated his choice of a "way out." The social reformers of his day also recognized the same dilemmas, but their "ways out" involved exercises of the human will. For the YMCA activist or the GMD physician, China's physical deficiencies were to be escaped by exercising and developing the body. According to foreign and modern Chinese educators, the inability to think scientifically *(kexue nengli)* was to be escaped by fostering "belief" in science. For political reformers, the inability to organize or develop a social consciousness was to be escaped by emphasizing the importance of individual contributions to society. All of these "ways out" assumed that China's problems were problems of will *(yizhi)*, not problems of ability *(nengli)*. Pan predicted that social reformers would be sorely disappointed when they realized that their programs did not work. They would inevitably discover that the main problem of the Chinese people was in their biological inheritance—their *xiantian*. A biological way out was needed, and this way out lay through the path of racial hygiene.[49]

CASE IV. THE CHINESE PHYSICIAN

Not all medical observers in Tianjin desired the same kind of hygienic modernity. During the first third of the twentieth century, Ding Zilang, a Tianjin physician of Chinese medicine, filled the city's newspapers and journals with his thoughts on the *weisheng zhi dao*. Ding's path to hygiene elevated "Chinese learning" and resisted the hegemony of the microscopic. He was outraged by modern methods of epidemic control used by Chinese and foreign authorities in the Tianjin area. For Ding, these techniques represented little more than a travesty of *weisheng*. His numerous essays and books promoted his own vision for hygienic modernity, a vision that combined minimal government involvement with Chinese traditions of guarding life.

Ding launched his attack on hygienic modernity from a position firmly grounded in the places, language, and people of Tianjin. Ding Zilang was a member of Tianjin's Hui community, the Chinese Muslims who lived for centuries in the northwest corner of the old city near Tianjin's huge mosque. Ding was acquainted with many of Tianjin's early social reformers and was himself a frequent contributor to the city's early-twentieth-century press. He was one of Tianjin's main proponents of the *baihua* movement for vernacular language and wrote essays in an earthy style that frequently included Tianjin dialect. Ding was also dedicated to the survival of Chinese medicine, which he sensed had come under attack with the arrival of the international relief force in 1900 and the subsequent official support for Western medicine in the city.[50] In 1905 he established the Tianjin Medical Research Association (Tianjin yiyao yanjiu hui) in the Muslim quarter to provide a forum for the development of a more rigorous Chinese medicine.[51]

Although Ding exhibited a willingness to learn about Western medicine, he was particularly vehement in his resistance against what he saw as the hegemony of the germ theory of disease. In Ding's understanding, bacteria was nothing more than a Western word for what the Chinese had long described as *yiqi*, or pestilent *qi*, and as such was nothing new or wonderful. According to Ding, Western medicine overemphasized the role of bacteria in generating illness, and therefore neglected other obvious pathogenic factors such as weather, eating habits, and lifestyle. Not only did this hegemony of germs constitute misguided medicine, but it was also used as the basis for politically harmful criticism of Chinese medicine. In Ding's opinion, the germ theory of disease was not a superior, modern philosophy of pathogenesis, but instead represented a naively mechanistic view of the human body. By comparison, Chinese medical diagnosis was a complex and sophisticated system that, if properly understood and employed, was superior to that of Western medicine. This contrast was most clearly highlighted in Ding's discussion of Western versions of *weisheng*, which he read about in the works of one of Shanghai's major promoters of Western medicine, Ding Fubao:

> I have read in Mr. Ding pamphlet "Weisheng wen da" [Questions and answers about hygiene] where he talks about the pathology of *shanghan*. He states that in China, this disease is called *shanghan*, while in the West it's called "a bacterial infection of the small intestine." [According to his explanation] sores form on the inside of the small intestine, and somehow these sores rot through and then the intestinal lining gets inflamed. . . . Now if only a way could be found to make these sores develop a coating, and if that coating could get thicker and thicker, then voilà, the disease would be cured. Ha ha! This Western "infection of the small intestine"—I don't understand this at all. I simply don't understand this pathology. At any rate, what in China is called *shanghan bing* has an entirely different set of explanations, and the cures are not that simple either. It is difficult to find a unified approach to these illnesses. . . . Even if I had ten days to talk about [all the various pathogenic combinations and cures], I wouldn't be able to finish.[52]

For the Shanghai popularizer of germ theory, Ding Fubao (no relation to Ding Zilang), *shanghan* referred to the specific infectious disease known as typhoid.[53] For Ding Zilang, the Tianjin doctor of Chinese medicine, *shanghan* was Cold Damage, a term that described a variety of febrile diseases, each exhibiting different pathological processes. In Ding's conception, there was a possibility that bacteria contributed to conditions like cholera *(huoluan)*, but such illnesses were always the result of a combination of factors, including abnormal weather, filth, and the ingestion of foods inappropriate to the season. *Huoluan* was a common disease that fell within the same category as other common seasonally related gastrointestinal disturbances such as *sha* and *li*, and represented no great cause for alarm. Ding's expansive approach to nomenclature and etiology was exactly the sort of thinking that health department medical officers tried so hard to eliminate during the Nationalist era. Physicians of modern biomedicine had pleaded with Tianjiners to abandon the use of concepts like *sha* and *li* and replace them with one terrifying word, *huoluan*. In contrast, Ding counseled his readers that "cholera" was not "cholera."

Ding warned his readers not to get excited by rumors of new epidemic disease and mocked those who followed the fashion of using exotic foreign words to describe common ailments. "Listen carefully, everyone: the "cholera" we're experiencing now is just the same *huoluan* we used to get every summer. . . . But once you give the illness the name *hulila* [the Japanese kanji compound for cholera], then that's really worth something!" For Ding, the names given to diseases were not simply a matter of fashion. In Ding's estimation, not only did the germ theory of disease mislead practitioners of medicine into hoping for simplistic cures; it also misled governments into thinking that *weisheng* simply meant controlling the spread of bacteria. Because Western medicine was convinced that cholera was caused by the fearful *hulila* vibrio, then governments reacted to the disease with rash and unreasonable measures:

> Foreigners take this set of symptoms most seriously. As soon as they hear "cholera!" their faces go white and they undertake especially severe precautions. . . . In Lushun and Yingkou, foreign authorities covered those who had not yet died with lime. Those who appeared only a little sick were condemned as cholera carriers and were thrown out of the city. Ai! This is not a "chaotic disease," but a "chaotic government!" [Fei huoluan bing, huoluan zheng ye!] [54]

For Ding Zilang, the germ theory of disease led foreign authorities to employ unnecessary violence against the Chinese population. He punned on the word for cholera, literally "sudden-chaotic disease," transferring the modifier to render the government's policy during cholera epidemics as chaotic as the disease itself. In Ding's mind, the most misguided and violent policy of foreign-style hygienic modernity was quarantine. [55] During the Manchurian plague epidemics of 1911 and 1918, Ding stated, more people died from the effects of quarantine than from the plague itself. Foreign soldiers removed innocent people from their homes at gunpoint. Once they were thrown into decrepit quarantine huts, victims suffered from starvation, isolation, and the harmful effects of Western medicines. After the victims died, families were not allowed to conduct proper burial rites. Instead corpses were treated like anonymous logs, thrown into trucks and transported to crematoriums where they were burned and their ashes scattered. The result, lamented Ding, was that Chinese "no longer fear epidemics, but fear the measures the government takes to 'prevent' epidemics" (bu pa yi er pa fang). In a more conspiratorial tone, Ding actually suggests that foreigners intentionally introduced epidemic prevention policies in order to kill the Chinese people and weaken Chinese cultural traditions. Foreign *weisheng* was not a method for saving China, but was instead a part of a larger plan for China's demise. [56] One can imagine how infuriated a Nationalist-era health department official would be to hear Ding's portrayal of quarantine. Chinese health officials pleaded with their compatriots to submit calmly to state intervention during epidemics, while Ding insisted that quarantine was part of a plan for a Chinese holocaust.

For Ding, it was clear that *weisheng* was a matter of guarding life through individual adherence to Chinese health precepts. Ding's precepts, with their emphasis on the circulation of fresh air and the avoidance of pestilent *qi*, are obviously influenced by developments in the Warm Factor school, but they might just as easily have been influenced by Ding's reading in late-nineteenth-century translations of American hygiene texts such as John Fryer's *Huaxue weisheng lun* (Chemistry and hygiene), which Ding had kept at his Chinese Medicine Association library. In his essay "On Guarding Health in the Summertime" *(Lun xiatian de weisheng),* Ding set out his formula for the prevention of epidemics during the hot weather, which included getting out into the countryside, breathing fresh air, and getting plenty of sleep.[57] Diet for Ding was the other main culprit that created summertime epidemics. Ding tells Tianjiners that they must give up their love of oily fried foods and eat more "light and bland" *(qingdan)* dishes in the summer. A dinner consisting of fried dough patties stuffed with mutton and Chinese chives or an oily fried shrimp and egg omelet, followed by a night spent sleeping on a warm *kang,* would guarantee a host of Hot discomforts in the morning, including red eyes, sore throat, dry nose, painful teeth, and constipation.[58] Gastronomic caution was not simply a matter of individual restraint, however. Ding believed that the municipal health department should regulate food vendors, restaurants, and butchers to make sure that no rotten or diseased meat was sold. But only education and individual willpower could keep Tianjiners away from the Hot fried foods that tasted good but were harmful to health.

The publication of Ding Zilang's writings generated considerable debate in Tianjin's medical world in the 1920s. Critics of Chinese medicine and supporters of government public health initiatives derided Ding's writings, saying they contained "not one sentence of real *weisheng* knowledge." Some remarked that Ding's treatises were not simply misguided, but represented a real threat to public health. They were filled with erroneous information about medical theory and promoted the use of ineffective therapies, including useless herbal formulas and ridiculous manual techniques such as *guafa,* the method of scraping the skin as a treatment for acute disease. In the eyes of his critics, Ding's writings would only confuse the Chinese people and incite opposition to much-needed epidemic-prevention efforts.[59] Ding refuted his critics by launching a counterattack against Western medicine in terms that hearken back to Zheng Guanying's nineteenth-century critique of Western *weisheng:*

> The principles of Western medicine come from a materialist civilization. Western medicine is quite precise when discussing things related

to form, but sketchy and imprecise when it comes to things without form. . . . Chinese medicine is superior in internal medicine. This is the opinion of the entire country. The vast majority of Chinese have come to this conclusion after a long period of practical experience.[60]

For Ding, Western medicine's ability to parse the workings of the body, to break down natural functions and pathologies into smaller and smaller discrete, concrete, and visible entities, was in no way an indication of Western medicine's superiority. Western medicine's fixation on determining "form," whether on the anatomist's dissecting table or in the bacteriologist's laboratory, was in and of itself nothing more than an interesting intellectual exercise. The problem with this new hygienic modernity was that the pursuit of biological "form"—particularly the microscopic form of bacteria—had become linked with political and military power, giving birth to a destructive new definition of *weisheng*. The alliance between Western medicine and political power was at its strongest during epidemics, when *weisheng's* attacks on human beings were justified as attacks on bacteria.

Throughout the late 1920s and into the 1930s, other Tianjin physicians of Chinese medicine echoed Ding's critique of hygienic modernity. Angered by the Nationalist government's embrace of Western medicine and subsequent criticism of Chinese medical traditions, some doctors made very explicit connections between the germ theory of disease and the forces of imperialism:

> The most laughable thing is how Western medicine mistakenly takes bacteria as the cause for all illnesses. Their diagnosis centers entirely around culturing bacteria and identifying what kind of bacteria is present, this kind or that kind, A form, B form, rod shaped, spherical, spindle shaped, gram positive, gram negative. . . . Western medicine is drunk and has fallen into a vat of germs, it swims in a veritable world of germs. . . . And now it dares to invade this land of the Yellow Emperor?[61]

For these men, Western modernity had brought with it a powerful government that violently interfered in the lives of the people in pursuit of a chimera. Their own visions of hygiene presented a picture of men and women relaxing (separately, in order to follow the rules of propriety) under the cool shade of trees on a hot day, eating healthful foods, and not worrying too much. The government would protect them by regulating food vendors and providing sanitation services, but representatives of the state had no need to touch the bodies of sufferers. As long as Chinese people educated themselves in Chinese forms of *weisheng*, they would be exceedingly well off without the interference of Western medicine. Searching for the source of Chinese deficiency within a microscopic germ, for Ding and other Chinese medicine activists, would amount to the destruction of the Chinese people.

CONCLUSION

In the 1920s and 1930s, reformers, physicians, bureaucrats, and consumers all turned to *weisheng* as a solution to the problems of China's twentieth-century predicament of high mortality rates, frequent epidemics, and imperialist incursions. Just how *weisheng* could provide a way out was fiercely debated. Actors in this debate differed in the degree to which they ascribed to foreign models, and yet comparison with foreign examples had all triggered within them an intense longing for modernity. Consumers purchased *weisheng* products in order to make themselves strong, decisive, and odor free, but such solutions would only be temporary. The anxieties of sexual decay and inherent weakness of Chinese "blood" would remain even after the product had been consumed. Physicians trained in Western medicine found China lacking in both the public and private aspects of hygienic modernity. The ignorance of China's people was an obstacle to the realization of individual health in China, but even more vexing was the failure of the Nationalist government to realize the hygienic dreams of foreign-educated elites. Eugenicists such as Pan Guangdan criticized any attempt at improving the health of the nation that did not involve his hygienic ideal: racial hygiene, or the purification of the genetic stock of the Chinese people. In all of these examples, comparison with a foreign standard showed the Chinese people to be lacking. This lack was so dire that it necessitated the discovery of an escape route, a "way out," a method for breaking free from the inferior state of being Chinese. There was little agreement on the best route, yet *weisheng* formed both the center of the predicament and the essence of escape. Few commentators active in Tianjin in the 1920s and 1930s noted any ambivalence about this pursuit. The presence of imperialism or the persistence of racial hierarchies within formulations of *weisheng* were invisible and ignored, or in the case of Pan Guangdan, even embraced as inevitable truth.

In her recent work on the creation of modern subjectivities among modernist writers in semicolonial Shanghai, Shu-mei Shih has examined the "strategies of displacement through bifurcation" that Chinese intellectuals employed in order to try to imagine themselves as equal partakers of a transcendent global cosmopolitanism.[62] The first basic move was an elevation of the West/Japan as a liberating metropolitan imaginary and a suppression of its identity as a colonial exploiter. The second move entailed separating Shanghai as a site of capitalism and modernity from Shanghai as a site of imperialist racism. The result was a group of elites who embraced modernity while side-stepping or ignoring the role of imperialism and inequality in the construction of that very modernity. I have suggested that these strategies of displacement were facilitated through another important and related bifurcation, as urban elites extricated themselves from association with the "backward" unhygienic masses.

In the field of *weisheng* it is perhaps the modern middle-class consumer of hygienic commodities who most closely replicated the seemingly ambivalence-free modernist position of Shu-mei Shih's Shanghai writers. By purchasing imported hygienic goods that circulated on a global market (Dr. William's Pink Pills, Lysol, American Standard toilets), the moneyed treaty-port resident could easily imagine herself as an equal partaker of a global hygienic modernity. All citizen of the modern world suffered from tired blood, a fear of germs, and a longing to be sexy in a hygienic way. By coating themselves inside and out with international supplements and disinfectants, Chinese could easily meet global standards for health and happiness. The ease of obtaining this liberation (for those with the money to buy it) belied the underlying ambivalence of the project and the pronounced strategies of bifurcation it required. Consumers, it seems, rarely contemplated the explicit racial hierarchies clearly embodied in the advertisements for hygienic products. Standards of health and vigor were set by Japanese and Western products that helped overcome implied Chinese deficiencies of weakness and filth.

Elites who wrote about health from the treaty ports employed similar strategies of displacement, but an analysis of their strategies is complicated by the difficulty of critiquing the benefits of modern biomedicine. Although cosmopolitan modernity for the Shanghai writer may have represented bourgeois values of individual liberation shaded by a patina of degeneracy and Eros, for the elite who contemplated health in treaty-port China, cosmopolitan modernity represented saving the lives of newborn infants and rescuing humans from physical suffering. For many reformers, *weisheng* was a perfect embodiment of reason and science, and as such, there was no possible basis for resisting it as a foreign imposition. Hygienic modernity in republican China was a "derivative discourse" par excellence.[63] Its origin in the West (and Japan) was taken for granted, and its introduction to China, even in the accompaniment of violence and racism, was ultimately a blessing.

The strategy of bifurcation that most elite writers on *weisheng* were unable or unwilling to execute was the split from "unmodern" Chinese. The elite physicians and leaders of the Nationalist era had internalized foreign discourses of deficiency, but at the same time they positioned themselves in the burdensome position of being saviors and educators of the deficient masses. Elites who wrote about *weisheng* were not able to embrace fully a separate cosmopolitan existence. For many, education abroad had linked them to a global modernity, but there was no transcendent space in which they could imagine themselves free of the "deficient" members of their race. It was this inability that made Western/Japanese-defined modernity seem even more frustratingly remote and unattainable than the immediately available modernity of Shanghai modernists, writers, or consumers. Unlike the protagonist in Liu Na'ou's "Hygiene and Etiquette," who uses the poor as a foil for his own superiority and then moves on, Nationalist-era physicians and reformers—even the eugenicist Pan Guangdan—take up the poor, even if in an ambivalent and dismissive embrace.

On the other hand, elite "displacement" or distancing from the imperialist and racist origins of Western medicine seemed complete and total. *Weisheng* was the ultimate global good. Remarkably few Western-trained physicians in Tianjin who wrote about the subject seemed to offer what Ashis Nandy has called an "empirical critique" of Western medicine and hygienic modernity, a critique that could focus on the political economy of medicine, particularly the unequal distribution of its benefits.[64] Such a critique might easily have entailed a consideration of the effects of imperialism and the foreign concessions on Tianjin's health, or may have questioned the emphasis on bacteria over the debilitating effects of poverty and malnutrition. Instead, the Western physicians who wrote on hygiene in the 1920s and 1930s placed blame on the deficiencies of the Chinese people and the inefficiencies of the Chinese government. In spite of Tianjin's position as a city marked by traumatic experiences with the violence of imperialism, medically minded elites had distanced themselves extraordinarily far from the events of 1860 or 1900. The violence that accompanied *weisheng*'s new epidemic control procedures was unavoidable and benevolent—it was simply better executed by Chinese themselves.

It is the physician of Chinese medicine, Ding Zilang, who invoked the violence of imperialism in his critique of modern *weisheng*. His awareness of the violent origins of Western medicine in Tianjin blended with his theoretical skepticism to produce what Nandy has termed "an ecology of knowledge" critique of modern biomedicine.[65] Ding suggested that there was "another reason" about the human body besides that which had generated

Western medicine.[66] Ding held out Chinese medicine as a rational, complex system superior to what he perceived as the reductionism inherent in biomedicine. Ding resisted the logic of the microscope, the modern propensity to parse life into smaller and smaller units of analysis. His critiques of imperialism and biomedicine met in his resistance to the germ theory. For Ding, germs were primarily a fetish, an obsession of foreign governments who turned microbes into a vehicle for corporal control. Ding did not deny the existence of bacteria. Instead, he rejected them as an instrument that, in the hands of foreigners, would eventually lead to the destruction of the Chinese people.

In Ding's writings it is difficult to discern any attempt at "indigenizing" Western medicine or creating a hybrid form of medical modernity that lay somewhere between Chinese and Western forms. He did not attempt to produce the synthesis of Chinese medicine and germ theory that Bridie Andrews observed in the writings of many other physicians of the same period.[67] Rather his approach is more analogous to how Gyan Prakash has proposed one should see Gandhi's move to use sexual asceticism as a form of national resistance. In Gandhi's insistence on *brahmacharya* as a source of strength for the nation, Prakash sees an acceptance of the colonizers' ideology of modern governance.[68] For proponents of Chinese medicine in the 1920s and 1930s, an indigenous form of *weisheng,* practiced privately within the home and centered on the body of the individual, was now brought into the "outer arena" of race and nation. Perhaps Ding's move to assert a Chinese *weisheng* was in fact "to acknowledge that something was lacking in the nation's present" and to embrace the hegemony of colonial modernity. Nevertheless, when compared with other discourses of *weisheng* in republican-era Tianjin, Ding located health far closer to the Chinese condition: it had not "fled to a remote place," but resided within knowledge possessed by the Chinese people themselves.

By the late 1930s, few elites would be willing to see Ding's type of resistance as a viable "way out" for China. The control of germs and the control of populations had become the model for national health and national sovereignty. That foreign regimes seemed to be so much more proficient at controlling germs—in the West, and in Japan—remained a dominant element in the Chinese elite's desire for hygienic modernity.

9 Japanese Management of Germs in Tianjin

On July 7, 1937, fighting broke out between Chinese and Japanese troops at Marco Polo Bridge outside of Beijing. By July 31, Japanese forces had occupied all of Chinese-administered Tianjin. Japanese military officers and Chinese civilians collaborated to form a new government for the city. The new government was embedded in a system formed by the far-flung Japanese military, local Japanese Concession concerns, and a network of Tianjin elites, many of whom had been educated in Japan.

Tianjin's memory of the Japanese occupation—as told by official PRC chroniclers—is one of unrelenting hardship and humiliation. The picture of city life from the fall of north China in 1937 to the end of the Japanese empire in 1945 includes images of barbed wire, bayonets, economic exploitation, drug proliferation, the murder of civilians, and random violence. Although Japanese military control of Tianjin brought with it a host of new forms of cruelty and exploitation, it can also be seen as a continuation of a variety of more mundane Japanese programs that were designed to facilitate colonial life in China. Central to Japan's goals was the carving out of a hygienically safe niche within the biologically threatening environment of the Asian mainland. The control of bacteria had been an integral part of Japan's presence in Tianjin, and indeed throughout all of its formal and informal imperial locales, since the birth of the Japanese empire around the turn of the century. Japanese goals, cast as cruel and exploitative by Chinese observers, were in fact similar to the goals of all modernizing regimes in China's twentieth-century history. If modern medical technology combined with enhanced enforcement ability had been the goal of *weisheng* in Tianjin since 1900, then the years of the Japanese occupation might have been seen by some as the culmination of hygienic modernity.

THE FRAMEWORK OF JAPANESE COLONIALISM

In 1936, Japanese in Tianjin policed and controlled only the fifty square blocks of the Japanese Concession. The next year, Japanese controlled the entire city exclusive of the remaining French, British, and Italian Concessions. By 1941, the Japanese controlled all parts of Tianjin, and along with it, a substantial proportion of the Chinese coast stretching from Manchuria in the north to Hong Kong in the south. The military expansion of Japanese control in Tianjin was a stage in the long, discontinuous, and highly complex process of expansion of the Japanese empire in East Asia. Beginning with the establishment of Taiwan as a formal colony, Japan gradually added to the blurred outlines of its empire through a combination of formal annexations (Korea), de facto control (Kwantung leased territories, the South Manchuria Railway corridor), spheres of political and economic influence (Fujian, north and northeast China, Inner Mongolia), and then, in the prelude to world war and during the war itself, occupation through the establishment of "puppet" regimes in Manchuria, China, and Southeast Asia. Peter Duus, Mark Peattie, and a host of other scholars of Japan have begun to trace the shifting contours of this ever-changing system: the "formal empire" in Taiwan and Korea, the "informal" empire represented by southern Manchuria and the Japanese Concessions in Chinese treaty ports, and the "wartime empire" that extended from the permafrost of northern Manchuria to the rubber plantations of Indonesia.[1]

Recent scholarship on this fifty-year experience of empire (1895–1945) has highlighted the distinctiveness of Japanese imperialism. Unlike the imperial experience of England, France, Germany, or the United States, Japan colonized peoples who lived nearby, shared the same religious and intellectual traditions, lived in a similar climate, and shared a common bond of "race" with the colonizer. The boundaries between colonized and colonizers, which scholars such as Ann Laura Stoler and others have described as fraught with tension in the European/non-European colonial context, were even more complex, more porous, and more baffling in the situation of "Asian on Asian" imperialism.[2]

Within the Japanese empire, cultures of superiority and dominance had to be manufactured from within a position of sameness. Japanese intellectuals in the main islands and abroad conducted the mental machinations necessary to separate a Japanese "race" from Japan's "Orient."[3] Japan may have shared common blood with Koreans or Polynesians, and may have borrowed its culture from China, but a combination of distinctive, essential Japanese traditions and a unique Japanese ability to master the secrets of the West's power had created a separate people poised to lead the rest of Asia to modernity. Significantly, Japan's own homeland project of tutoring its populations in modes of modern existence took place simultaneously with its project of pacifying and governing indigenous populations in the colonies. As Barbara Brooks has observed, historians of Japan have even more reason to see colonies as "laboratories of modernity" than do historians of Europe or the United States. Boundaries between "metropole" and "periphery" were constantly blurred as administrators, military officers, scientists, and capitalists were posted back and forth between Tokyo and nearby colonies with remarkable frequency. Likewise, millions of Japanese farmers, petty traders, laborers, entertainers, and sex workers took the short boat ride from Japanese ports to seek their fortunes in Taipei, Shanghai, and Seoul, resulting in a transient diaspora of "proletarian colonizers" who occupied some of the same economic and social niches as the colonized. Japanese regimes of discipline, education, and economic development were worked out simultaneously through intersection with similar populations on the main islands and in the colonies.[4]

Within the vaguely defined empire itself, degrees of perceived difference between colonizers and colonized resulted in different colonial policies. In Taiwan and Korea, Japanese authorities allowed indigenous populations to become a type of citizen of the Japanese empire, albeit citizens with a special designation. For a certain period of time in the history of the Japanese empire, official policy looked forward to and encouraged the assimilation of the Taiwanese and the Koreans: the possibility of "becoming Japanese" was held up as a terminal goal for the progress of indigenous people.[5] Rather than police the sexual boundaries between colonizer and colonized, official Japanese policy actually encouraged intermarriage as a form of racial uplift, especially for Koreans.[6] Colonial administrations worked on the cultural and physical advancement of colonials through education and public health: the school and the clinic became symbols of assimilationist rule. Indigenous populations formed the bulk of lower echelon positions in the administration: links between local society and colonial government were solidly formed by thousands of Taiwanese and Korean elites who negotiated their identities between the colonizer and the colonized.[7]

Not all "benefits" of Japanese colonial rule were distributed equally throughout the empire, and not all Japanese were as optimistic about the goals of assimilation. In outposts of the "informal empire" such as Manchuria and treaty-port concessions, education, public health, and career advancement were not extended to the general Chinese population. There was less of an official emphasis on bringing "civilization" to the indigenous population. In China, separation and the policing of boundaries was more the norm, and administrative emphasis was on protecting Japanese populations from a dangerous and diseased Chinese environment while extracting economic gains for the homeland. But even within the formal colonies, not all Japanese shared the early official sentiment that boundaries between the colonizers and the colonized should fade away. Strident discourses of Korean and Chinese inferiority, often based in the rhetoric of cleanliness, disease, and hygiene, abounded among Japanese observers and residents in both the informal and formal colonies alike. Some intellectuals who visited Manchuria took one look at Chinese, pronounced them "very dirty," and spent their entire time in China in a constant state of anxiety about health and the vectors of disease lurking around them.[8] Even in Korea, amid an official policy of assimilation, middle-class Japanese residents created racist discourses of Korean hygienic inferiority and criticized the Japanese authorities for not doing enough to protect the well-being of Japanese settlers.[9]

Within this complex system of formal and informal empires, health and hygiene were combined to produce a cornerstone of modern civilized identity: *eisei*. *Eisei* as hygienic modernity was a central element in shaping and defining the nature of Japanese colonialism. Japanese medical elites reconfigured *weisheng* as a powerful tool to transform domestic governance and used it as a key strategy to advance Japan's military endeavors abroad (see chapter 5). Tianjin's medical experience under Japanese authorities between 1900 and 1937, when Japanese only governed one small corner of the city, and during the 1937–1945 occupation, when the city formally entered the Japanese "wartime empire," is best understood within the shifting boundaries of *eisei* in the empire at large.

EISEI AND JAPAN'S "EMPIRES"

Like colonial medicine elsewhere, Japan's colonial health policies emerged as its military encountered epidemic disease during the acquisition of its first colony. In the initial conquest of Taiwan in 1895, approximately eight thousand Japanese troops contracted cholera.[10] Within a year of establishing rule on the island, the south China bubonic plague epidemic spread from Hong Kong to Taiwan. These two massive health crises, following one after the other, compelled the new rulers of Taiwan to make *eisei* and disease prevention a top priority. In 1897, the chief of the Army Medical Department, Ishiguro Tadanori, established strict guidelines for maintaining the health of the new colony. First and foremost, water treatment facilities and underground sewers for military bases were to be immediately established. Cleanliness, both public and personal, had to be maintained, and boundaries between Japanese and Chinese residential areas would be monitored by Japanese troops. The number of health workers had to be increased, and opium use was to be eliminated from the island. From Ishiguro's perspective boundaries of cleanliness, policing, and safe water would protect the Japanese community from the dangerous environment and people of Taiwan.[11]

Gotô Shinpei brought a different approach to the hygienic governance of Taiwan. When Gotô became governor of Taiwan's civil administration in 1896, he brought to the colonies decades of experience of managing the health of the "national body" in Japan. Rather than emphasize segregation and policing, Gotô sought the "uplift" of the local population through a gradualist colonial rule. Based on his experience in Japan proper, Gotô felt that it was preferable to rule through preexisting indigenous structures than to force foreign systems upon the colonized population. To this end, Gotô established a version of Japan's local hygiene committee organization in Taiwan, utilizing the traditional Chinese *baojia* (Japanese, *hôkô*) system of organizing local society that had already been in place on the island. The elected heads of each group of one thousand families worked with Japanese administrators to implement public health policies such as the reporting of contagious disease and the administration of vaccines.[12]

Scholars of British imperialism have pointed out the intense contradictions between the enlightenment values of modernity in the metropole and the despotic policies of governance in the colonies.[13] Unlike the highly centralized British colonial public health administration in India, which diverged significantly from its domestic policy of local self-governance, Japanese colonial administration in Taiwan did not diverge that much from practices within Japan proper. However, less contradiction existed between Japanese domestic and colonial health policies because self-governance was exercised within a framework of strong central leadership both at home and in the colonies. This centralizing tendency, combined with the different racial dynamic of the Japanese empire, produced a colonial medicine that diverged in many ways from the regimes established in India.

Gotô's policies were used to great effect in the colonial administration's malaria prevention program. Rather than attempt to separate themselves from indigenous carrier populations, the Japanese implemented Robert Koch's method of testing the blood of suspected carriers and treating positive cases with quinine. "Progressive" Taiwanese *hôkô* heads were instrumental in persuading Taiwanese families to submit to the government blood testing and medication schedule. Western observers were highly impressed by the rates of compliance that the Japanese colonial government achieved without an overreliance on brute force.[14] By cultivating indigenous bridges between the local population and the Japanese authorities, Gotô Shinpei's approach to *eisei* helped make Taiwan become a "hygienic zone" for the habitation of Japanese citizens—and helped some Taiwanese elites begin the long journey to "becoming Japanese."

In Korea, Japanese authorities placed emphasis on the development of medical education and public health infrastructure as part of a conscious policy of civilizing and potentially assimilating the Korean people. Hundreds of Japanese physicians moved to Korea, and Japanese institutions trained hundreds of Korean physicians in Western medicine. By 1938, Korean physicians of Western medicine outnumbered Japanese. Contagious disease control operated on a combined basis of direct state intervention and hygiene education. Colonial administrators saw Koreans, like Japanese, as a malleable population that could be transformed by government education and mobilization policies into hygienically modern subjects of the empire.[15]

The average Japanese settler in Korea was not as optimistic and assimilationist as colonial authorities. They perpetually decried the unsanitary habits of their Korean neighbors and criticized the government for not doing enough to ensure the hygienic security of Japanese. Brooks attributes this anxiety to the relative lack of clear boundaries of class or race between the colonizer and the colonized in Korea, citing the illustrative example of the large number of Japanese women who worked as prostitutes in the colony and who often intermarried with Korean men.[16] In a colony run by officials from the metropole, however, these anxieties were often glossed over by the rational "scientific" plans of administrators from Tokyo.

Finally, it must be noted that Japanese health policy in the colonies did not remain the same throughout the colonial period. Liu Shiyong has demonstrated a significant change in Japanese approaches to *eisei* in Taiwan within the first three decades of the twentieth century, a shift that reflected worldwide changes in modern biomedicine. Disease prevention in the first decades of Japanese rule focused on the techniques of quarantine and isolation. By the 1910s, a new generation of colonial administrators turned away from the management of populations toward the management of blood. This increasing confidence in the ability of the laboratory to solve the problem of disease was foreshadowed in the adoption of Koch's blood screening/quinine therapy approach to malaria control on Taiwan. Japanese public health policy increasingly ordered the use of vaccinations at the onset of outbreaks of cholera, plague, dysentery, and any other disease that had any sort of vaccine available, even if the vaccine was of questionable utility and limited effectiveness. Pharmaceutical and immunological means to disease control epitomized Japan's attempt at being among the world's most "scientifically advanced" colonizers.[17]

In Japan's "informal empire" in mainland China, *eisei* played a central role, but its characteristics were decidedly different from *eisei* in Taiwan or Korea. Formal Japanese health administration operated within small enclaves of military and settler activity, and rarely extended beyond Japanese communities to include Chinese populations, except when they became the object of sanitary policing. As early as 1899, when plague hit the Liaodong peninsula treaty port of Yingkou, Japanese physicians and Japanese police were called upon by foreign consulates to play a role in maintaining sanitary order.[18] Japanese troops and military medical officers were essential in establishing China's first public health bureau in Tianjin in 1902. With the establishment of Japanese management over the southern Manchuria leased territories in 1906, a full-fledged *eisei* network spread in the Liaodong peninsula. The presence of the Kantô Army meant that military medical officers were perpetually present in Manchuria. But for the most part the region's *eisei* was managed not by a military or colonial administration but by a company, the South Manchuria Railway (Mantetsu). Beginning with a massive mobilization of Japanese sanitary police during the devastating 1910–11 Manchurian plague epidemic, the Mantetsu *eisei* infrastructure grew to include a state-of-the-art bacteriological laboratory in Dalian (which produced massive amounts of vaccine), two medical schools, a series of railway hospitals, sanitary infrastructures in major cities and towns, and sanitary policing capabilities in locales all along the railroad.[19] Within the city of Dalian itself, under the administration of the Kantô government, *eisei* administration included sanitary police to enforce quarantine of potentially dangerous populations of Chinese dock laborers, but it also included sanitary associations on which both Chinese and Japanese elites served.[20] Japanese authority in Manchuria exhibited many of the same characteristics as Japanese *eisei* in the colonies: an important role for the military, the establishment of sanitary infrastructures, a large sanitary policing capacity, cooperation from Chinese elites, and an increasing reliance on laboratory breakthroughs to stem epidemics. However, one major difference existed between the formal and informal empires. In Korea and in Taiwan, colonial authorities undertook the hygienic "uplift" of the indigenous population through basic education, medical services, training Taiwanese and Korean physicians, and establishing sanitary infrastructures. In Japan's "informal colonies," there was no such official optimism that Chinese would become as hygienically modern as the Japanese.

EISEI AND THE TIANJIN CONCESSION

Very little has been written on the Japanese Concession in Tianjin, in spite of its central role as "the jewel of Japan's privileged territories in China."[21] PRC histories portray the Japanese Concession as a fifty-square-block den of iniquity, full of nothing but sordid brothels, opium dens, Chinese gangsters, and murderous Japanese secret police. In contrast, Japanese writings from the time provide a portrait of a virtuous merchant community increasingly threatened by the looming specter of violent Chinese nationalism. Much more research needs to be done in Japanese newspapers, memoirs, and foreign ministry archives to fully illuminate the role of the Tianjin Japanese Concession in the larger story of China's experience with imperialism. The Japanese Concession's official record reveals that the Japanese military, commercial concerns, and public health services distinguished this section of the city. Other sources reveal that the Japanese Concession was also the central site for the trade in flesh and drugs in Tianjin—and perhaps all of north China. This complex picture highlights some of the paradoxes of Japanese imperialism in China, and the central role that hygiene played within those paradoxes.

Official prewar histories of the concession Residents' Association admit that the first Japanese residents of Tianjin were small-time merchants and petty traders who tended to adopt the lifestyles and mindsets of the Chinese "petty urbanites."[22] But these sources then narrate the gradual elevation of concession life, a process intimately connected with the arrival of more prosperous merchants and the creation of an *eisei* infrastructure.

Sandwiched in between the French Concession and the Chinese city, the Japanese Concession began in 1898 with the construction of a few streets along the shore of the Hai River. After World War I, a real estate boom took off in the concession, financed in part by the successes experienced by Japanese shipping and trading companies while Britain and France were distracted with the war in Europe.[23] By the mid 1920s, the overall shape of the concession had been set. Approximately five thousand Japanese, two hundred Koreans, a handful of Taiwanese, and more than thirty thousand Chinese lived within the fifty square blocks of the concession, making it one of the most densely populated areas of the city. Japanese residents lived primarily clustered around three streets: Asahi Street, Kotobuki Street, and Sakae Street, the most flourishing sector of the concession. Few Japanese lived in the areas of highest Chinese population: the concession's northwestern perimeter (bordering the Chinese city) or southeastern perimeter (near the French Concession).[24] This residential segregation pattern reflected an extreme domestic insularity on the part of Japanese residents that was even more profound than that found in the European concessions. Although Europeans relied on Chinese servants, drivers, and storekeepers to provide services, the small number of prosperous Japanese families of the Chinese treaty ports could avail themselves of a large population of Japanese working-class sojourners to provide the services they needed.

The concession's Chinese residents showed a similar partitioning of social classes. It included an elite community of merchants, scholars, and former Qing officials, some of whom interacted with Japanese as members of the Residents' Association. Perhaps the most illustrious non-Japanese resident of the Japanese Concession was the "last emperor," Pu Yi, who resided in the concession's "Quiet Garden Villa" after he was evicted from the Forbidden City in 1924 and before he became the "emperor" of Manchukuo in 1934. But the Chinese population also included tens of thousands of workers, peddlers, and service providers. The poorest Chinese neighborhoods were concentrated in the northwest corner of the concession, along streets that bordered the Chinese city's "South Market." This area possessed a large concentration of small restaurants and "lower-class" brothels that catered primarily to a Chinese clientele.

The Japanese Concession was not without its own impressive architecture and sites of imperial dignity. Representatives of the major Japanese trading and shipping companies housed their offices in Western-style buildings along Yamaguchi Street. The Japanese consulate, police headquarters, public park, and kendo hall off of Fukushima Street were all visually impressive reminders of the Japanese presence. But in the eyes of many Chinese, what distinguished the Japanese Concession were the many brothels and "entertainment clubs" that flourished openly in the center of the concession, along its most prosperous thoroughfare, Asahi Street. It was also an open secret that the many "pharmacies" on Asahi Street were places where one could easily obtain morphine, heroin, and opium. As early as 1923, Chinese guidebooks described the Japanese Concession as a place where a tourist could go to enjoy hedonistic pleasures in a vaguely foreign yet Chinese-friendly environment. The welcoming nature of the Japanese Concession was symbolized by the concession's park, where, unlike the British Settlement's Victoria Park, Chinese were free to enter and stroll about at will. But it was unlikely that most visitors to the concession spent much time in the park when there were other attractions to be seen behind the closed doors of Asahi Street's "houses."[25]

A significant sector of the Japanese Concession's economy may have thrived on vice, but the concession government was run by dignified career diplomats of impeccable education and social background. The highest authority in the Japanese Concession was the consul, who was appointed directly by the Ministry of Foreign Affairs in Tokyo and had the power to administer justice, investigate crimes, and mediate between the Japanese community and Chinese authorities.[26] But the day-to-day business of the concession was administered by the Japanese Residents' Association, the Tensin Nihon kyoryûmindan.[27] In this concession where more than 85 percent of the population was Chinese, Chinese tax payers were granted the right to vote and run for Residents' Association office much earlier than in the European concessions. Nevertheless, positions of power in the day-to-day workings of the administration were reserved for Japanese residents. Chinese could hold up to half of the seats in the association, but Chinese names do not appear in the published lists of responsible citizens and officials involved in the Japanese Concession's civic enterprises. Schools, social services, and police were run at the top by local Japanese elites. *Eisei* was no exception.

As in other locales in Japan's formal empire, *eisei* organization in Tianjin began with military conquest and disease—the international relief expedition in 1900 and the cholera outbreak of 1902. After the suppression of the Boxers, the Japanese army made the Temple of Oceanic Radiance, at the southern tip of the concession, into a permanent garrison.[28] No major outpost of the Japanese military was without its modern hospital and laboratory, and the Tianjin headquarters built impressive facilities next to the garrison. The hospital's extensive laboratory and medical staff were crucial to the *eisei* of the Japanese Concession, and even aided in maintaining the health of the other foreign concessions by supplying them with vaccines.

The experience of the 1902 cholera outbreak made Japanese Concession residents and the Foreign Ministry particularly anxious to establish adequate *eisei* organization for the civilian population. In 1908 the Residents' Association established a health department *(eisei ka, eisei bu)* and hired an *eisei* expert from the Japanese Ministry of the Interior's Infectious Disease Research Institute as its head. The department kept vital statistics, oversaw the sanitation of the concession, tested the concession's water supply, inspected food vendors and markets, managed the concession's crematorium, and intervened in the case of epidemics. This very busy part of the local government frequently benefited from the advice and the resources of the military: soldiers helped in times of epidemic crisis, and the military hospital laboratory frequently conducted biological assays for the civilian authorities. During health emergencies, the consul, police, and military came together with health department personnel to coordinate epidemic control measures.

What was the terrain of sanitation, health, and disease in the Japanese Concession? As of 1928, only half of the concession population used treated running water, and less than one-quarter of the population had flush toilets. More than half used nonflush privies, and more than three hundred families used chamber pots alone. Sanitary facilities statistics are not broken down according to nationality, but anecdotal evidence suggests that the majority of people without running water or toilets were Chinese.[29]

Health department statistics on disease focus almost exclusively on the incidence of acute infectious diseases (cholera, typhoid fever, scarlet fever) among the Japanese population. In spite of this obsession with acute diseases, it is possible to conclude from statistics that tuberculosis was the leading killer. Childhood diseases such as diphtheria and scarlet fever were common among the concession's Japanese population, and the Japanese had not managed to banish smallpox from the concessions borders. From 1927 to 1933, however, the concession seemed to be bringing some of these childhood diseases under control through the use of vaccines and antitoxins. Similarly, with improvements in sewer and water supply systems, incidents of typhoid fever and dysentery were nearly halved during the same period. Mortality rates in the first few years of the Showa era (1925–89) decreased rather dramatically from approximately twenty-two to sixteen deaths per thousand. This trend toward decline mirrored that experienced in Japan during the same years, making living in the Japanese Concession in Tianjin as healthy as living in Osaka (and slightly less healthy than living in Tokyo) during the same period—at least for Japanese.[30]

Chinese residents were not offered the same type of access to the life-saving vaccines and antitoxins that protected Japanese residents. Vaccination statistics (usually for smallpox) for the years before 1937 show that Japanese recipients usually outnumbered Chinese recipients by as many as five to one. Those Chinese who received vaccinations probably represent the Chinese children who were enrolled in Japanese schools and adults employed by the concession authorities or Japanese companies. Outside of the small number of vaccinated elites, the Residents' Association statistics are silent about the health of the Chinese. The concession was served by one public hospital, but the majority of its patients were Japanese, the exception being the occasional Chinese policeman or employee of the Residents' Association.[31] Chinese are not even counted among the concession's dead: cause of death figures only reveal the diseases that ended Japanese lives.

Only when health crises threatened the Japanese population of the concession did Japanese authorities show more interest in enforcing the health of the Chinese through the application of laboratory technologies. An early example of a citywide public health crisis demonstrated how Japanese Concession authorities were even more willing than other foreign concessions to trust the power of disinfectants and vaccines to eliminate threats to health that seemed to stem from the indigenous population. During the plague crisis of 1911, Japanese applied the epidemic control techniques learned in semitropical Taiwan to the northern port of Tianjin. The plague episode contrasts a European impulse toward segregation from indigenous populations with the Japanese belief in the possibility of effecting the sanitization of the indigenous population through the "scientific management" of germs and people.

JAPANESE "SCIENTIFIC MANAGEMENT" OF GERMS: THE 1911 PLAGUE IN TIANJIN

As in Taiwan and Dalian, one of the first major challenges to Japanese *eisei* systems in Tianjin was an outbreak of plague.[32] Beginning in the fall of 1910, pneumonic plague ravaged Manchuria, leaving as many as sixty thousand fatalities in its wake. Tianjin faced a particularly complicated situation as this epidemic moved south. The city was the largest treaty port close to the epicenter of the outbreak. The main railroad lines from Manchuria converged on Tianjin, and steamships often stopped in Taku on their way from Manchurian ports to points further south. In addition, eight different foreign concession administrations and the native city government were all responsible for the public health situation within their own borders. For the foreign concessions, the major question was how to coordinate plague prevention efforts and at the same time deal with the "native" presence both within their borders and in the Chinese-administered city.

In 1911 Tianjin's foreign administrations convened an All-Concession Epidemic Committee in order to plan a united strategy. The committee consisted of the consuls, heads of police, and health officers of all of Tianjin's concessions. As they had in the 1900 occupation of the city, European authorities looked to Japanese *eisei* experts for guidance in how to manage health in China. Concession representatives elected the newly hired head of the Japanese Concession's health department, Dr. Fukuda Sakusaburô, to be the leader of the All-Concession Epidemic Committee.[33]

The convening of the 1911 committee marked the first time that representatives of Tianjin's major foreign powers had come together to decide on policy for the city as a whole since the TPG of 1900–1902, but in 1911 the task of coordination proved impossible. Although each concession adhered to the doctrines of hygienic modernity and understood the plague's mode of transmission, there was disagreement from the start about the best method of halting its spread. The French and British representatives proposed a ban on any Chinese movement into the foreign concessions, and suggested using police and military forces to enforce a strict *cordon sanitaire* around the concessions. The German and Russian representatives agreed. This approach mirrored the steps taken by foreigners in Shanghai during the plague threat. Bryna Goodman's study of Shanghai highlighted the anxiety foreigners in Shanghai felt about the presence of Chinese in their midst during the plague year. The International Settlement police took the dramatic step of erecting a wall between the Chinese district and the foreign enclave, an action that provoked riots and left lingering animosity on both sides of the wall after the end of the threat.[34] Fukuda protested the European plan, arguing that it would be impossible to cut off all traffic between the Japanese Concession, with its large Chinese population, and the Chinese-administered populations on the concession's border. Fukuda called for the use of "scientific methods" of surveillance, disinfection, and education to stem the plague, and argued that crude military methods would only harm Tianjin's business and anger the Chinese. In the end, no agreement was reached, and the committee was disbanded. Each settlement chose to deal with the plague in its own way.

The Japanese authorities were confident that their "scientific methods" could track individual residents and pinpoint carriers of disease without shutting down concession commerce and society. Japanese authorities issued passes to all Chinese residents of the concession who had to travel beyond the concession borders. Police established checkpoints at all roads that led in and out of the concession. Chinese were allowed to enter the concession borders from the Chinese city, but they were physically inspected for any signs of plague and had to undergo full-body chemical disinfection with a potent carbolic acid spray. Those suspected of having plague were forcibly isolated and tested for the presence of plague bacteria.[35] Within the concession, a hygiene committee was set up on every street to conduct rat-catching contests and facilitate door to door inspections, which were carried out by the combined forces of the health department, the police department, and the Japanese army stationed in Tianjin. The entire population of the concession, both Chinese and Japanese, was required to attend a series of compulsory lectures on *weisheng* given by the head of the army hospital and Dr. Fukuda himself.[36]

After the plague threat passed, the Japanese Residents' Association applauded the success of its "scientific methods." Other concessions had used their police forces to cut off all traffic with the Chinese, an action that was denounced by the Chinese Chamber of Commerce and had serious repercussions for business within those concessions. In contrast, the Japanese had allowed traffic across their borders to continue in a regulated fashion. The authorities were vindicated when statistics showed that in contrast to the total of seventy-three plague deaths reported in the Chinese city, the Japanese Concession suffered only one death from plague.[37] In contrast with the European impulse to segregate themselves from the "unsanitary" Chinese, the Japanese had instead attempted to make the Chinese sanitary, and felt that they had succeeded. The Japanese plague policy reflected Japanese confidence that it could, even if only temporarily, bring other Asian groups into the embrace of hygienic modernity. The successful deployment of scientific administration techniques in Tianjin echoed Japanese government efforts to turn Taiwan, the southern Manchurian leased territory, and the new colony of Korea into "hygienic zones," safe for Japanese colonization and economic activities. As health threats in Tianjin continued unabated, the health department turned more attention to the concession's Chinese residents, a trend that coincided with the increasing number of Chinese in the Residents' Association. But this attention came not in the form of health services, but in the form of sanitary inspectors who scrutinized the interiors of residences and the bodies of prostitutes.

ROUTINE INTERVENTIONS

Although Japanese authorities claimed to place their trust in carbolic acid sprays and vaccines in health emergencies, everyday health in the concessions was maintained on a regular basis through the vigorous employment of more mundane administrative technologies: surveillance, inspecting, and therapeutic interventions. Postwar Chinese histories of Tianjin may represent the Japanese Concession as a sea of crime and social disorder, but from the perspective of *eisei*, the Japanese Concession may have been the most thoroughly monitored area in all of Tianjin.

Japanese Concession authorities intervened in the private lives of concession residents more aggressively than did authorities in other locales in the city. Beginning in the 1920s, biannual domestic cleanliness inspections became a regular part of concession life. Every spring and fall, the supervisors of the concession's Sanitation Section *(hôjo ka)* conducted week-long cleanliness inspections in all ten districts of the concession. Resistance to inspection was met by doubling the number of policemen accompanying the civilian inspection team, and by undertaking more aggressive *eisei* propaganda campaigns.[38] By the 1930s, the number of households inspected during the spring and fall campaigns surpassed ten thousand. Reports neither disclose the nationality of the inspection committee nor the nationality of the violators of the regulations, but both Japanese and Chinese residents were expected to let officials in to their homes to inspect kitchens, examine privies, and look for unhygienic clutter under family beds.

Prostitutes were subjected to the closest hygienic scrutiny of all. The proportion of female residents of the concession who worked in sex trades was astounding. In 1933, the five-by-ten-block concession boasted a population of more than three thousand sex workers, including 2,306 Chinese, 402 Japanese, and 314 Koreans. In the Japanese Concession, one out of six Japanese, one out of four Chinese, and one out of two Korean women worked as a licensed prostitute.[39] The Japanese Concession followed the homeland policy (and continental European practice) of regulating prostitution through the collection of taxes on licenses and the examination of prostitutes for venereal disease.[40] Brothels produced considerable tax income for the concession, providing at one time the third largest single tax amount for the Residents' Association, behind property taxes and taxes on rickshaw licenses. By the late 1920s, government inspection of prostitutes had become a highly standardized practice in the Japanese Concession. Health officers examined prostitutes once every seven to ten days. Japanese prostitutes, most of whom worked on Asahi Street, had to travel down to the concession's public hospital for their examination; Chinese and Korean prostitutes were examined in the more conveniently located Fugui hutong clinic, located in the western extreme of the concession, near the Chinese city. Early statistics show that Chinese prostitutes were less healthy than their Japanese and Korean counterparts. In 1933, Japanese prostitutes had a venereal disease infection rate around 10.7 percent; Korean prostitutes, 16.4 percent; and Chinese prostitutes exhibited an infection rate of 35 percent.[41] Those who were found to be infected were prevented from working and treated (as outpatients) by doctors of the concession government. The rates of "cure" were quite low, around one out of four. The frequent inspection of the brothels most likely ensured that a woman with venereal disease, once discovered, would have to leave the brothel, providing new opportunities for new arrivals to the city to take their place.[42]

Residents' Association statistics suggest that Japanese Concession physicians efficiently and thoroughly examined thousands of prostitutes fifty-two times a year, yet the state of "sanitary sex" in the concession may have been quite different. Other sources reveal that gangs and drug smugglers exerted considerable influence over both the concession police and its brothels. One of the most infamous opium den owners was Yuan Wenhui, a local gang leader who founded the Deyi lou, a multi-floor "all-purpose" entertainment center on Asahi Street. Yuan was reputed to have run protection rackets for the neighboring brothels. Like Huang Jinrong in Shanghai's French Concession, Yuan held an official position in the Japanese Concession police force. Yuan was also known to have made his thugs available to Japanese military and diplomatic officials, who used them in machinations to undermine Guomindang control in the Chinese city. As Frederic Wakeman, Brian Martin, and others have shown, the intertwining of the Chinese underworld and the world of foreign concession officials was one of the main features of life in Shanghai during the 1930s and 1940s.[43] The involvement of Chinese gangsters in the Japanese Concession police, the collusion between concession officials and Chinese gangs, and the involvement of Japanese officials in the north China drug trade suggest that the Residents' Association health department inspections were not as efficient as statistics imply. Still, it is quite possible that even the nefarious elements that influenced the sex business in the Japanese Concession would have a vested economic interest in making vice sufficiently disease free. In a Chinese treaty port, hygienic modernity and the violent underworld of gangs, opium dens, and drug lords might not have been mutually exclusive realms.

THE MEDICAL OCCUPATION OF TIANJIN: EXTREME INTERVENTIONS

On July 7, 1937, a brief skirmish flared between Chinese and Japanese troops at the Marco Polo Bridge outside of Beijing. In spite of ongoing low-level negotiations between Nanjing and Tokyo, major fighting began again around Beijing on July 27. Two days later, Japanese troops captured Tianjin. The brief but intense attack had a tremendous impact on certain parts of the city. Among the casualties of the conquest was Nankai University, one of China's premiere institutions of higher learning. The day before they took Tianjin, Japanese forces bombed this center of Chinese nationalism, destroying all but one of the buildings on the school's American-funded, Western-style campus.[44] Tens of thousands of Japanese troops continued their advance southward into Shandong and Henan, and thousands of troops stayed on to occupy the Chinese city of Tianjin. As Europeans hunkered down within their politically neutral concessions, the Japanese population of Tianjin skyrocketed. In 1936, approximately nine thousand Japanese lived in Tianjin, almost all of them in the Japanese Concession. By 1941, more than fifty thousand Japanese soldiers, suppliers, prostitutes, and medical personnel lived scattered in locations throughout the city, a number that would grow to more than seventy thousand by the end of the war.[45] Occupying a city the size of Tianjin required massive manpower, and the able-bodied population of Japan poured into the Chinese mainland to support the occupation.

Japanese did not run Tianjin by themselves. Three days after the fall of the city, the Tianjin Security Preservation Committee announced its authority over the city. This committee was composed of approximately ten Chinese members, most of whom were former officials in the Beijing government during the warlord period. All of these men had long-standing close ties to Japan.[46] Under the supervision of the Japanese military, the collaborationist committee began to assume police and other government functions in Tianjin. This new government embraced the old Guomindang government apparatus, including a department of social welfare, education, finance, and hygiene *(weisheng)*.

Reestablishing the function of the municipal health department was a top priority for the Security Preservation Committee. As had happened time and time again over the past fifty years in Tianjin, fighting in the countryside led to a massive influx of refugees. More than one hundred thousand people from the area around Tianjin crowded into the city, and collaboration officials and Japanese military alike were fearful of the outbreak of epidemic disease. Many of Tianjin's health department physicians stayed at their posts even after the occupation. All of the Guomindang regime's units—the municipal hospitals, the contagious disease hospital, the police hospital, and six neighborhood health stations—were back to work within a few days of the invasion. But the health department saw significant changes in its administration and staffing.[47] Physicians with experience in Japan or an ability to speak Japanese rose to the top of the department hierarchy. Dozens of doctors and nurses from the Japanese Imperial Army were positioned at hospitals, clinics, and epidemic inspection centers throughout the city.[48] At least according to department records, the Chinese and Japanese health personnel seemed to work together in relative harmony.

Less than a month into the occupation, cholera was discovered in Tianjin.[49] Female factory workers, flour sack transporters, Chinese laborers who had been impressed into service for the Japanese military, and a family of Russian Jews were among the unfortunate victims of the epidemic who were brought to the Municipal Contagious Disease Hospital.[50] To try to contain the epidemic, the Japanese army ordered a door-to-door sanitary inspection of the entire city. Less than two months after the beginning of the occupation, one thousand armed soldiers and more than five hundred vaccinators descended on Tianjin's neighborhoods in search of dirt and disease. The vaccinators wore white coats and carried black bags filled with medical supplies. At least one soldier for every team stood beside the doctors, garbed in the uniform of the Imperial Japanese Army and carrying a rifle at the ready, bayonet attached. Some of these teams included Chinese medical personnel from the health department.[51]

The inspections were swift, thorough, and frequently violent. As an armed soldier stood in the doorway of each residence, inspectors scoured the house for signs of disease. They recorded the names of everyone in each household, made general observations about their state of health, and noted if anyone needed medical treatment. Inspectors filled out forms detailing the cleanliness and condition of kitchens, living areas, toilets, and courtyards. After conducting cursory examinations of family members and their environment, the teams gave cholera vaccine shots to all the men, women, and children of each family.[52] By the second day word had gotten out in Tianjin that the Japanese were forcing their way into homes and injecting men, women, and children with an unknown substance. Chinese attempted to escape the visitations. In one incident, thousands of Chinese living in the former German Concession tried to escape the vaccinations by fleeing into the British Settlement. Unable to enter the neutral British area to pursue the escapees, the Japanese army simply cut off traffic between the two areas and trapped fleeing Chinese at the border.[53]

While the Japanese army conducted its violent inspections, a few Chinese physicians with the health department went around the city, giving public lectures on *weisheng*. Audiences for the lectures were drummed up by local collaborationist neighborhood security committees, known as "Support the Government Associations" (Fu zhi hui). In their content and tone, these lectures, given during the Japanese occupation, differed little if at all from public health lectures that had been delivered under the Nationalist government since 1928, or by reformers and educators in Tianjin since the turn of the century. The lectures reminded people of the horrors of past cholera epidemics such as the outbreak of 1902. They then explained in sim-

ple terms the cause of cholera, and assured the listener that the cholera vaccine was the best way to avoid another disaster in Tianjin. The lectures proclaimed the harmlessness of the cholera vaccine itself and emphasized that
the "authorities" were demonstrating their benevolence by providing medical assistance to the masses. There was no mention at all of the presence of
the Japanese army.[54]

When not inspecting homes for cholera, Japanese medical personnel were
busy inspecting the city's new "army" of women designated as prostitutes.
With the occupation of the city, the number of sex workers who came under Japanese hygienic jurisdiction skyrocketed. This was in part because the
Japanese now administered the Chinese city and thus brought previously
unregulated prostitutes into the Japanese "sanitary sex" system. However
the number of Chinese prostitutes was equaled and then surpassed by the
number of Japanese women designated as *shôgi* (prostitutes, a category tal-
lied separately from geisha or other female entertainment workers). By 1939,
the Japanese authorities had set up prostitute examination stations at nine
points around the city. There they processed the inspections of more than
thirty-seven thousand women: approximately sixteen thousand Chinese,
sixteen thousand Japanese, and five thousand Koreans. By 1943, this number
had decreased to twenty-nine thousand, primarily because of the tremendous decrease of Chinese women in the trade.[55] These figures were presented
as a matter of course in the reports of the concession's Residents' Association, not by military authorities; thus it is not immediately clear if these
vast numbers represented women trapped in the Japanese Imperial Army's
system of military sexual slavery, or if some were camp followers who established themselves in Tianjin in the wake of the occupying army. More
research needs to be done on the conditions for female populations of Chinese cities under the Japanese occupation. What is clear is that these women
were under the constant scrutiny of government/military authorities and
underwent health inspections on the average of thirty times a year at the
hands of Japanese medical personnel.

As the war dragged on, Japanese and Chinese physicians in Tianjin fre-
netically generated a never-ending cycle of examinations, inspections, and
vaccinations of the native populace. Microscopes, hypodermic needles, and
swabs were joined by rifles and bayonets to effect the inspection and sanitization of hundreds of thousands of individuals. In 1939, the combined
forces of the Japanese military, the Japanese Concession health department,
and the collaborationist government health department conducted 213,000
cholera vaccinations, 217,000 smallpox vaccinations, and 9,000 typhoid
fever vaccinations. Laboratories in the Japanese Concession examined thou-

sands of samples of feces, blood, spinal fluid, and sputum in an attempt to pinpoint cases of intestinal parasites, scarlet fever, cholera, meningitis, and tuberculosis among increasingly ailing Japanese soldiers and Chinese residents alike.[56] Japanese health department personnel, supplemented by the Japanese Army, scrutinized the bodies of Tianjin in ways never before experienced in the city. The Chinese city no longer provided anonymity or refuge from government intervention. Individuals were located, named, recorded, and injected by a determined network of soldiers and doctors. If visibility and accessibility of the body is a goal of modern biomedicine, then the Japanese occupation of Tianjin brought with it an unprecedented regime of hygienic modernity.

MEANINGS OF THE OCCUPATION FOR CHINESE DOCTORS

Anecdotal evidence indicates that many physicians affiliated with the GMD health department remained in Tianjin during the occupation and worked under the collaborationist regime. No memoirs or writings of these men have come to light, so it is difficult to understand their positions or motivations. But to call all of these physicians collaborators is perhaps an oversimplification. R. Keith Schoppa has suggested that local collaborationist regimes were part of a long continuum of political trends, nurtured under violent warlords and corrupt GMD officials, which blurred the line between "morally legitimate and illegitimate elites." For Schoppa, the collaborationist regimes during the war simply represented "a difference in degree, not of kind" from previous local administrations. Under such conditions, remaining in town to work with Japanese occupiers might not have appeared much different from working with constantly shifting warlord regimes or GMD officials. Analyzing the defenses put forth by collaborators during their postwar trials, Lo Jui-jung has suggested that individuals collaborated in the hopes of assuring various types of survival: survival for a political or military position, survival for a family, or survival for an imagined group such as a local community, a region, or a people.[57] All of these approaches might illuminate the motivations of Tianjin's physicians. Many had lived in Tianjin through the multiple shifts in warlord regimes during the 1920s. Even after the establishment of the Nationalist regime in Nanjing, their city government continued to change hands between rival warlord factions. The Japanese occupying force permeated the Chinese city in ways unlike any previous warlord regime, yet exchanging one invading force for another had been a way of life in Tianjin for years. Given that many physicians had strong commitments to the health of the city, it is also easy to imagine that Tianjin's doctors of Western medicine worked with the occupying regime in order to ensure the very survival of Tianjin's people. To abandon the ill or to refuse to work for an occupying force for moral reasons would only serve to put more lives in jeopardy. Physician may have been highly ambivalent about taking orders from an alien regime, and yet the goal of survival would compel the physician to comply in order to save lives.

Going beyond the political economy of collaboration, Prasenjit Duara has suggested that the project of the Japanese empire contained compelling strains of a "redemptive transnationalism" that genuinely appealed to certain Chinese audiences. Invocations of a traditionalist, vaguely Confucian, "kingly way" inspired many elites in Manchuria to subscribe to Japanese visions of empire. Similarly, Poshek Fu has characterized the collaborationist "Gujin" group of Shanghai writers as men immersed in nostalgia who sought to preserve the traditional essence of Chinese culture. In these analyses, the transnational meanings that linked China and Japan were generated from a shared construct of "traditional East Asian culture." Beliefs that tied China to Japan were those that made them unique from the West—indeed, they offered an aggressive alternative to the penetration of Western cultural and social ideologies.[58]

Although nostalgia for a virtuous East Asian past may have played a part in mobilizing support for the Japanese project of empire, many Chinese elites may have also looked to the Japanese occupation as a harbinger of a long-awaited modernity. This may have been particularly true for the significant segment of the Chinese medical elite who had been educated in Japanese-led medical institutions in China or in Japanese medical schools in Japan.[59] Indeed several of the physicians active during the Japanese occupation of Tianjin had received medical degrees from the Tokyo University Medical School, regional medical schools in Japan, the Mantetsu Medical School in Mukden (Fengtian), the Manchukuo Medical School in Harbin, and, of course, the Beiyang Army Medical School in Tianjin.[60]

Many of the leaders of the health department during the occupation were men who had spent considerable time in Japan and were fluent in Japanese. There was perhaps no better example than the director of the contagious disease hospital, a young doctor named Hou Fusang. From a family originally from Wuxi (near Shanghai), Hou practiced medicine with his father, Hou Ximin, in a private practice in Tianjin's Italian Concession. Both the elder and younger Hous' medical degrees were from Japan, and there is clear evidence that the younger Hou was fluent in Japanese. Hou's reports to the head of the health department are written in Japanese, an interesting exercise considering that both he and the bureau chief were Chinese. Even his given name, Fusang (Japanese, Fusô) is an ancient name for Japan, a remarkably clear marker of cultural affiliation with the city's new overlords.[61] Hou was only twenty-five when he became head of the contagious disease hospital. The picture that emerges from his neatly penned reports is of an energetic, ambitious young man who was very serious and enthusiastic about his job of controlling epidemics for the Japanese occupation government.

It is possible that for men like Hou, the combination of medical technology and military effectiveness possessed by the health department under the Japanese occupation may have represented an ideal of public health organization. Never before in Tianjin's history had it been possible to wage such an effective war against harmful germs in the city. The mass vaccination of Tianjin residents, the health inspection of individual homes, and the rigorous enforcement of quarantine was made possible through the policies, priorities, organization, and power of the Japanese military. For some, the new political order may have represented an opportunity for the realization of long-hoped-for medical modernity in Tianjin. Like Chinese elites who invited Japanese to their homes during the 1900–1902 occupation of Tianjin, medical elites like Hou Fusang seemed to have been able to distance themselves from the violence inflicted upon their compatriots by the Japanese military. Certainly Hou's identification with the Japanese—embodied in language, education, and even in name—was far deeper than anything achieved by earlier Tianjin elites. Three decades of Japanese influence had created a stratum of Chinese who shared the Japanese colonial medical world's obsession with eliminating bacteria. The crises of war may have justified in these men's minds the use of unprecedented force to accomplish a certain kind of hygienic modernity in the city. Yet these distancings and bifurcations, even for a goal as "redemptively transnationalist" as modern medicine, must have become increasingly untenable as the deprivations of the occupation drained the city of its health.

MEANINGS OF THE OCCUPATION FOR CHINESE SUFFERERS

In June of 1938, cholera struck Tianjin once again.[62] The report below, written by Tianjin Contagious Disease Hospital director Hou Fusang, details the first case of cholera that came to the attention of city authorities. This remarkable case history reveals how the state intersected and influenced the medical choices of Tianjin's common people in unprecedented ways during the Japanese occupation. It also suggests how thirty years of hygienic modernity in Tianjin may have shaped the meanings and experiences of illness for Tianjin's people:

> On the afternoon of June 30, we received at the hospital a suspected case of cholera, Mrs. Sun (maiden name Yang), aged 28, of Tianjin county, Zheng Village, Li Family Alley number 11. Her mother's home is in Zhang Da Village. Seven days ago the patient went to visit her mother. On the evening of the 29th, she had crabs for dinner, and then drank untreated water from the Hai River. At around 11 P.M. she suddenly experienced several bouts of vomiting and diarrhea. She did not take any medicine. On the 30th, at approximately 10 A.M., she sought the help of a doctor of Chinese medicine. The doctor treated her with acupuncture and also administered an "emergency-rescue"–type liquid medicine. Then a doctor of the Japanese army unit stationed in that area administered medicine in liquid and tablet form, but there was no improvement in the patient's condition. She thereupon returned to Zhang Village and sought the help of another doctor of Chinese medicine, who treated her with acupuncture. At 3 P.M., a doctor of western medicine in Dazhigu administered injections twice (the name of the medicine was unknown to the patient). Thereupon she was discovered by the head policemen of that district, who sent her to the Contagious Disease Hospital.
>
> On examination we found that she had a weak pulse and a temperature of 37 degrees Celsius. The patient was experiencing severe pain in all four limbs. The patient was moaning, her eyes were sunken, her fingers were purple and black. She was severely dehydrated, her heart weak. She vomited once, passed loose stools five times. A sample of her stool was sent to the Japanese Military Hospital for examination. Since her arrival at the hospital the patient has been undergoing treatment and at the present her condition is good. The disinfection squad has been dispatched to the patient's home to conduct a thorough search and disinfection. We submit this report for your inspection.[63]

Mrs. Sun's struggle with cholera reveals the complex matrix of political, social, and military elements that surrounded disease and cure in occupation Tianjin. The cholera victim, a young married Chinese woman, lived in a neighborhood on the outskirts of the city, just south of the former Belgian Concession. This area along the Hai River was never directly administered by Belgium and had become a sort of free zone of industrial development during the 1920s. By the occupation period, the area was a jumble of scattered textile factories and worker dormitories. Contagious diseases that traveled up the Hai River from the main port at Taku often hit this area and its factory worker population first.[64]

The workers' lives were enriched by simple pleasures. Crabs from the mouth of the Hai River were a special treat, perhaps eaten to celebrate Mrs. Sun's return to mother Yang's home. Probably stir-fried until just tender, then topped with scallions and a little bit of rice wine, the undercooked crabs provided a perfect vector for cholera infection. The potency of the crabs was undoubtedly augmented by a dose of water from the Hai River. The residents along the lower reaches of the Hai took their water from a river that had already passed by the Chinese city, the Japanese, French, British, and Italian Concessions, and the neighborhoods of the former Austro-Hungarian, Russian, German, and Belgian Concessions. An international mix of garbage and sewage unified by its essentially foul nature flowed untreated into the Hai River, eventually to be washed out to sea or imbibed by unsuspecting Chinese. Water pipes laid by the privately owned Tianjin Native City Waterworks carried heavily chlorinated water through the Chinese city and most of the concessions, but the network stopped before it reached Zhang Da Village. The political fragmentation of Tianjin resulted in an inadequate patchwork of public health services, which combined with poverty to create ideal conditions for the outbreak and spread of epidemic diseases. These various byproducts of imperialism and capitalist development all shaped the sufferings of Mrs. Sun.

Faced with the sudden, wrenching symptoms of cholera, Mrs. Sun cast about for an effective treatment. She switched quickly from practitioner to practitioner without concern about debates over medical theory or national culture. However, these choices were exercised within a system of constraints, at the pinnacle of which stood the Japanese military. Mrs. Sun first turned to a doctor of Chinese medicine, perhaps the most trusted option, but also possibly the most readily available and cheapest option available to her. By 1939, licensed physicians of Chinese medicine outnumbered physicians of Western medicine by a ratio of four to one.[65] In spite of the regulatory efforts of decades of modernizing regimes, even more unlicensed healers could be found in poorer neighborhoods. The first practitioner who encountered Mrs. Sun used a method for treating *huoluan* that had been recommended in Chinese medical classics since the beginning of the common era. Particularly acute cases of sudden chaotic disorders could be treated by applying acupuncture needles to particular points on the surface of the skin. Nineteenth-century physicians such as Wang Shixiong had preferred treatment with liquid foods, drugs, and the scraping technique, but desperate situations called for the immediate application of acupuncture. This particular physician, however, had added a "modern" medicine to his repertoire, an "emergency rescue fluid" that was quite likely the kind of electrolyte replacement fluid that was commercially available in Tianjin's "Western medicine" drugstores. Perhaps the emergency rescue fluid was of dubious quality, or perhaps Mrs. Sun's violent vomiting had rendered such treatments useless, but Mrs. Sun received no relief from her experience with this healer.

Remarkably, Mrs. Sun then turned to the Japanese military stationed in her area for a cure. Just how Mrs. Sun encountered the Japanese medical officer is unclear, but the report suggests that she voluntarily sought him out. The fact that this remote industrial area of the city possessed a unit of the Japanese army illustrates the extensive reach of the Japanese occupation, and how much manpower was required to maintain it. The Japanese occupation had brought advanced modern biomedicine to this working-class district of Tianjin, but surprisingly, the Japanese doctor did not seem to respond to Mrs. Sun's illness with the most appropriate therapy available in the biomedical repertoire. Rather than immediately connect Mrs. Sun to a saline drip, he instead gave her oral electrolyte replacement in liquid and tablet form and sent her on her way. The blasé reaction of the Japanese medical officer is puzzling: He not only did not seem to care about Mrs. Sun's condition, but he also apparently did not notify military or civilian authorities about the presence of a potential cholera case, a certain breach of military discipline and public health regulations.

Disappointed in the results of her encounter with Japanese medicine, Mrs. Sun returned to her mother's home and sought out the help of a different doctor of Chinese medicine. Her actions mirrored the old Tianjin adage, "*You jibing qing san shi*" (If you are seriously sick, hire three different doctors to attend to you). More than just the solicitation of a "second opinion," Mrs. Sun's actions reflect an acceptance of different skill levels, different schools of thought, and different therapeutic approaches among healers. Physicians like Ding Zilang had sought to standardize Chinese medicine in Tianjin, and since the advent of the GMD regime, Chinese physicians desiring to be licensed by the government had to pass a standardized test that included questions on topics ranging from the Yellow Emperor's *Inner Cannon* to bacteriology.[66] Nevertheless, sufferers might value a family medical lineage more than a government license, and reputation among healers was built through association with hoary traditions or through advertised "proven success" in healing. The third healer, however, proved no more successful than the first one in his acupuncture technique.

Mrs. Sun then turned to a "doctor of Western medicine in Dazhigu" who did the right thing according to modern biomedicine and the public health directives of the city: He injected her with electrolyte solution and notified the local police. Given that he had no hesitation about interacting with local authorities, this physician was most likely a Chinese doctor of Western medicine who was licensed by the city government. Located not in the impressive neighborhoods of the French, British, or Italian Concessions, but in a peripheral location, this unnamed physician was most likely not one of Tianjin's medical elite, and may have been an employee of a nearby factory clinic. It is quite likely that the actions of this humble doctor, who had remained in Tianjin in spite of the Japanese occupation, saved Mrs. Sun's life.

The Chinese police, whose duties for the sanitary inspection of the city had begun along Japanese lines in 1902, came to the doctor's office and took the declining Mrs. Sun to the contagious disease hospital. There she was treated by Chinese doctors trained in Japanese medical schools, and her stool samples came under the scrutiny of Japanese bacteriologists at the Tianjin garrison hospital laboratory. Mrs. Sun survived, but it was probably not the end of suffering for her family. The police dispatched a medical squad to Mrs. Sun's mother's home "to conduct a thorough search and disinfection." This squad, which probably included Japanese soldiers, would have forced Mrs. Sun's relatives to an area isolation unit, where they would undergo observation and have to render up three stool samples to the doctors. Mrs. Sun's (most likely very meager) clothing, bedding, and possessions would be gathered up and burned. If perchance any of her relatives succumbed to cholera, their corpses would not be returned to the family, but would be quickly cremated by the Japanese military.

Timely intervention in Mrs. Sun's struggle with disease by agents of the Chinese collaborationist government and the Japanese military clearly resulted in her survival. Nevertheless, it is difficult to known how Mrs. Sun and her family may have interpreted these interventions. Mrs. Sun had first turned to Chinese medicine. She either had never heard or did not heed a decade of health department lectures warning that cholera could only be treated by Western medicine. It is quite likely that Mrs. Sun did not even call her illness *huoluan,* the "official" name for cholera, but may have called it *sha* or *li,* disorders marked by vomiting and loose stools but whose cause may have arisen from food, the environment, or pestilent *qi.*

In spite of an apparent preference for Chinese medicine, Mrs. Sun did not hesitate to turn to Western medicine, moreover, she went directly to a physician who was part of the invading force occupying her city. Perhaps it would be a mistake to assume that Mrs. Sun would be automatically adverse to being treated by an officer in the Japanese army. The Japanese military had occupied the city for a year, and her home had probably already been visited by Japanese sanitary inspectors. Perhaps Mrs. Sun had already been vaccinated for smallpox and for cholera by the Japanese military in the previous year (cholera vaccine only imparts a partial and temporary resistance to the cholera vibrio). In contrast to the Chinese who had tried to escape vaccination the previous year, Mrs. Sun did not seem to see the Japanese as a terrifying alien force. Perhaps the Japanese detachment in her area had become a fairly familiar presence, one seen as a potential source of medical services.

Through the course of this ordeal, Mrs. Sun finally found relief through encounters with needles and injection. In the past decade, the hypodermic needle had become a symbol of two disparate phenomena in treaty-port China: Western medicine and drug abuse. Police and health authorities in the 1920s and 1930s attempted to regulate the sale of hypodermic needles because of the potential for their abuse not only by drug addicts, but also by unlicensed healers claiming to be doctors of "Western medicine." If herbs and acupuncture needles typified Chinese medicine, then in the minds of many Chinese, Western medicine was marked by the knife and the syringe. With their propensity toward injection of vaccinations on a mass scale at the slightest indication of an impending epidemic, the Japanese military furthered the equation of *weisheng* with the needle-wielding, white-coated physician. In 1937, many Chinese had attempted to flee the advance of Japanese syringes, fearing they might contain a less than benevolent substance. Mrs. Sun, suffering from the devastating symptoms of cholera, in the end was saved by a Japanese intravenous drip. The course of Mrs. Sun's search for effective treatment complicates any assumptions about popular understandings of medical modernity. At the same time, it highlights how the benevolence of modern health was inextricably intertwined with a legacy of physical coercion.

Of all the forceful interventions practiced in the name of hygienic modernity by the occupation forces, only one aspect triggered violent resistance from the residents of Tianjin. Soon after the first cholera deaths at the contagious disease hospital in the summer of 1938, the health department held an emergency meeting to discuss the issue of corpse disposal. Those present, including Hou Fusang, department director Fu Ruqin, and five medical officers from the Japanese military, concluded that the most hygienic way to dispose of the corpses of cholera victims was to cremate them. A small crematorium for this purpose was quickly built near the contagious disease hospital in the former Russian Concession. All subsequent deaths were followed by cremation, and corpses that had already been buried were disinterred and burned.[67]

The first indication of resistance to this policy came from the Tianjin branch of the Chinese Islamic Association (Zhongguo huijiao hui). The leaders of Tianjin's Hui community petitioned the mayor and the health department, stating that cremation was a violation of their religious practice and requesting exemption for any Muslim victims of cholera. Considering the zeal with which other aspects of germ eradication were pursued by the occupation forces, it seems surprising that the petition request was granted. The bodies of all Han victims of the epidemic were burned, but two Hui victims were spared the crematorium.[68]

Resistance was also expressed through less formal channels. On the night of September 4, 1938, the ovens of the unguarded crematorium were secretly attacked and destroyed. There is no record of any investigation or prosecution in the health department records. But by this time, the cholera epidemic was already over, and the crematorium had served its purpose.[69]

CONCLUSION

Tianjin's memory of occupation under the Japanese is one of unrelenting hardship and humiliation. The picture of city life from the fall of north China in 1937 to the end of the Japanese empire in 1945 includes images of barbed wire, bayonets, cruel soldiers, and random murders. Rampant inflation and food shortages emmiserated previously comfortable families, and pushed poorer residents into malnutrition and starvation. Japanese military officers and functionaries of the Japanese army took over schools, public bureaus, and private companies. The drug smuggling, gambling, and prostitution associated with the Japanese Concession before 1937 became more open and widespread in the city, elevating local gang leaders to new heights of power. Male peasants and urban laborers were conscripted into coolie gangs and forced to work as slave labor on secret construction projects for the Japanese military. After their labor was no longer needed, the men were executed and their bodies dumped into the Hai River.

Although the occupation was undeniably a period of mass suffering and misfortune, for some it may have represented a high point in Tianjin's experience with a certain kind of hygienic modernity. The control of epidemic disease in occupied cities was an important priority for the Japanese military. Expertise in the technologies of Western biomedicine, including bacteriology and epidemiology, made the Japanese army well equipped to manage epidemics. Years of experience in military medicine and hygiene, traceable back to the first Sino-Japanese War, gave the Japanese strengths in organization and information management that were essential to the implementation of a successful modern epidemic control policy. Finally, this medical and organizational expertise was accompanied by a resolute policing capacity that made the management of germs swift and relatively unimpeded by competing interests. If modern bacteriological technology plus enhanced enforcement ability was a goal of hygienic modernity, then the Japanese army can be seen as representing the culmination of government-administered *weisheng* in treaty-port China.

This observation is both ironic and controversial, given that Japanese forces also used their ability to manage germs to inflict epidemic disease on the Chinese civilian population during the war. In the past two decades Japanese and American scholars have exposed the horrors of Japanese biological warfare experiments and campaigns in Manchuria and in central China, particularly the infamous activities of Unit 731.[70] In China the legacy of Japanese bacterial expertise is thoroughly dominated by the specter of germ warfare. Suggesting that Japanese public health enforcement in occupied China was the culmination of a specific stage of hygienic modernity is deeply offensive to some, an unworkable paradox to others.

One way of understanding this paradox is to allow that the Japanese military sought total control over bacteria in any area they occupied. This control may have meant the ability to prevent disease—or it may have entailed the ability to cause it. If one removes the moral dimension from a consideration of bacteriological sciences, then these abilities appear as two sides of the same coin. It may seem rather perverse that the official name for the Imperial Army's germ warfare unit was the Epidemic Prevention and Water Supply Department *(bôeki kyusui bu)*. Yet it is helpful to remind ourselves that Unit 731's infamous leader, Ishii Shirô, was a bacteriologist originally best known for his development of an individual water filtration system for field use by the Japanese military. Ever since the conquest of Taiwan in 1895, the Japanese army had been bedeviled by problems with gastrointestinal disease and had made the development of safe water supplies a top military priority. Ishii's water filtration apparatus was so effective that the scientist reportedly demonstrated the device by urinating into it and then drinking the filtered product.[71]

This confidence in the ability to cause and prevent epidemics at the same time may have been a form of fatal hubris for the Japanese military. The Japanese military was not entirely successful at protecting itself from intentionally spread germs. Japanese troops were among the victims of their own biological warfare campaign in Zhejiang in 1942, and it is possible that similar mistakes occurred at other points during the war.[72]

Opinion persists among some Chinese that the Japanese military intentionally spread epidemic disease in Tianjin during the war. Cholera rocked the city at least three times during the Japanese occupation, in 1937, 1938, and 1943. It is easy to see how the frequency of epidemics, the spread of stories about germ warfare in Manchuria, and the invasive vaccination and quarantine methods used by the Japanese during the occupation might have given rise to such suspicions. No solid evidence in support of this opinion has come to light. Nevertheless, it is difficult to state with confidence that the Japanese army would not have attempted to cause epidemics in a city like Tianjin, even if such a strategy would have seemed ill-advised. According to confessions recorded as late as 1954 from Japanese prisoners of war in Chinese Communist custody, a major branch of Unit 1855, the Japanese army's north China Epidemic Prevention and Water Supply Unit, was situated in Tianjin.[73] If this unit engaged in biological warfare in Tianjin, the personnel who oversaw the city's health department did not seem to have been informed of their intentions.

Had Tianjin been rendered a safe "sanitary zone" by the Japanese occupation? Was the period from 1937 to 1945 a culmination of hygienic modernity in Tianjin? If hygienic modernity entails both the effective interventions of government health policies and the effective internalization of the goals of the state, then the results of the occupation period are mixed. The resistance to the 1937 health inspections demonstrates that the Imperial Japanese Army had to negotiate its vigorous vision of hygienic modernity with a recalcitrant and suspicious population. At the same time, however, Chinese doctors complied with collaboration health department objectives and lectured Tianjin's residents on the benevolence of Japanese forced vaccinations. At least some working-class residents may have seen Japanese military physicians as local representatives of modern medicine. Coercion and desperation may have left Tianjin's people with little choice but to accept the presence of the Japanese doctors, soldiers, and vaccinators. And yet it is telling that after 1949, working-class residents of Tianjin faulted the new Communist health department for not coming to vaccinate them often enough. Previous regimes, they argued, had come to their neighborhoods to vaccinate them all the time, but the Communists seemed to have neither the will nor the resources to "pay attention to them" in the same way (see chapter 10). Might these "previous governments" have also included the Japanese occupation regime?

From another perspective, however, Japanese occupation-era *weisheng* policies fell decidedly short of a hygienic ideal. Vaccinating hundreds of thousands of individuals with cholera vaccine was an easier proposition for the Japanese army than ensuring that everyone in the city had a disease-free water supply. Conducting forced health inspections at gunpoint may have temporarily produced the transparent "governmentality" so desired by Japanese administrators, but it was of dubious utility in preventing or combating epidemics. Although powers of inspection and the resources for vaccination were desired by health administrators since the turn of the century, the enforcement of such a sanitary regime during the occupation instead represented the highest degree of convergence between hygienic modernity and the specter of Chinese victimhood at the hands of imperialism. The management of germs at gunpoint, ostensibly for the purpose of protecting the health of the Chinese people, coincided (in time, if not in location) with the use of germs as weapons in a war against them. Rumors that injections given by white-coated doctors caused, rather than prevented, disease was a common response to the role of the needle in modern biomedicine throughout the world.[74] Only in China during the 1930s and 1940s were such fears justified by the very real existence of an extensive enemy germ warfare program. During the Japanese occupation, the role of *weisheng* as a marker of inherent Chinese deficiency turned on the pivot of China as victim of violent imperialism. It was a moment that would establish *weisheng* as a potent basis for Chinese resistance against imperialism after the treaty ports had ceased to exist.

10 Germ Warfare and Patriotic *Weisheng*

March tempo, vigorously, with intense anger:
American imperialism, monstrously evil!
As it approaches the edge of doom,
It dares to use germ warfare against the people of China and Korea!
crescendo to fortissimo:
American imperialism, monstrously evil!
For the sake of the future of mankind,
We resolve to wipe out germ warfare.
Wipe out germ warfare!
Wipe it out!
Wipe it out!
Wipe out germ warfare, capture the germ warfare criminals,
Finish off the American imperialists and their stinking bugs
    and flies!
Wipe out germ warfare, capture the germ warfare criminals,
All of China, the whole world, must mobilize as one! Must mobilize
    as one!

"Wipe Out Germ Warfare!"
Words by GUO MORUO, Tune by LU JI
To be performed at Patriotic Hygiene Campaign mass meetings

In the winter of 1952, reports of American use of germ warfare in the Korean War hit the front pages of newspapers throughout the People's Republic of China. Government sources accused "American imperialists" *(Mei di)* of using biological weapons against innocent civilian populations in Manchuria. Radio addresses, banners, posters, and public announcements urged the populace to rise and fight against the evil insects, spiders, and bacteria that threatened to spread pestilence within China's borders. The weapon the Communists wielded against germ warfare was *weisheng*. Like the vision that had been embraced before by regimes throughout the twentieth century, this *weisheng* included personal cleanliness, environmental sanitation, compulsory vaccinations, suspicion of insects, and the scrutiny of germs. To a greater degree than any other public health movement in China, this *weisheng* also entailed mass mobilization through an unprecedented appeal to nationalism through the "Aiguo weisheng yundong": the Patriotic Hygiene Campaign.

The threat of germ warfare and the Patriotic Hygiene Campaign provided an opportunity for the Communist government to mobilize multiple levels of society. Workers, housewives, professors, and doctors dredged sewers, swatted flies, picked up garbage, and submitted to vaccinations in order to eliminate germs and defend the nation. If modernity for the Chinese Communist Party (CCP) meant that all citizens should be hypervigilant, intensely aware, and physically involved in the life of the nation, then hygienic modernity under the conditions of a biological threat was an excellent vehicle for the realization of this vision.

Whether the Patriotic Hygiene Campaign was launched in response to a real threat or was part of an elaborate hoax orchestrated by Communist leaders matters little from the perspective of this study.[1] The Patriotic Hygiene Campaign remains significant as both a continuation and culmination of the history of *weisheng* in urban China. The campaign was in many ways a continuation of the lectures, movements, and programs that treaty-port elites, Christian missionaries, and governments had been supporting for decades. The post-1949 *weisheng* message was a continuation from previous years, its content on germs and disease remarkably similar to the content of education programs from the 1910s, the Nanjing decade, and the Japanese occupation period. As in every period before 1949, the Communist government maintained an ideal of hygienic modernity, then struggled to achieve it with limited resources and personnel.

At the same time, the 1952 *weisheng* campaign represented an extreme version of the hygienic modernity that had gone before. In the past, hundreds of thousands of urban Chinese had been exposed to the message of *weisheng*. In 1952, millions of urban Chinese actively did *weisheng*. "Doing *weisheng*" included killing flies, dredging sewers, and picking up trash. Through the Patriotic Hygiene Campaign, consciousness of dirt and germs became manifest through an official language that became part of daily life, and *weisheng* became inextricably locked into association with cleanliness. Government agents monitored hygienic performance through public rallies and household inspections. Though a part of hygiene campaigns in the past (for example, the door-to-door inspections in Tianjin's Japanese Concession and under Japanese occupation), the penetration of state agents into private life became an accepted and routine part of life under the Communists.

The documentary record of alleged germ warfare attacks and the Patriotic Hygiene Campaign in the city of Tianjin provides a unique window into the governance and society of the early PRC. The germ warfare allegations and Patriotic Hygiene Campaign emerged within the highly charged political context of the early 1950s urban environment. During this uncertain, transitional time, the Communist government sought ways to modernize and rationalize urban society—to make it transparent and more permeable and to bring individuals into direct contact with the state. The Communist goal was aided by the powerful metaphor of germs as invisible enemies. This metaphor had been used since the early republican period, but China's experience during the Japanese occupation made it far more evocative of a potential reality. By waging war against germs throughout northern China's cities, the rural-based CCP could portray itself as a wielder of modern scientific knowledge, able to visualize, classify, and contain enemy germs hidden in insects, dirt, and in the bodies of individual Chinese. They did so not in the name of ruthless control and tyranny, but in the name of national defense and the pursuit of modernity.

HIDDEN DANGERS AND THE PURSUIT OF POLITICAL PURITY

On January 15, 1949, the Nationalist Army defending Tianjin surrendered to the People's Liberation Army (PLA). Compared to many other cities in China over the previous twelve years, Tianjin had been spared the ravages of war. Tianjin had exchanged hands three times since the Japanese invasion, but much of the fighting had taken place in the outer reaches of the city. Realizing they could not protect the city's core from the tens of thousands of troops the Communists had amassed outside the city, the Nationalists surrendered without fighting. This quick surrender meant that Tianjin's industries, banks, and mansions were spared the destruction of war. The new regime's task was not to rebuild a city, but to understand and ultimately control a city that had survived in all its complexity.[2] This complexity no longer included foreign concessions: The last of the imperial outposts were officially dissolved in 1943, and after the defeat of Japan, Tianjin became a city entirely administered by Chinese.

Tianjin was an important challenge for the rural-based Chinese Communists' shift to urban administration. Tianjin was north China's largest port, a finance and transportation hub that served as the link between the sea and Beijing, and between the south and Manchuria's vast resources. By the time it was "liberated," Tianjin's population of approximately four million had swelled with two hundred thousand civilian refugees and over one hundred thousand Nationalist troops, including thousands of undisciplined army deserters who had fled to Tianjin from battle zones in Manchuria. Landmines lurked under fields and roads, city neighborhoods remained blockaded in anticipation of street-to-street combat, and residents were fearful of the all-too-familiar postwar combination of rogue soldiers, commodity shortages, and hyperinflation. Into this confused and tense situation, the CCP dispatched a minute force of approximately seventy-four hundred civilian cadres, many of whom had just recently received crash courses in urban administration. This small core of small-town students, ex-farmers, and CCP underground operatives was charged with taking over all of Tianjin's urban functions and bringing the chaotic city under control.[3]

It is not surprising that the CCP was suspicious of Tianjin. Tianjin's defenses had collapsed in a remarkably short time, leaving many Nationalist troops, administrators, and sympathizers trapped within the city. For the Communists, GMD spies lurked everywhere: among poverty-stricken refugees, army deserters, students, clerks, and bureaucrats.[4] For this countrified Communist force (which had yet to capture Shanghai and other southern cities), Tianjin also represented the first encounter with a large treaty-port society, the very definition of foreign-influenced danger and decadence against which the Communists claimed to be fighting. Under the Japanese occupation, Tianjin had been the center of opium trade in north China, and certain neighborhoods within the city still teemed with opium shops and dealers. Tianjin had long been a center for various "heterodox" religious movements, many of which had elaborate hierarchies of command and membership. Guild/gangs, such as those that organized transportation workers, controlled many of Tianjin's most important services. All of these elements were suspicious, not only because they represented alternate networks of power to the government, but also because they represented the anathema of the Communist vision of a pure, New China. Although they had gained experience dealing with cities in Manchuria, Tianjin's urban landscape represented a new level of complexity and obscurity.

Adding to the complexity of the situation, hostilities broke out between U.N. (American) forces and North Korea less than eighteen months after Tianjin had been "liberated." By the fall of 1950, Chinese troops were fighting Americans on the bitter Korean front, across the Bohai Gulf from Tianjin. War in Korea intensified the CCP dread of internal enemies lurking in inscrutable and impenetrable urban spaces.

The fear of political impurity and invisible enemies shaped CCP actions in Tianjin from Liberation through the early 1950s. Immediately after taking the city, PLA troops and cadres set about rounding up Nationalist soldiers and shipping potentially disruptive refugees back to their homes in the countryside.[5] The great "cleanup" of Tianjin continued in 1950–51 with the Campaign to Suppress Counterrevolutionaries (Zhenya fangeming yundong).[6] In this campaign, the CCP arrested thousands of gang leaders,

TABLE 3. Major Political Campaigns in Tianjin, 1949–53

Campaign	Date
Suppress Counterrevolutionaries I	Spring–Fall 1949
Resist America, Aid Korea	October 1950–July 1953
Suppress Counterrevolutionaries II*	February–July 1951
Three-Anti Campaign	December 1951–June 1952
Five-Anti Campaign	January–June 1952
Thought Reform Campaign	November 1951–June 1952
Patriotic Hygiene Campaign	February–July 1952

*This campaign included movements against prostitutes, drug dealers, and religious sects.

drug smugglers, religious sect leaders, and alleged Nationalist spies, and executed hundreds. A wide-scale program was launched to crack down on petty criminals, beggars, and prostitutes.[7] Several new campaigns arose in 1952 that were aimed at the professional classes. The Five-Anti Campaign was designed to undermine the authority of China's capitalists and managers by targeting the five "crimes" of bribery, tax evasion, theft of state property, cheating on contracts, and stealing state economic information. The Three-Anti Campaign sought to rectify three "common defects" of Communist cadres: corruption, waste, and "obstructionist bureaucracy." Finally, the Thought Reform Movement (Sixiang gaizao yundong) penetrated institutions of higher education and professional services. Intellectuals who had previously thought of themselves as benignly progressive or politically neutral now had to announce their allegiance to the masses publicly and undergo "consciousness raising" to ensure a proper outlook.[8]

All of these campaigns sought to eliminate the strength of nonstate organizations and replace diffuse hierarchies of authority in civil society with direct ties of loyalty (and control) between the individual and the state. Ultimately the overlapping of so many campaigns resulted in a concentrated atmosphere of suspicion and confusion in many sectors of Chinese society (see table 3 for a detailed chronology). In mass meetings, radio broadcasts, and daily newspapers, the state called upon the populace to expose evildoers, confess crimes, and eliminate "poisonous germs" *(dujun)* from the body politic. Constant media repetition of the words *tanwu* (corruption) and *tanbai* (confession) made aural and visual messages of pollution *(wu)* and purity *(bai)* the predominant motifs of the early 1950s. From 1949 to 1952, as the state executed GMD spies, compelled businessmen and bureaucrats to confess to crimes, and purged cadres of incorrect thoughts, vectors of political contagion were eliminated, and society was inoculated against internal pathogens.

THE HEALTH OF THE CITY

While the Communists tended to the political "health" of the city, the corporal health of the city was also a major concern. Alleviating the illnesses of the poor was one of the commitments of the Communist Revolution. In Tianjin, cadres consciously pursued health policies that would visibly demonstrate the benefits of their regime to the masses. The Communists inherited a city whose health was divided. In certain areas, most residents drank tap water and had adequate nutrition. In other areas, people drank water out of stagnant ponds and faced starvation. In 1949, infectious diseases such as tuberculosis, neonatal tetanus, dysentery, and encephalitis were the most common causes of death in Tianjin, the result of poverty, poor nutrition, inadequate housing, contaminated water supply, and a dearth of obstetric services and infant care. Epidemics still loomed even after Liberation. A small but alarming outbreak of bubonic plague in Manchuria threatened Tianjin in the winter of 1949. In the summer of 1950, a cholera epidemic swept through the city.[9]

Although Communist histories suggest that the CCP brought public health to cities that had previously been devoid of any organizational infrastructure, the Communists in Tianjin actually inherited a system of district health stations, public hospitals, and isolation hospitals from the Nationalists, who had in turn built their infrastructure on warlord and concession governments from previous decades.[10] Tianjin was a city with relatively abundant medical resources. The problem was their unequal distribution. To solve these all-too-familiar public health problems, a great deal of work would have to be done to raise basic standards of living and to build up a public health infrastructure; improvements that would require a tremendous investment of time, money, and personnel from the new government.

The new Tianjin municipal health bureau tackled these problems with considerable enthusiasm but limited resources. The bureau adjusted its priorities to reflect the realities of the situation: (1) place prevention above treatment; (2) promote a "serve the people" mentality in health workers; (3) cultivate more health workers with a basic level of education; and (4) pay attention to the laboring masses.[11] The way the bureau attempted to fulfill these goals can be summarized by examining their actions at two sites of *weisheng:* water supply and the management of hospitals.

The new municipal health bureau placed considerable emphasis on the provisioning of water for the city's poor. The Communists had taken over the Native City Waterworks, but tens of thousands of people in the city were not serviced by this network. According to a water-use survey conducted in the spring of 1950, 1,619,922 people in Tianjin, or 89 percent of the city's population, used treated water, mostly water purchased from neighborhood water shops. But 96,921 people still drank water that came directly from the river, and 4,761 poverty-stricken people drank from local ponds/cesspools. The survey paid particular attention to the south branch of the Grand Canal, traditionally the source of Tianjin's drinking water. The Communists were appalled by what they found. Water carriers still took water from the canal at dozens of locations, but more than one hundred sewage ditches drained into the canal near these sites. Toilets, pigpens, and garbage lined both sides of the canal.[12]

The health bureau recognized that it would be impossible to extend the water supply network to serve everyone in Tianjin before the next summer "cholera season" arrived. Instead, they devised a plan to use boats with water tanks aboard to distribute clean water to the poor living along the banks of the Grand Canal. The inexperienced cadres who had devised the plan had not thought through all the details of the actual execution. It took several months to find the funding to rent the boats and pay the laborers necessary to launch the scheme. Once the huge water tanks were hoisted aboard, the boats rocked so violently that they almost tipped over. It took several more weeks before this engineering problem could be solved and water could finally be distributed to the city's poor.[13]

People were grateful, progress reports stated, and yet the poor had other complaints. The Communists had put their emphasis on the provisioning of clean drinking water and the management of the urban infrastructure, the very things that had been relatively neglected by previous administrations. But when cadres went into the poor neighborhoods, they were surprised to find that people complained about the Communist's lack of commitment to the poor. Remarkably, their criterion for a concerned government revolved around the hypodermic needle. "Before Liberation," poor residents were reported as saying, "the government was constantly coming here and vaccinating us. But after Liberation we don't have the chance to be 'hit by the needle' [da zhen]. The government is not paying as much attention to us."[14] Through the Nationalist and Japanese occupation regimes, *weisheng* became associated with vaccination. It would take several more months before the Communist health infrastructure would produce enough vaccines to resume the type of mass vaccination schedules that the poor had begun to see as a marker of government benevolence.

At the opposite end of the public health hierarchy, the Communists gradually took over Tianjin's foreign hospitals. This phase involved the judicious handling of the most sophisticated medical elites in the city: the Chinese physicians who worked in Tianjin's various missionary hospitals and the large Mackenzie Memorial Hospital in the British Settlement. In preparation for making the hospitals part of the state-owned public health network, the CCP sent cadres to take inventories of all the equipment and staff of each hospital. The Communists then secretly cultivated informants within the hospitals to collect information on any anti-CCP comments or appearance of any *qin Mei* (close with America) attitudes among hospital staff.[15] Communists were particularly suspicious of the political sentiments of Chinese physicians who had worked with foreigners. Not only were they solidly bourgeois, but they also saw the foreign presence in China as a benevolent phenomenon. *Qin Mei* attitudes were considered highly subversive in the environment of the Korean War and the recent germ warfare attacks in Manchuria.[16]

Communist suspicion of Western-trained physicians was a theme of *Minglang de tian* (Bright skies), a 1954 play by the famous Tianjin playwright, Cao Yu. Cao Yu spent his career criticizing foreign imperialism; his best known work, *Richu* (Sunrise, 1935), was a drama, set in the Tianjin French Concession's Grand Hotel, that exposed the decadent ways of foreign-influenced Chinese. *Bright Skies* is set in an American-founded hospital in Beijing (obviously modeled on Peking Union Medical College). There Communist cadres try to guide foreign-trained Chinese physicians to understand the evil nature of foreign imperialism. The hospital's chief bacteriologist, Dr. Ling, refuses to believe that his former colleagues were evil until he is convinced by evidence of American germ warfare. Inspired to patriotism, he takes up his microscope to serve his country by joining medical workers on the Korean front. "This microscope has been keeping me company for thirty years, all for nothing," muses Dr. Ling. "Now . . . the time has come for me to render some real service to my country and make my microscope really useful."[17] Dr. Ling's recalcitrance and his eventual embrace of the Communist spirit of "serving the people" reflected one of the major goals of the Patriotic Hygiene Campaign: the mobilization of the entire nation— including the nation's medical elites—to fight against imperialism through the vehicle of health and hygiene. The metaphor of "enemies as germs" had shaped and sustained the Communist's first attempts at intervening in local society—the campaigns that focused on specific groups such as prostitutes, capitalists, and cadres. Now the idea of "germs as enemies" would offer a new vehicle for an even more widespread intervention, one that would encompass both housewives and professors, factory workers and physicians.

GERM WARFARE AND THE PATRIOTIC HYGIENE CAMPAIGN

The first official news of germ warfare in the Korean War came on February 23, 1952, when the *People's Daily* carried a front-page editorial denouncing "the appalling crime of the American aggressors in Korea in using bacteriological warfare." Daily reports of germ warfare activities continued throughout February. The campaign against the United States gained worldwide recognition on March 8, 1952, when Zhou Enlai issued a statement through the Hsinhua News Agency calling upon all nations to condemn the "U.S. Imperialists' War Crime" of germ warfare *(xijun zhan)*. The inflammatory rhetoric heightened in intensity after reports announced that the United States had extended germ warfare into China as far south as Qingdao.[18]

Internal documents of the Tianjin municipal health bureau record eight germ-warfare attacks experienced by the city in the summer of 1952. The case presented below is particularly rich in detail, but is typical in most aspects:

> Case #4: June 9, 1952. Insects were first discovered at noon near the pier at the Tanggu Workers Union Hall. At 12:40 P.M., insects were discovered at the New Harbor Works Department, and at 1:30, in Beitang town. Insects were spread over an area of 2,002,400 square meters in New Harbor, and for over twenty Chinese miles [approximately ten kilometers] along the shore at Beitang. Insect elimination was carried out under the direction of the Tianjin Municipal Disinfection Team [Xiaodu dui; literally, Poison Eradication Team]. Masses organized to assist in catching insects included 1,586 townspeople, 300 soldiers, and 3,150 workers. Individual insects were collected and then burned, boiled, or buried. Insect species included inchworms, snout moths, wasps, aphids, butterflies . . . giant mosquitoes, etc. Samples of the insects were sent to the Central Laboratory in Beijing, where they were found to be infected with typhoid bacilli, dysentery bacilli, and para-typhoid.[19]

Many of the Tianjin cases displayed a heightened visual scrutiny of nature in action. According to internal reports, the initial sightings of potential germ-warfare vectors came from vigilant citizens. Internal reports indicate that these sightings were not the result of plants or hoaxes, but that citizen-activists spotted what they considered to be biological anomalies in the natural environment. To these vigilant observers, insects not only suddenly appeared before the eye, they loomed large and menacing as inherently evil carriers of deadly germs.

Months of reports, accusations, and propaganda that saturated the Chinese media during the germ warfare allegations seemed to have produced this heightened visual awareness of the natural environment. New ways of seeing the smallest of insects—and imagining in the mind's eye the existence of invisible bacteria they might contain—had been fostered by a barrage of microscopic representations in the national media. Newspaper reports also prominently featured entomological descriptions of antennae, wings, and mandibles of the insects that threatened China. Close-up photographs of invading flies, fleas, mosquitoes, and other less-recognizable species were published together with numerous political cartoons featuring insects and rodents.[20] These cartoons depicted U.S. imperialism as a Grim Reaper riding the back of a housefly (see Fig. 10), or showed Western political leaders releasing diseased rats upon the Chinese population. In addition, a large-scale exhibit on the "American war crime of germ warfare" toured major cities throughout China in the spring of 1952. The national exhibit arrived in Tianjin on March 12, 1952, and was seen by almost two hundred thousand individuals. Among its many images, the exhibit featured large magnifications of insect heads with hairy antennae and multicompartment eyes, looming dark and menacing over audiences of school children and workers.[21]

Exhibits and newspapers also rendered microbes visible to a mass audience. Depictions of bacteria appeared in a variety of manifestations: as streaks on the surfaces of petri dishes, as cloudy masses suspended in test tubes, and as stained rods appearing in the circular field of a microscope. These images invited viewers to come face to face with invisible agents of death. Colonies of anthrax and plague bacteria, captured and cultured by Communist authorities, simultaneously alarmed viewers and assured them that the People's science had the skill to contain the threat. Seen by millions of people throughout China, such images defined an insect, rodent, and bacterial menace. Objects once unseen or unnoticed in nature now threatened the very existence of the new nation.

There is no direct evidence that the Patriotic Hygiene Campaign was launched in order to improve shortcomings in domestic public health. The fear of germ-warfare attacks was palpably real. And yet in Tianjin, it is clear that the Patriotic Hygiene Campaign helped to rectify, at least temporarily, the problems of the city's public health administration. Hygiene education became the main subject in newspapers, radio addresses, and public lectures. Officials at the highest levels placed priority on public health work. Build-

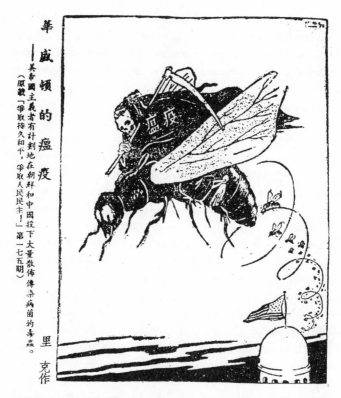

Figure 10. "The Washington Plague." Korean-War era cartoon depicting the Grim Reaper leading a swarm of pestilential flies out of the U.S. Capitol building. *Fujian ribao* (Fujian daily), 30 March 1952.

ing on republican-era precedent, the government established its own system of public health stations *(weisheng zhan)*, thus providing a higher profile for the new government's public health bureau in the city's more peripheral neighborhoods. The CCP took advantage of the patriotism of the moment to harmonize relations between the relatively uneducated cadres who administered the health department and the city's more sophisticated medical professionals who chafed at being under their direction. Yet most important for a cash-strapped and personnel-deficient program, the mass mobilizations of the Patriotic Hygiene Campaign turned average citizens into an army of volunteer public health and sanitation workers. By the summer of 1952, hundreds of thousands of men, women, and children stood poised to annihilate the biological and environmental enemies of New China.

The Patriotic Hygiene Campaign consisted of two major phases: the Five

Annihilations (Wu mie) and the Big Cleanup (Da qingsao).[22] The Five Annihilations resulted in the formation of mass armies arrayed against nature's
tiny vectors of imperialism. In the spring of 1952, China's citizens were called
upon to eliminate the Five Pests: flies, mosquitoes, mice and rats, lice, and
bedbugs.[23] Even when germ warfare attacks were not suspected, individuals in factories, offices, and schools throughout China were expected to kill
and count any creeping or flying life-form they encountered.

The insect extermination teams detailed in Tianjin's germ-warfare-
attack reports exemplify the grand scale of the Five Annihilations mobilizations. In these public performances, thousands of workers and soldiers
were equipped with gauze masks, cotton sacks, gloves, and chopsticks and
then directed to scour hundreds of acres of land for suspicious insects. Individuals picked up insects one by one from the ground with their chopsticks and stuffed them into their collection sacks. The bug harvest was then
turned over to public health officials for counting, analysis, and destruction.
Rodents, too, were targeted for systematic annihilation. Unlike insects, which
were to be captured by hand, rats were killed with traps and poisons. In spite
of this distancing from the actual death of larger vermin, rat annihilation
did contain a hands-on element. Today elderly Tianjin residents still recall
chopping off the tails of hundreds of dead rats—the harvest from one neighborhood's Five Annihilations exercise—to facilitate tabulation by public
health authorities.[24]

In the Big Cleanup phase of the campaign, women and others who labored inside the home were mobilized to clear, dredge, and sweep the city
clean. In Tianjin, hundreds of thousands of housewives, joined by university and high school students, helped to clear miles of the city's stagnant
and odiferous drainage canals.[25] Residents supplied with picks, shovels, and
shoulder-poles filled in more than seven hundred cesspools, one bucketful
of soil at a time. Neighborhood cleanups removed tons of trash from domestic interiors and from public spaces: old derelict temples, opera halls, and
street corners.

A combination of peer pressure, sociability, and patriotism created this
unprecedented mobilization of the undermobilized. The government employed neighborhood committees, household visits, and persistent "sleeping platform" *(kangtou)* discussions to convince housewives, retirees, and
others to concern themselves with domestic hygiene. Household labor was
monitored through committee inspection of domestic interiors. At the same
time, neighborhood committees also organized women to sweep streets and
do washing out of doors. These neighborhood groups may have had a certain social appeal, as they resembled more convivial rural settings for

women's domestic work. Without a certain element of patriotism and a sense of contributing to the nation, however, it is difficult to see how so many housewives could have labored shoulder to shoulder with high school and college students in Tianjin's numerous sewer-dredging bucket brigades.[26]

As the Patriotic Hygiene Campaign came to a close, cadres evaluated its success. Hundreds of thousands of people had been vaccinated, tons of garbage had been removed, and tens of thousands of people had participated in mass insect killings and cleanups. Nevertheless, officials were disappointed at the rates of participation and realized that more had to be done to maintain the hygienic vigilance of the population. In 1953, Tianjin's Patriotic Hygiene Campaign Committee developed newer, more tempting incentives to encourage participation in the second round of annihilations and cleanups. Individuals who achieved the designation of "hygienic exemplar" *(weisheng mofang)* would be offered more money, more attractive crimson banners, and more privileges than in the previous year.

The Patriotic Hygiene Campaign was born at a moment when the CCP portrayed germs as foreign enemies rather than as a part of an indigenous Chinese terrain of deficiency. For a moment, the enemy that had to be overcome in order for China to achieve sovereignty and modernity was one from without, not one from within. The path to *weisheng* became indigenized, represented by a healthy cadre whose years in the countryside had given him robust features and a genuine concern for the Chinese people. Nevertheless, the standards taken up by the Chinese Communists for the new nation were still primarily those of modern biomedicine. Moreover, from the perspective of the new regime, the campaign ultimately failed to produce an adequately hygienic populace: deficiencies still lurked beneath the surface of patriotism. During the 1952 mobilizations, there was considerable foot dragging and ignoring of the government's objectives. For every *jiji fenzi* (activist from local society) who joined a neighborhood domestic hygiene inspection team, there were many more who failed to see any connection whatsoever between sweeping the floor and defending the nation against germs.[27] Apparently fear of biological weapons was not an entirely adequate motivation to compel the masses to become hygienically modern.

For the CCP, the gap between an individually internalized state of hygienic modernity and China's reality continued to exist well past the 1950s. The Patriotic Hygiene Campaign outlasted the Korean War germ warfare allegations and extended into the years of the Great Leap Forward and the Cultural Revolution. The campaign continues even today in a postsocialist China. Its basic goal remains to "change habits, improve customs, and transform the nation," a massive task accomplished by simultaneously promoting hygiene and eradicating the Four Pests. Officials still hold that the Patriotic Hygiene Campaign had not only been necessary in the past, when China's economy and culture were "backward," but is necessary even today in an era of "improving livelihoods and advancing levels of civilization."[28] In the eyes of the Communist regime, *weisheng* is still something that resides at some distance away from the Chinese people.

CONCLUSION

The goals of the Patriotic Hygiene Campaign represented the culmination of the goals of *weisheng* since Nagayo Sensai first used the word to summarize an essential technology of modernity. In the Patriotic Hygiene Campaign the health of the individual was equated with the health of the nation. The threat to the corporal nation was portrayed as a threat to the individual body as "foreign" germs penetrated New China's borders. In order to maintain the integrity of the nation's health, individuals were mobilized to act as though their own health was inseparable from the health of the collective. This was a vision of hygienic modernity held dear by Japanese bureaucrats, late Qing reformers, GMD modernizers, and CCP cadres alike: a system that combined government institutions and individual participation to form the basis of a national health. Achieving this national health would in turn guarantee the status and sovereignty of the nation against the threat of foreign imperialism.

The Patriotic Hygiene Campaign's technique of intensive intervention into society in the name of *weisheng* was not a new Communist phenomenon. The government-mandated lectures and propaganda meetings of 1952 would have been familiar to anyone who had lived through the GMD's New Life Movement. Government-mandated inspections of homes, conducted by local elites on behalf of the state, would have been biannual occurrences for anyone who had lived in the Japanese Concession of Tianjin during the 1920s and 1930s, and was experienced by everyone in the city during the Japanese occupation. The mass vaccinations of hundreds of thousands of people during the Patriotic Hygiene Campaign were also nothing new to Tianjiners; voluntary vaccination against smallpox had begun in the mid-nineteenth century, and the administration with hypodermic needles of mandatory vaccinations to the masses was a phenomenon that had begun as early as the warlord period and reached a high point during the Japanese occupation. Indeed, by the end of the first half of the twentieth century, the intervention of the government in policing and promoting health—one crucial aspect of *weisheng*—was not something that automatically inspired resistance in Tianjin, but had instead become a basic criterion that determined a government's legitimacy.

Urban residents may have clearly expected their governments to have a responsibility for the *weisheng* of the city by 1952, but it is not entirely clear to what extent their participation in the Patriotic Hygiene Campaign represented an internalized embrace of the state's hygienic goals. All hygiene education, from the programs of the YMCA to the policies of Japanese colonial administration, had sought to produce new citizens through the inculcation of new modes of decorum and cleanliness. It would be a sign of desirable modern governmentality if the state no longer needed to "enforce *weisheng [eisei]* where it was lacking," as determined Japanese administrators vowed to do in the aftermath of Japan's 1877–79 cholera epidemic. Armed soldiers attempted to force young men to relieve themselves in designated spots during the 1900–1902 occupation of Tianjin and similar indiscretions remained a crime under Chinese administration, but generations of reformers still hoped that education could ultimately supplant policing to produce hygienically modern individuals and a hygienically modern society. Embattled modernizers of the Nationalist era questioned the progress that common Chinese had made toward this goal, in spite of various efforts at generating hygienic "uplift" like Chiang Kai-shek's New Life Movement. Some thinkers, such as the eugenicist Pan Guangdan, proclaimed the entire "uplift" enterprise a folly: China's governments would be doomed to forever indoctrinating an unfit Chinese Everyman in a hygienic modernity that he was incapable of achieving. Rather than pursue a course of altering behaviors, Pan counseled the alteration of genetic material as the only way out for China. The CCP has proved itself an inheritor of both the optimistic program of the GMD New Life reformer and the hardnosed scientific pessimism of republican-era eugenicists. As Frank Dikötter has pointed out, the present-day government of the PRC combines massive propaganda campaigns on health and well-being with explicit eugenics laws that require the sterilization of married individuals deemed genetically "unfit."[29] *Weisheng* once tutored individuals in the art of producing healthy and numerous progeny through the imbibing of medicines and the nurturing of vitalities. In the twentieth century, *weisheng* compelled the state to create a hygienically modern nation in order to counter the specter of national deficiency.

Conclusion

Throughout the twentieth century, *weisheng* became an instrumental discourse informing the Chinese elite's vision of a modern ideal, a vehicle through which they hoped state, society, and the individual would be transformed. As grasped by Meiji bureaucrats, late Qing reformers, and Guomindang modernizers, *weisheng* centered concerns of national sovereignty, institutional discipline, and government administration on the site of the body. In an uncanny way, the single modern Chinese term *weisheng* encompasses what Foucault called " biopower," a series of techniques through which the state undertakes the administration of life, and "governmentality," the idea that individuals internalize disciplinary regimes and thus harmonize their own behaviors with the goals of the state. I am not suggesting that Nagayo Sensai, Yuan Shikai, and Mao Zedong were all prescient poststructuralists. Rather, beginning with Meiji reformers, modernizing elites in East Asia, from their perspective on the outside of the European Enlightenment project, quickly grasped some of the core elements that made the West appear "modern" and sought to employ them as "full kits" to transform their own societies. Scholars have debated whether or not modernity actually functions in the ways described by Foucault. The point here is not whether or not Chinese modernity worked along Foucauldian lines. Rather, the goal has been to understand how Chinese elites envisioned modernity and sought to transform the nation.

I have only occasionally hinted at how subalterns intersected with this vision: as objects of police control during the 1900–1902 occupation, as Dark Drifters who foiled plans for hygienic water and sewer solutions for Tianjin, as glue boilers and sheep slaughterers who offended the hygienic sensibilities of elites and the state, and as suspicious masses who attempted to escape from advancing Japanese vaccinators. Occasionally intriguing actions and voices emerge from the reports of collaborationist physicians or Communist health officers—textile factory workers who sought out medical assistance from the Japanese army, urban poor who complained about not getting vaccinated—evidence that further complicates our emerging understanding about the relationship between Chinese common people and foreign (particularly Japanese) imperialism.

But in general this has not been a study of the popular reception of *weisheng,* but a glimpse at how *weisheng* was used, by a segment of the elite, to transform a city and to establish their own identity as "moderns." The acquisition of *weisheng* by the elite—manifest in domestic plumbing, flush toilets, foreign underwear, and a knowledge of germs—allowed them both to distinguish themselves from the masses and at times to unify their interests with the foreign presence in China. In the eyes of many elites, the hygienic transformation of the common man and thus of the nation was never complete. Modernizers embraced *weisheng* as the basis for a discourse of Chinese deficiency: it was that which the Chinese lacked, and that which the foreign Other possessed.

An elite embrace of hygienic modernity came through several simultaneous paths: education in missionary schools or Western-influenced Chinese schools, exposure to YMCA programs, the purchase of imported *weisheng* commodities. Ironically it also seemed to manifest itself at moments when the foreign presence was most violent. Some Tianjin elites could applaud the way that the foreign occupation government brought hygienic order to the city even as Japanese soldiers were beheading accused Boxers. After suffering defeat at the hands of Meiji Japan in the Sino-Japanese War and after ten thousand Japanese soldiers had stormed the gates of Tianjin, Qing reformers employed Japanese advisors and a Japanese model of hygienic modernity in the city's new government. These events, played out in Tianjin but not unique to that city, question the assumption that Chinese elites may have enthusiastically embraced modernity (in contrast with the ambivalence and resistance of India) because semicolonialism in China was less violent and the colonizer less of a constant presence than in colonialisms elsewhere.

The seemingly unambivalent embrace of a foreign-defined modernity by dominant Chinese elites has recently been taken up by a several scholars, including John Fitzgerald, Shu-mei Shih, and Prasenjit Duara. Fitzgerald has suggested that this embrace occurred in large part because Chinese elites took to heart the colonial representations of a deficient John Chinaman. Denying claims that semicolonialism was less onerous than colonialism, Fitzgerald argues that the "psychological" effects of the foreign portrayal of Chinese deficiencies were as significant for Chinese as similar racist representations were for indigenous people elsewhere (as described in the works of Ashis Nandy and Frantz Fanon), even if the influence of these representations "happened to be felt in different ways."[1] Fitzgerald suggests that Chinese elites embraced this discourse of deficiency because it allowed them to position themselves as "awakeners of the people" and by extension, as the builders and controllers of a powerful centralized state.[2] Shu-mei Shih has suggested that elites embraced colonial modernity through two processes of bifurcation: first by suppressing the foreign as colonizer in favor of the foreign as cosmopolitan, and second, by separating Shanghai as a site of colonial exploitation from Shanghai as a site of global capitalist modernity. Significantly, Shih adds a consideration of the role that Japan plays in facilitating these strategies. Chinese modernists embrace the West through Japan, a place at once foreign but familiar, modern yet bearing underlying similarities to China.[3]

In this study the embrace of discourses of deficiency—and a discovery of methods for escaping this deficiency through the "awakening of the people" and the establishment of a strong state—coalesced around the term *weisheng*. A focus on life and events in a specific locale has highlighted the frustrations, violence, and everyday hardships that attended this embrace. It also provides other insights into the mystery of why "Chinese History," using Duara's formulation for the master narrative generated by Chinese elites and the state, is so "unabashedly modern"; or, in other words, why China produced a modernizing Mao, and not a Gandhi who questioned the very underpinnings of "Western civilization."[4]

The first insight is that a great deal of the rhetoric of Chinese deficiency and Western superiority revolved around modern biomedicine, science, and the body: the very items encompassed by the term *weisheng*. China was made into the Sick Man of Asia, his deficiencies measurable in terms of mortality rates and the number of bacteria (from a sample of indigenous feces or sputum) that could be cultured in a laboratory petri dish. For most Chinese elites, science became an irresistible universal way of perceiving the world and judging themselves, perhaps, as Prasenjit Duara has suggested, because religion for Chinese elites had far more political than religious significance, thereby enabling them to disregard religious for secular authority.[5] But one must also take into account that science and biomedicine appealed widely to Chinese elites at a specific time in the history of imperialism. Chinese disregard for the medical component of imperialism before 1900 stemmed in part from the inability of "Western" medicine or public health to offer much in the way of instrumental knowledge, not only for cure of individual bodies, but for the organization of governments or the ordering of society. It is perhaps not a coincidence that Chinese nationalism in its most familiar form only emerged after 1900, at a time that coincided with the violent arrival of a politicized sanitary science that was used to reconstruct cities, order society, and transform human beings.

A second insight that is provided by a focus on health and hygiene in Tianjin is to highlight the importance of Japan. If most Chinese elites embraced modernity without suspicions (in comparison with India), this embrace was in great part a result of the mediating role played by Japan. Japan gave Chinese observers a model of nonwhite modernity, a successful copy of the European way of progress produced by a fellow Asian nation. A consideration of Tianjin highlights the significant role played by Japan in shaping the ways Chinese imagined modernity. Tianjin was home to Japan's most active concession. The Japanese involvement in the Boxer suppression brought Japanese soldiers as well as Japanese advisors to the city. The twentieth century began with the adoption of Japanese models to transform the city's police, hospitals, and public health. The very term for health and hygiene was the product of the physician-bureaucrats of the Meiji regime, something true not only for Tianjin, but for the rest of China as well. Many elites in Tianjin welcomed Japanese as sympathetic tutors who offered a bridge between a shared Asian past and a promising decolonized future. The presence of a "yellow modernity" may have eliminated for some Chinese the alienating distance between themselves and a distant "white modernity." Shu-mei Shih has called this strategy, as employed by Shanghai intellectuals, "loving the Other through Japan."[6] Prasenjit Duara has drawn attention to the persuasive power of transnational rhetoric that emphasized common cultural and historical ties between China and Japan.[7] Perhaps ties created through a shared vision of modernity—based on an ideal of strong states, science, and hygienic modernity—linked China with Japan as strongly as ties that rested on reminders of a common cultural past. Such ties of common modernity, cultivated between Chinese and Japanese over a brief period at the beginning of the twentieth century, even survived the devastating war between the two countries and helped determine the characteristics of the Chinese revolution and the modern Chinese nation. This connection between Japan and the PRC can be traced vividly through an examination of *eisei/weisheng* as hygienic modernity, from Nagayo Sensai's 1875 reinvention of *eisei*, to the mass mobilizations of the Patriotic Hygiene Campaigns.

. . .

Throughout the one-hundred-year existence of China's treaty ports, the creation of hygienic modernity entailed a considerable amount of linguistic forgetting. By 1952, the term *weisheng* would no longer be associated with quotations from *Zhuangzi*, methods of circulating *qi*, or herbal medicines that bolstered vitality. By the mid-twentieth-century, *weisheng* had become an official discourse on health, one that brought the body and its conditions directly under the knowing regimes of science and the state. In a process begun through translations undertaken in Shanghai, Osaka, and Tokyo in the late nineteenth century and put into effect by armies, missionaries, and Chinese modernizers in the early twentieth century, *weisheng* shifted away from Chinese cosmology and was realigned to reside in chemistry, physiology, and anatomy. Bodies and environmental influences were now quantified, measured, and tested. This way of envisioning health and disease as outcomes of chemicals and bacteria possessed legitimacy because it was based on universal standards of science rather than culturally specific (and scientifically questionable) Chinese methods of ordering the natural world.[8]

Other ways of talking about health and illness certainly continued to exist in twentieth-century China: the rise of a "scientific" *weisheng* as hygienic modernity did not at all entail a simultaneous demise of the Chinese approaches to health detailed in the first two chapters of this study. Thinking about food in terms of correlative cosmology, taking herbal medicines and supplements based on unique individual bodily configurations, and practicing meditative movement to circulate vitalities remain as widely dispersed forms of knowledge, possessed in various forms by different strata of the population. These manifestations of a former Way of Guarding Life also remain the object of study, veneration, and elaboration for hundreds of thousands of scholars and practitioners of Chinese ways of healing. The rise of *weisheng* as hygienic modernity, however, effectively pushed these approaches to health to a realm just outside of the legitimate public discourses of science. From the PRC government's perspective, they now exist primarily under the rubric of *yangsheng*, literally "nurturing life," related to a newly configured "Traditional Chinese Medicine." Marked as part of "Chinese tradition," they retain an aura of cultural legitimacy, but in order to become publicly legitimate forms of knowledge about health, they must be submitted to the universalizing logic of science. Traditional Chinese Medicine and its attendant arts live on (in an altered state) within officially sanctioned schools and hospitals, but they are constantly subjected to government-funded investigations into the "scientific" nature of traditional Chinese medicines or the "actual" mechanisms underlying the beneficial effects of *daoyin* exercise (or *qigong*).[9] Official attempts at combining Chinese and Western medicine *(zhongxi jiehe)* under the PRC demonstrate both the cultural/national value of Chinese medicine and the impossibility that Chinese "traditions" can exist unambiguously in the modern era.[10] Millions of Chinese, believing in the empirical and time-tested value of *yangsheng,* happily maintain dual approaches to health—"scientific" and a "semiscientific"—seemingly with little sense of conflict. But the fact that *yangsheng* traditions are officially separated from a universalized *weisheng*—separated through institutions, government regimes, and through language—means that original Chinese paths to health exist in an uneasy space. Especially from the perspective of the government, *yangsheng* traditions and their associations with religion, alternative cosmologies, and "superstition," remain suspiciously dispersed in the population and thus potentially unruly. In spite of massive effort to contain them within official institutions and sanctioned learning, they exist just outside of the realm of state monitoring, where they can be utilized by "backward" elements to destabilize the modern Communist regime.

This study has traced how *weisheng* gained its universalizing legitimacy through the efforts of reformers under conditions of a frequently violent imperialism. It has highlighted moments when practitioners of Chinese pathways to health used Chinese cosmologies to critique the parsing tendencies of modern biomedicine and the emergence of a state that policed health. But significantly, the voices of men like Zheng Guanying and Ding Zilang were not incorporated in the construction of an officially sanctioned hygienic modernity. Claims of the superiority of a distinctly Chinese *weisheng* were effectively drowned out by invading armies, foreign-trained health professionals, and a modernizing elite that sought modes of knowledge for the construction of an autonomous nation within the context of imperialism.

To adequately explore the continued existence of Chinese hygiene in *yangsheng* and the political significance of the bifurcation between *weisheng* and *yangsheng* would require a companion volume to the present study. Several scholars of contemporary Chinese medicine are actively exploring the creations, transformations, and continuations of health and healing "traditions" in China.[11] Considered together, this scholarship may illuminate the crucial role of the body in the construction of China's modern existence. It would create the sort of "bifurcated" history that Prasenjit Duara has suggested would open up new understandings of the suppressions and continuities that lie beneath the metanarrative of the rise of the Chinese nation. Such a history would require collaborative effort between modernists and premodernists, historians and anthropologists, and scholars of different colonial histories. In recognition of the remarkable complexity of the relationships among the body, medicine, imperialism, and modernity in China, these essential collaborations are emerging on the near horizon. The present study's contribution lies in outlining a history, specific to Tianjin but evocative of a larger process, of how *weisheng* emerged as a term used by Chinese elites both to name and to shape "the condition of their existence" in the modern world.

Glossary

Aiguo weisheng yundong	愛國衛生運動
Akiyama Yoshifuru	秋山好古
Anguo shi	安國市
ba da jia	八大家
ba gua	八卦
Baguo lianjun	八國聯軍
baihua	白話
Banzhen niangniang	班疹娘娘
Baochi tang	保赤堂
baojia	保甲
baojing ke	保淨科
baowei minsheng	保衛民生
Beiyang fangyi chu	北洋防疫處
Beiyang junyi xuetang	北洋軍醫學堂
Beiyang yixue tang	北洋醫學堂
bencao	本草
Bian	卞
Bian Chufang	卞楚芳
bôeki kyusui bu	防疫給水部
Bohai	渤海
bu	補
bu pa yi er pa fang	不怕疫而怕防
Bu qiu biaozhun de Zhongguo ren	不求標準的中國人
bu weisheng	不衛生
bu xue	補血

bu zu	不足
bu zun weisheng guiding	不尊衛生規定
Buzhu wenyi lun	補注瘟疫論
Cao Kun	曹坤
Cao Yu	曹禺
chang sheng zhi yao	長生之藥
Changlu	長蘆
cheng yao	成藥
chouqi	臭氣
chu lu	出路
Chuxue weisheng bian	初學衛生編
ci zhimindi	次殖民地
cimao wen sha	刺蟊溫痧
da	大
Da gong bao	大公報
da qingsao	大清掃
Da Shi Zong	大師宗
da zhen	打針
Dagu [Taku]	大沽
dahuang	大黃
dan bai zhi	蛋白質
dan tian	丹田
dang gui	當歸
Dao de jing	道德經
daoyin	導引
dasao weisheng	打掃衛生
diandao	顛倒
diaojiao sha	吊腳沙
dihuang	地黃
Ding Zilang	丁子郎
Dôjinkai	同任會
dong shi	董事
du	毒
Du xixueshu fa	讀西學書法
duanchang	短長
dujun	毒菌
eisei	衛生

eisei chôsa	衛生調査
Eisei hanron	衛生凡論
eisei keisatsu	衛生警察
eisei kumiai	衛生組合
Eisei kyoka	衛生局
Eisei shinhen	衛生新編
Eisei shinron	衛生新論
Eiseigaku tai i	衛生学大意
fan	翻
fan	礬
Fan Bin	樊彬
fang	方
fasha	發痧
Fei huoluan bing, huoluan zheng ye	非霍亂病霍亂政也
feng	瘋
Fengshan miao	峰山廟
Fengwo	峰窩
Fu Lanya	傅蘭雅
Fu Ruqin	傅汝勤
Fu zhi hui	復治會
fugu	河豚
Fukushima Yasumasa	福島安正
gaige kaifang	改革開放
gan	甘
gao weisheng	搞衛生
ge lu deng	哥路登
Gengsang Chu	庚桑楚
geren weisheng	個人衛生
Gezhi huibian	格致彙編
Gezhi shushi	格致書室
Gezhi shuyuan	格致書院
gong fei	公費
gonggong kuaizi	公共筷子
Gotô Shimpei	後籐新平
gu ren yu xin ze gua wei sheng zhi dao ze jin ye	古人慾心則寡衛生之道則盡也

guafa	刮法
guasha	刮沙
guance	官廁
guniangzi	姑娘子
guo	過
Guo Moruo	郭末若
Hai (River)	海河
Haiguang si	海光寺
Haitong weisheng bian	孩童衛生編
hetu	河圖
hetun	河豚
hoken	保健
hojôka	保淨課
Hong Tianxi	洪天錫
Hou Fusang	侯扶桑
Houjia hou	侯家後
Hua Guangwei	華光韋
Hua Hengfang	華衡芳
Hua Xuelan	華學蘭
huan jing bu nao	還精補腦
Huang Jinrong	黃金榮
Huang hui	皇會
Huaxue weisheng lun	化學衛生論
Hui	回
hui qi	穢氣
hui yin	會陰
hunhunr	昏昏兒
huoluan	霍亂
Huoluan lun	霍亂論
Ishiguro Tadanori	石黑忠眞
Ishii Shirô	石井四郎
ji yi	疾醫
jian bing (gao)	煎餅 (糕)
Ji'an zilaishui gongsi	濟安自來水公司
Jiang Shi	蔣詩
jiang weisheng	講衛生
jiaochangsha	腳長痧

Jie Yuan	芥園
jiemo wen	假莫溫
jiji fenzi	積極分子
jing (Seminal Essence)	精
jing (warp)	經
jing (fright)	驚
Jinmen hao	津門好
jinshi	進士
jintaiteki kokka	人体的国家
Jintan	仁丹
jiu gong	九宮
jiucai yangrou xianrbing	韭菜羊肉餡兒餅
jiuji shui	救濟水
jiujing	酒精
jue	絕
Juzhai weisheng lun	居宅衛生論
ka fei yin	咖啡因
kang	炕
kangtou	炕頭
keng	坑
kenkô	研究
kexue nengli	科學能力
Kitasato Shibasuburô	北裏柴三郎
Kokka eisei genri	国家衛生原理
kongqi	空氣
korera byô ari	コレラ病アリ
Kosôso hen	庚桑楚編
ku	苦
kuhai	苦海
Kyoryû mindan	居留民団
lao	勞
Laozi	老子
li	理
Li Gao	李杲
Li Hongzhang	李鴻章
Li Jinghan	李景漢
li qi	厲氣

Li Shizhen	李時珍
Li Yunke	李允可
Liang Qichao	梁啓超
Lihua weisheng yaozao	力華衛生藥皂
ling zhi hua fen er bian qi xing	令之化分而變其性
liu jing	六經
Liu Kui	劉奎
Liu Na'ou	劉吶鷗
Liyi he weisheng	禮儀和衛生
Long wang	龍王
Longshunrong	隆順榕
Lu Dongbin	呂洞賓
Lu shan zhen mian mu	盧山真面目
luan	亂
Lun xiatian de weisheng	論夏天的衛生
Lunyu	論語
Lunyu jing yi	論語精意
Luo Hongxian	羅洪先
Luo Tianyi	羅天益
luotuo sha	駱駝瘦
mai	脈
Mantetsu	滿鐵
mantou	饅頭
Mawangdui	馬王堆
Mazu	媽祖
Mei di	美帝
Meiyou shenjing de Zhongguo ren	沒有神經的中國人
Mengzi	孟子
minzu jiankang	民族健康
Minzu texing yu minzu weisheng	民族特性與民族衛生
minzu weisheng	民族衛生
Minzu weisheng de chulu	民族衛生的出路
Mori Ôgai	森鷗外
Nagasaki	長崎
Nagayo Sensai	長与専斎
Nanjing	南京
Nankai	南開

Nanrong Chu	南榮趎
nei dan	內丹
nengli	能力
ni wan	泥丸
nian jing wen	拈頸溫
Niang niang gong	娘娘宮
niangdu	釀毒
Niu dou ju	牛痘局
Ogata Kôan	緒方洪庵
Ogata Koreyoshi	緒方維準
Pan Guangdan	潘光旦
Pan Wei	潘爵
ping	平
Pu Yi	溥儀
putao yi	葡萄疫
qi	氣
Qi Bo	岐伯
qian niu zi	牽牛子
Qianlong	乾隆
Qifu	祁阜
qihai	氣海
qin Mei	親美
qing dan	清淡
Qing Dao Wan	清導丸
Qiu Changchun (Changchun zhen ren)	邱長春(長春真人)
qu jiang	曲江
Quan Shaoqing	全紹清
Rangaku	**蘭學**
re	熱
ren mai	任脈
riben diguo shunmin	日本帝國順民
san	散
Sanbuguan	三不關
sha	痧
Shadi shen	傻弟神
shamie	殺滅

shanghan	傷寒
Shanghan pai	傷寒派
shao yao	芍藥
shaoyang jing	少陽經
shen	神
Sheng shi wei yan	盛世危言
shi yi	時疫
shiliao	食療
shina jin	支那人
shinkei suijaku	神経衰弱
shizhi	食治
shôgi	娼妓
shuidian	水電
si	私
Song feng shuo yi	松峰説疫
Sôshi	莊子
Su Shi	蘇軾
suan	酸
suidao	髓道
Sun Chuanfang	孫傳芳
Sun Simiao	孫思邈
Suzhou	蘇州
taidu	台毒
Taiping	太平
Taiyi	太醫
Taku	大沽
tanbai	坦白
Tang Shaoyi	唐紹儀
Tanggu	塘沽
tanwu	貪污
Tekijuku	適塾
Tekitekisai juku	適適斎塾
tian gan di zhi	天干地支
Tianjin	天津
Tianhou gong	天後宮
Tôa dôbunkai	東亞同文會
Tongren hui	同任會

tonza	頓挫
Tsuzuki Jinnosuke	都築甚之助
tugun	土棍
Wan shou xian shu	萬壽仙書
Wang hai lou	望海樓
Wang Shixiong	王士雄
Wei lian shi da yisheng hong se bu wan	韋廉氏大醫生紅色補丸
Wei sheng bao jian	衛生保健
wei sheng bao xun	衛生寶訓
wei sheng zhi dao	衛生之道
weisheng	衛生
weisheng bu	衛生部
weisheng chu	衛生處
weisheng jian	衛生間
weisheng ju	衛生局
weisheng qiu	衛生球
weisheng tang	衛生湯
Weisheng wen da	衛生問答
Weisheng yao shu	衛生要術
weisheng yi	衛生衣
Weisheng zazhi	衛生雜誌
weisheng zhan	衛生站
Weisheng zhenjue	衛生真決
weisheng zhi jing	衛生之經
Wen bing pai	瘟病派
wenming weisheng chengshi	文明衛生城市
wu da jia	五大家
wu ling san	五苓散
wu mie	五滅
wu xing	五行
Wu Youxing	吳有性
wu zhi	無質
xiantian	先天
xiaodu dui	消毒隊
xiaofen	小粉
xie	惡

xiezi wen	蟹子溫
Xiguo	西國
xijun zhan	細菌戰
xin	辛
Xin shenghuo yundong	新生活運動
xing	性
xingzhi	性質
xu	虛
Xu Jianyin	徐建寅
Xu Shou	徐壽
xue	血
xue yi bu ming, an dao sha ren	學醫不明暗刀殺人
Yan Xiu	嚴修
yang	陽
yang wu	洋務
Yang Yide	楊以德
yangsheng	養生
Yanguang niangniang	眼光娘娘
Yangzhou yi	揚州忆
yao	藥
Yaowang (miao)	藥王廟
Yihetuan	義和團
yindao	陰道
Yingkou	營口
yinshi	飲食
yisheng zuojiao, qiong jia bu dao	醫生作轎窮家不到
yongyi	庸医
Yongding he	永定河
you jibing qing san shi	有急病請三士
You si wu gong de Zhongguo ren	有私無公的中國人
yousheng	優生
Youtong weisheng bian	幼童衛生編
yu zhi hua he er cheng xin zhi	與質化合而成新質
yuan qi	元氣
Yuan Shikai	袁世凱
Yuan Wenhui	袁文會
Yue Fei	岳飛

yûkitaiteki kokka	有機体的国家
za qi	雜氣
Zha Riqian	查日乾
Zhang Ji	張機
Zhang Tao	張濤
zhangqi	瘴氣
zheng	爭
Zheng Guanying	鄭官應
Zhenya fangeming yundong	鎮壓反革命運動
Zhibao	直報
Zhong wai weisheng yaozhi	中外衛生要旨
Zhongguo huijiao hui	中國回教會
zhongxi jiehe	中西結合
Zhou li	周理
Zhou Xuexi	周學熙
Zhu Xi	朱熹
zhuangyuan	狀元
Zhuangzi	莊子
Zi sun niang niang	子孫娘娘
zui yi ru fang	醉以入房

Notes

ABBREVIATIONS USED IN THE NOTES

Adm.	Great Britain, Admiralty. Archives. Public Record Office, London.
BYGDLZ	Gan Houci, ed., *Beiyang gongdu leizuan* (Classified collection of public documents of the commissioner of trade for the northern ports)
CXTJFZ	Shen Jibian et al., eds., *Chongxiu Tianjin fuzhi* (Revised gazetteer of Tianjin prefecture)
DECYPZZ	Qi Shihe, ed., *Di'er ci yapian zhanzhen* (The second opium war)
DTYMHYJY	*Dutong yamen huiyi jiyao* (Minutes of the meetings of the Tianjin Provisional Government)
DYYY	Tianjin shili diyi yiyuan (Tianjin Number One Municipal Hospital), record group 123, Tianjin Municipal Archives, Tianjin
FO	Great Britain, Foreign Office. Archives. Public Record Office, London
GX	Guangxu reign period
JA	Ji'an zilaishui youxian gongsi (Tientsin Native City Waterworks Company, Ltd.), Tianjin Municipal Archives
NCH	*North China Herald* (1850–67); *North China Herald and Supreme Court and Consular Gazette* (1870–1941)
PRO	Public Record Office, London
TJWSZL	*Tianjin wenshi ziliao* (Tianjin historical materials)

TJXXZ   Gao Lingwen, ed., *Tianjin xin xianzhi* (A new gazetteer of Tianjin county)

TJZSYGJ   Wang Shouxun, *Tianjin zhengsu yan'ge ji* (Record of changes of the government and customs of Tianjin), 1938

TMA   Tianjin Municipal Archives

WSC   Tianjinshi weisheng chu (Tianjin Municipal Health Department)

ZAWSJ   Tianjinshi zhi'an weichi weiyuanhui weisheng ju (Health Department of the Tianjin Security Preservation Committee)

PROLOGUE

1. "Sun zhenren weisheng ge" (Sun the Perfected One's song of guarding life), in Hu Wenhuan, comp., *Lei xiu yao jue* (Essential formulas for self-cultivation, divided in categories), in Hu Wenhuan, *Lei xiu yao jue* (c. 1600; Shanghai: Shanghai zhongyi xueyuan chuban she, 1989); reprinted in Zhou Shouzhong (fl. 1208), comp., *Yang sheng lei zuan* (Compilation of nurturing life), and Hu Wenhuan, comp., *Lei xiu yao jue*.

INTRODUCTION

1. Lydia Liu, *Translingual Practice: Literature, National Culture, and Translated Modernity—China, 1900–1937* (Stanford: Stanford University Press, 1995), 28.

2. John Fitzgerald, *Awakening China: Politics, Culture, and Class in the Nationalist Revolution* (Stanford: Stanford University Press, 1996).

3. Several scholars, most notably Frank Dikötter, have already begun to explore the relationships among health, disease, and modernity in China. In his pathbreaking intellectual histories, Dikötter has uncovered premodern Chinese antecedents of hierarchical concepts of race and sex difference. At the same time, he has demonstrated the radical shifts that occurred when these concepts became part of a discourse of science. See Dikötter, *The Discourse of Race in Modern China* (Stanford: Stanford University Press, 1992); *Sex, Culture, and Modernity in China: Medical Science and the Construction of Sexual Identities in the Early Republican Period* (London: Hurst and Co., 1995); and *Imperfect Conceptions: Medical Knowledge, Birth Defects, and Eugenics in China* (New York: Columbia University Press, 1998).

4. For a genealogy of this term, see Jürgen Osterhammel, "Semicolonialism and Informal Empire in Twentieth-Century China: Towards a Framework of Analysis," in *Imperialism and After: Continuities and Discontinuities*, ed. Wolfgang Mommsen and Osterhammel (London: Allen and Unwin, 1986).

5. Li Chih-ch'ang, *The Travels of an Alchemist: The Journey of the Taoist Ch'ang Ch'un from China to the Hindukush at the Summons of Chingiz Khan,* trans. Arthur Waley (London: George Routledge and Sons, Ltd., 1931), 101. Translation slightly altered. The original Chinese may be found in Li Zhichang, *Chang Chun zhen ren xi you ji* (The journey to the west of the Perfected One Chang Chun), 1228, in *Kuo hsueh chi pen cong shu,* vol. 349, ed. Wang Yunwu (Taibei: Shangwu jin shu guan, 1968), shang juan 16.

6. Li Chih-ch'ang, *Travels of an Alchemist,* 24.

7. Andrew Wear, "The History of Personal Hygiene," in *Companion Encyclopedia of the History of Medicine,* vol. 2, ed. Roy Porter and W. F. Bynum (London: Routledge, 1993), 1283–1308.

8. For an excellent intellectual history of hygiene in Europe, see Heikii Mikkeli, *Hygiene in the Early Modern Medical Tradition* (Helsinki: Academica Scientiarum Fennica, 1999). Henry Sigerist, *Landmarks in the History of Hygiene* (Oxford: Oxford University Press, 1956), is a convenient summary of major texts. On shifts in regimens (primarily from hot to cold), see Virginia Smith, "Prescribing the Rules of Health: Self-Help and Advice in the Late Eighteenth Century," in *Patients and Practitioners: Lay Perceptions of Medicine in Pre-industrial Society,* ed. Roy Porter (Cambridge: Cambridge University Press, 1985).

9. For comprehensive narrative histories of public health in the West, see George Rosen, *A History of Public Health* (1958; reprint, Baltimore: Johns Hopkins University Press, 1993); and Dorothy Porter, *Health, Civilization, and the State: A History of Public Health from Ancient to Modern Times* (London: Routledge, 1999).

10. Norbert Elias, *The Civilizing Process* (London: Blackwell, 1993); Nancy Tomes, *The Gospel of Germs: Men, Women, and the Microbe in American Life* (Cambridge, Mass.: Harvard University Press, 1998).

11. See, for example, Roy Porter and Dorothy Porter, *In Sickness and in Health: The British Experience, 1650–1850* (London: Fourth Estate, 1988).

12. Morris J. Vogel and Charles E. Rosenberg, eds., *The Therapeutic Revolution: Essays in the Social History of American Medicine* (Philadelphia: University of Pennsylvania Press, 1979).

13. Emily Martin, *The Woman in the Body: A Cultural Analysis of Reproduction* (Boston: Beacon Press, 1987); Roger Cooter, *Studies in the History of Alternative Medicine* (Basingstoke: Macmillan, in association with St. Antony's College Oxford, 1988); Andrew Wear, *Health and Healing in Early Modern England: Studies in Social and Intellectual History* (Brookfield, Vt.: Ashgate, 1998); W. F. Bynum and Roy Porter, eds., *Medical Fringe and Medical Orthodoxy* (London: Croom Helm, 1987).

14. Examples of such works include David Arnold, ed., *Imperial Medicine and Indigenous Societies* (Manchester: Manchester University Press, 1988); Roy MacLeod, ed., *Disease, Medicine, and Empire* (London: Routledge, 1988); Mark Harrison, *Public Health in British India: Anglo-Indian Preventive Medicine, 1859–1914* (Cambridge: Cambridge University Press, 1994); David Arnold,

Colonizing the Body: State Medicine and Epidemic Disease in Nineteenth-Century India (Berkeley and Los Angeles: University of California Press, 1993); Ken De Bevoise, *Agents of Apocalypse: Epidemic Disease in the Colonial Philippines* (Princeton, N.J.: Princeton University Press, 1995); Megan Vaughan, *Curing Their Ills: Colonial Power and African Illness* (Cambridge: Cambridge University Press, 1991).

15. See especially Vaughan, *Curing Their Ills;* and Warwick Anderson, "Excremental Colonialism," *Critical Inquiry* 21, no. 3 (1995): 640–69.

16. David Arnold, *Colonizing the Body,* 4, 8, 211.

17. For this approach, see Dagmar Engels and Shula Marks, eds., *Contesting Colonial Hegemony: State and Society in Africa and India* (London: I. B. Taurus, 1994); Bridie Andrews and Chris Cunningham, eds., *Western Medicine as Contested Knowledge* (Manchester and New York: Manchester University Press, 1997); Bridie Andrews, "Tuberculosis and the Assimilation of Germ Theory in China, 1895–1937," *Journal of the History of Medicine and Allied Sciences* 52, no. 1 (1997): 114–57.

18. Andrews, "Tuberculosis and the Assimilation of Germ Theory in China."

19. Gyan Prakash, *Another Reason: Science and the Imagination of Modern India* (Princeton, N.J.: Princeton University Press, 1999).

20. Ashis Nandy, "Modern Medicine and Its Non-modern Critics," in *The Savage Freud and Other Essays on Possible and Retrievable Selves* (Princeton, N.J.: Princeton University Press, 1995).

21. Partha Chatterjee, *Nationalist Thought and the Colonial World: A Derivative Discourse* (Minneapolis: University of Minnesota Press, 1986).

22. Ann Laura Stoler, *Race and the Education of Desire: Foucault's History of Sexuality and the Colonial Order of Things* (Durham, N.C.: Duke University Press, 1995).

23. Mark Harrison, *Climates and Constitutions: Health, Race, Environment, and British Imperialism in India, 1600–1850* (Oxford and New York: Oxford University Press, 1999).

24. Warwick Anderson, "Immunities of Empire: Race, Disease, and the New Tropical Medicine, 1900–1920," *Bulletin of the History of Medicine* 70, no. 1 (1996): 94–118.

25. Ann Laura Stoler's *Race and the Education of Desire* is perhaps the most significant work in this direction. Also of great interest is Gail Bederman's *Manliness and Civilization* (Chicago: University of Chicago Press, 1995), which explores formulations of race and class in turn-of-the-century America against the backdrop of America's expanding Pacific empire.

26. Warwick Anderson, "Where is the Postcolonial History of Medicine?" *Bulletin of the History of Medicine* 79, no. 3 (1998): 522–30.

27. The international scholarship on eugenics perhaps comes closest to this sort of project, although it is not closely linked to scholarship on colonial medicine. See Robert Proctor, *Racial Hygiene: Medicine Under the Nazis* (Cambridge, Mass.: Harvard University Press, 1988); Nancy Leys Stepan, *The Hour*

of Eugenics: Race, Gender, and Nation in Latin America (Ithaca: Cornell University Press, 1991); and Dikötter, *Imperfect Conceptions.*

28. The present study focuses primarily on only two of the concessions, the Japanese and the British. This focus is due to a variety of factors. Only the French, British, Italian, and Japanese concessions lasted beyond World War I. The Belgian concession was barely administered at all by Belgium, and reverted to the Nationalist government in 1930. Ultimately, this focus on the Japanese and British is due primarily to the limitations on sources available in Tianjin itself, where I conducted most of my research. Perhaps other intrepid scholars will produce more comprehensive studies on all of Tianjin's foreign zones, using sources housed within the home countries of each concession.

29. Sun Yat-sen, *Guofu quanji* (Taibei: Chung-yang wen-wu kung-ying she, 1961), vol. 1, *San-min chu-yi* lecture 2: 19.

30. Shu-mei Shih, *The Lure of the Modern: Writing Modernism in Semi-colonial China, 1917–1937* (Berkeley: University of California Press, 2001), 34.

31. Shih, *Lure of the Modern*, 373.

32. Bryna Goodman, "Improvisations on a Semicolonial Theme, or, How to Read a Celebration of Transnational Urban Community," *Journal of Asian Studies* 59, no. 4 (2000): 916.

33. Osterhammel, "Semicolonialism and Informal Empire in Twentieth-Century China," 295; Goodman, "Improvisations on a Semicolonial Theme," 889.

34. Mark Peattie, "Japanese Treaty Ports Settlements in China, 1895–1937," in *The Japanese Informal Empire in China, 1895–1937*, ed. Peter Duus, Ramon Myers, and Peattie (Princeton, N.J.: Princeton University Press, 1989), 166–209.

35. Ann Laura Stoler, *Race and the Education of Desire*, 2.

36. On nostalgia and historicity, see Susan Naquin, *Peking: Temples and City Life, 1400–1900* (Berkeley: University of California Press, 2001).

37. Nancy Rose Hunt, *A Colonial Lexicon of Birth Ritual, Medicalization, and Mobility in the Congo* (Durham, N.C.: Duke University Press, 1999); Luise White, *Speaking with Vampires: Rumor and History in Colonial Africa* (Berkeley: University of California Press, 2000); Prakash, *Another Reason;* Bridie Andrews, *The Making of Modern Chinese Medicine* (Cambridge: Cambridge University Press, 2004).

38. Liu, *Translingual Practice.*

39. Quote from Nagayo's autobiography, *Shôkô shishi* (Pine fragrance memoirs), in William Johnston, *The Modern Epidemic: Tuberculosis in Japan* (Cambridge, Mass.: Harvard University Press, 1995), 179. According to Johnston, the original word Nagayo was trying to translate was *Gesundheitspflege* (literally, health care). Commentary by Ban Tadayasu states the word was *hygiene.* Ban Tadayasu, *Tekijuku to Nagayo Sensai: eiseigaku to Shôkô shishi* (The Tekijuku and Nagayo Sensai: Hygienics and the fragrant pine memoirs) (Osaka: Sogensha, 1987), 151–57.

40. Foucault's ideas of biopower and governmentality are worked out primarily in *Discipline and Punish: The Birth of the Prison* (New York: Vintage,

1979); and *The History of Sexuality* (New York: Vintage, 1985). For a cogent critique of Foucault's concepts in the context of colonialism, see Ann Laura Stoler, *Race and the Education of Desire*. A remarkably clear summary of Foucault's sometimes obscure explications of these terms can be found in Timothy Rayner, "Biopower and Technology: Foucault and Heidegger's Way of Thinking," *Contretemps* 2 (May 2001), 142–56. (*Contretemps, An Online Journal of Philosophy,* http://www.usyd.edu.au/contretemps/2may2001/rayner.pdf)

41. A "return graphic loan" is a term, written in Chinese characters, that originated in a (usually ancient) Chinese text but was used by Japanese scholars to translate the meaning of terms in Western learning, then returned to China with a different meaning. See Frederico Massini, *The Formation of the Modern Chinese Lexicon and Its Evolution toward a National Language: The Period from 1840 to 1898* (Berkeley: Journal of Chinese Linguistics, 1993).

42. Lydia H. Liu, ed., *Tokens of Exchange: The Problem of Translation in Global Circulations,* (Durham, N.C.: Duke University Press, 1999); Michael Lackner, Iwo Amelung, and Joachim Kurtz , eds., *New Terms for New Ideas: Western Knowledge and Lexical Change in Late Imperial China* (Leiden: Brill, 2001).

43. Roger Hart, "Translating the Untranslatable: From Copula to Incommensurable Worlds," in Liu, *Tokens of Exchange,* 45–73.

44. The classic expression of this approach is Joseph Needham and Lu Gwei-djen, "Hygiene and Preventive Medicine in Ancient China," in *Clerks and Craftsmen in China and the West,* ed. Needham et al. (Cambridge: Cambridge University Press, 1970), 340–78. This article is reprinted in Needham's *Science and Civilisation in China,* vol. 6, *Biology and Biological Technology,* part 6, *Medicine,* ed. and intro. Nathan Sivin (Cambridge: Cambridge University Press, 2000).

45. Prasenjit Duara, *Rescuing History from the Nation: Questioning Narratives of Modern China* (Chicago: University of Chicago Press, 1995).

CHAPTER 1

1. The *Zhuangzi* assumed its form in the late third century C.E., compiled from texts that had been circulating as early as the third century B.C.E. "Gengsang Chu" was identified by late imperial scholars as one of *Zhuangzi's* "miscellaneous" chapters, pieces whose anecdotal, narrative style indicated a later authorship than the seven original "inner chapters." In spite of the questions of authorship cast upon it by later scholars, the Gengsang Chu chapter was certainly part of the *Zhuangzi* read and commented upon by Chinese scholars throughout the late imperial period On the structure of the *Zhuangzi*, see A. C. Graham, *Chuang-tzu: The Seven Inner Chapters and Other Writings from the Book Chuang-tzu* (London and Boston: Allen and Unwin, 1981). The following translation is from Victor H. Mair, *Wandering on the Way: Early Taoist Tales and Parables of Chuang Tzu* (Honolulu: University of Hawaii Press, 1994).

2. This metaphor in *Zhuangzi* echoes a well-known passage from the *Dao*

de jing where the infant can cry all day without becoming hoarse and possesses a firm grasp in spite of the softness of its bones. Despite its small size, the infant is brimming with vitality and never seems to tire. It is even invulnerable to attacks by poisonous insects and beasts. Lao-tzu, *Tao te ching,* trans. James Legge (Taipei: Ch'eng-wen Publishing Company, 1969), chap. 55.

3. Donald Harper, *Early Chinese Medical Literature: The Mawangdui Medical Manuscripts* (London and New York: Kegan Paul International, 1998), 53.

4. Ibid.

5. Ibid.; Vivienne Lo, "The Influence of Western Han Nurturing Life Literature on the Development of Acumoxa Therapy" (Ph.D. diss., London University, 1998).

6. Confucius, *The Analects,* trans. D. C. Lau (New York: Penguin, 1979), 103.

7. Zhu Xi, *Lunyu jingyi,* juan 5: 17a, *Electronic Si ku quan shu, Wenyuange edition* (Hong Kong: Digital Heritage Publishing, 1999).

8. *Zhouli jishuo,* juan 3: 5a, *Electronic Si ku quan shu, Wenyuange edition* (Hong Kong: Digital Heritage Publishing, 1999).

9. Cynthia Brokaw, "Commercial Publishing in Late Imperial China: The Zou and Ma Family Businesses of Sibao, Fujian," *Late Imperial China* 17, no. 1 (1996): 49–92. On medical texts, see Brokaw, "Field Work on the Social and Economic History of the Chinese Book" (paper presented at the annual meeting of the Association for Asian Studies, Chicago, Ill., Mar. 2001).

10. *Wan shou xian shu* (c. 1560), attributed to Luo Hongxian, Daoguang renzhen edition (1832), comp. Cao Ruoshui, in *Zhongguo yixue dacheng sanbian,* ed. Qiu Peiran, et al. (Changsha: Yuelu shu she, 1994), 8: 781–849.

11. Luo was the optimus in the imperial examinations of 1525. He is best known as an innovative thinker of the Wang Yangming school and a compiler of the *Guang yu tu* (Expanded terrestrial atlas), a geographical treatise on the Ming and foreign lands. See L. Carrington Goodrich, ed., *Dictionary of Ming Biography, 1368–1644* (New York: Columbia University Press, 1976).

12. Luo, *Wan shou xian shu,* juan 1, n.p., in *Zhongguo yixue dacheng sanbian,* 784–91.

13. For discussions on *qi,* see Nathan Sivin, *Traditional Medicine in Contemporary China* (Ann Arbor: Center for Chinese Studies, University of Michigan, 1987); Paul Unschuld, *Medicine in China: A History of Ideas* (Berkeley and Los Angeles: University of California Press, 1985); and Manfred Porkert, *The Theoretical Foundations of Chinese Medicine: Systems of Correspondence* (Cambridge, Mass.: MIT Press, 1974). For an examination of Qi that goes beyond the medical classics, see Elisabeth Hsu, *The Transmission of Chinese Medicine* (Cambridge: Cambridge University Press, 1999).

14. For various renderings of a number of Chinese medical terms, see the extremely helpful glossary in Hsu, *Transmission of Chinese Medicine.*

15. Sivin, *Traditional Medicine in Contemporary China,* 47.

16. Mark E. Lewis, *Sanctioned Violence in Early China* (Albany: SUNY Press, 1990), 213, quoted in Hsu, *Transmission of Chinese Medicine,* 80.

17. Graham (1981); Unschuld, *Medicine in China: A History of Ideas.*

18. Hsu has noted that in contemporary Traditional Chinese Medicine, the Five Phases have become conceived of more as entities than processes. See Hsu, *Transmission of Chinese Medicine*, 198–200.

19. Nathan Sivin, "State, Cosmos, and the Body in the Last Three Centuries B.C.," *Harvard Journal of Asiatic Studies* 55, no. 1 (1995): 5–38.

20. See Harper, *Early Chinese Medical Literature*, 110–11.

21. Guo Aichun, ed., *Huangdi neijin suwen jiaozhu yuyi* (Basic questions from the Inner Canon of the Yellow Emperor: Annotated with explanations in modern Chinese) (Beijing: Renmin weisheng chuban she, 1992).

22. John Henderson, *The Development and Decline of Chinese Cosmology* (New York: Columbia University Press, 1984); Benjamin Elman, *From Philosophy to Philology: Intellectual and Social Aspects of Change in Late Imperial China* (Cambridge, Mass.: Harvard University Press, 1984); Marta Hanson, "Inventing a Tradition in Chinese Medicine" (Ph.D. diss., University of Pennsylvania, 1997).

23. Frederick W. Mote, "Yuan and Ming," in *Food in Chinese Culture*, ed. K. C. Chang (New Haven: Yale University Press, 1977), 243.

24. Porkert uses "sapor" to distinguish from conventional sense of "flavor." Modern sources and practice also includes *dan*, or neutral. See Judith Farquhar, *Knowing Practice: The Clinical Encounter of Chinese Medicine* (Boulder, Colo.: Westview Press, 1994).

25. Ibid.

26. On the diversity of bodies in Chinese medicine, see Judith Farquhar, "Multiplicity, Point of View, and Responsibility in Traditional Chinese Healing," in *Body, Subject, and Power in China*, ed. Angela Zito and Tani Barlow (Chicago: University of Chicago Press, 1994).

27. For discussions of the Six Warps, see Farquhar, *Knowing Practice*, 71–74; Sivin, *Traditional Medicine in Contemporary China*, 80–87.

28. Meng Xian (c. 621–c. 713), *Shiliao bencao* (Pharmacopoeia of foods for treating illness) (reprint ed., Beijing: Zhongguo shanye chubanshe, 1992), 124. Similar discussions on sheep can be found in the "Shizhi" (Food therapeutics) chapter of Sun Simiao, *Beiji qianjin yaofang* (Prespcriptions worth a thousand gold for every emergency) (c. 652 C.E., reprinted as *Qian jin shi zhi* (Food therapies worth a thousand gold) (Beijing: Zhongguo shanye chubanshe, 1985), 55; Husihui, *Yinshan zhengyao* (Essentials of food and drink) (1330, reprint ed., Shanghai: Shanghai guji chubanshe, 1994); and Li Shizhen, *Bencao gangmu* (Great compendium of Materia Medica) (1596, 1885 ed.; reprint, Beijing: Renmin weisheng chubanshe, 1957), juan 55: 1724. On traditions of "food therapeutics," see Yuan-peng Chen, "Food and Healing in the Tang and Sung: The Shih-chih Chapter in Sun Szu-miao's *Ch'ien chin yao-fang*," *Bulletin of the Institute of History and Philology: Academia Sinica* 69, no. 4 (1998): 765–825.

29. The meat of southern sheep is not as tasty or as efficacious as the sheep meat of the north. In any region, the meat of white sheep with black heads, black sheep with white heads, and sheep of any color with only one horn are to be avoided, warnings that date back to the Han period. See Meng Xian, *Shiliao ben-*

cao, 124; Husihui, *Yinshan zhengyao,* 51. On the *Yinshan zhengyao,* see Paul D. Buell and Eugene N. Anderson, *A Soup for the Qan: Chinese Dietary Medicine of the Mongol Era as Seen in Hu Szu-Hui's Yin-shan cheng-yao* (London and New York: Kegan Paul International, 2000).

30. Husihui, *Yinshan zhengyao,* juan 8: 2a–b.

31. Ibid., juan 2: 26b–50a.

32. A combination of passages on crab from Sun Simiao, *Qianjin shizhi,* 92–93; Meng Xian, *Shiliao bencao,* 518–20; and Li, *Bencao gangmu,* juan 45: 1634–35.

33. Sun Simiao, quoting Wei Xun, in *Qianjin shizhi,* 12.

34. Luo was a student of the famous physician Li Gao (Li Donghuan, 1180–1251). One of the "Four Great Physicians of the Jin and Yuan," Li Gao's major contribution to medical culture was his *Pi Wei lun* (The treatise on the spleen and stomach). For Li, the Spleen and the Stomach were the most important of the body's Visceral Systems as they were responsible for transforming and distributing the *qi* derived from food. They were also the most vulnerable.

35. Luo Tianyi (fl. 1246–1283), *Weisheng baojian* (Beijing: Weisheng chuban she, 1987), juan 1: 1–2.

36. Sivin, *Traditional Medicine in Contemporary China,* 98; Guo, *Huang di nei jing,* 3–4.

37. Harper, *Early Chinese Medical Literature,* 400, 397.

38. Sun Simiao, *Qian jin yao fang, qian jin yi fang,* annotated by Liu Gengsheng et al. (Beijing: Huaxia chuban she, 1993), juan 27, *fang zhong bu yi:* 389.

39. Ibid., 388.

40. Ibid., 389. Different bedchamber manuals offer a different array of parameters, see Douglas Wile, *Art of the Bedchamber: The Chinese Sexual Yoga Classics, Including Women's Solo Meditation Texts* (New York: SUNY Press, 1992), 46–47. The point is that ejaculation (although not necessarily ejaculant) is quantified and regulated on a numerical basis.

41. For a summary of this economical approach to sex, see Ping-chen Hsiung, "More or Less: Cultural and Medical Factors Behind Marital Fertility in Late Imperial China," in *Abortion, Infanticide, and Reproductive Culture in Asia: Past and Present,* ed. James Z. Lee and Osamu Saito (Oxford: Oxford University Press, forthcoming).

42. Wile's *Art of the Bedchamber* is the most authoritative work on these texts to date.

43. Wile, *Art of the Bedchamber,* 47.

44. Joseph Needham, *Science and Civilisation in China,* vol. 2, *History of Scientific Thought* (Cambridge: Cambridge University Press, 1991), 199.

45. Hsiung, "More or Less"; James Z. Lee and Wang Feng, *One Quarter of Humanity: Malthusian Mythology and Chinese Realities, 1700–2000* (Cambridge, Mass.: Harvard University Press, 1999).

46. Hugh Shapiro, "The Puzzle of Spermatorrhea in Republican China," *positions* 6, no. 3 (1998): 550–96.

47. Frank Dikötter, *Sex, Culture, and Modernity in China: Medical Science*

and the Construction of Sexual Identities in the Early Republican Period (London: Hurst and Co., 1995); and Dikötter, Imperfect Conceptions: Medical Knowledge, Birth Defects, and Eugenics in China (New York: Columbia University Press, 1998).

48. Luo Hongxian (attrib.), Weisheng zhen jue (c. 1560; reprint, Beijing: Weisheng chuban she, 1987), 1.

49. Ibid., 2.

50. Henri Maspero, Taoism and Chinese Religion (Amherst, Mass.: University of Amherst Press, 1981), 456–57; Catherine Despeux, La Moelle du Phénix Rouge: Santé et longue vie dans la Chine du XVIe siècle (Paris: Guy Tredaniel, 1988), 34 (illus.); Needham, Science and Civilisation, vol. 2, 38–39.

51. What Needham refers to as the "enchyomoma" in Science and Civilization in China, vol. 5, Chemistry and Chemical Technology, part 2, Spagyrical Invention and Discovery: Magisteries of Gold and Immortality (Cambridge: Cambridge University Press, 1974), 27. Needham gives a detailed discussion of the importance of the yin within yang and yang within yin through their sequencing according to the eight trigrams (ba gua) in Science and Civilization in China, vol 5, part 2, 49–67.

52. See, for example, the Hu Wenhuan compilation Shouyang cong shu. In Beijing tushuguan guji zhenben chongkan, vol. 82 (Beijing: Beijing tushuguan guji chuban she, 1987).

53. On Ming prosperities and anxieties, see Timothy Brook, Confusions of Pleasure: Commerce and Culture in Ming China (Berkeley: University of California Press, 1998).

54. Luo Tianyi, Weisheng baojian, juan 2: 17.

CHAPTER 2

1. Pan Wei, Yishenji: Neigong tushuo (1858; reprint, Beijing: Renmin weisheng chuban she, 1982), 44.

2. Ibid., 45.

3. I have translated Tianjin literally as "The Ford of Heaven" or "Heaven's Ford." The two characters in the city's name mean heaven (tian) and ford or river crossing (jin). This literal form of translation has precedent in modern Chinese: for example, England's Oxford is rendered in Chinese as Niujin, literally "Ox Crossing." Suzhou and Hangzhou have long been considered China's most beautiful cities, as captured in the popular saying "Above there is heaven, below there is Suzhou and Hangzhou." On Suzhou in the late Qing, see Peter Carroll, "Between Heaven and Modernity: The Late Qing and Early Republic (Re)Construction of Suzhou Urban Space" (Ph.D. diss., Yale University, 1998).

4. Roy Porter and Dorothy Porter, In Sickness and in Health: The British Experience, 1650–1850 (London: Fourth Estate, 1988).

5. See, for example, Angela Leung, "To Chasten Society: The Development of Widow Homes in the Qing, 1773–1911," Late Imperial China 14, no. 2 (1993): 1–32.

6. Man-bun Kwan, *The Salt Merchants of Tianjin: State-Making and Civil Society in Late Imperial China* (Honolulu: University of Hawaii Press, 2001).

7. For floods and water control in eighteenth- and nineteenth-century Tianjin, see Man-bun Kwan, "The Merchant World of Tianjin: Society and Economy of a Chinese City" (Ph.D. diss., Stanford University, 1990), 31–56. For a discussion of floods, drought, and famine in Zhili province, see Li Wenhai, *Jindai Zhongguo zaihuang jinian* (Changsha: Hunan jiaoyu chubanshe, 1990) and *Zaihuang yu jijin* (Beijing: Gaodeng jiaoyu chubanshe, 1991).

8. Fan Bin, "Jinmen xiaoling," in *Zili lianzhu ji*, ed. Hua Dingyuan (1879; reprint, Tianjin: Tianjin guji chuban she, 1986), 106. The "three villages" here refer to the "Three Yangs": Yangliuqing to the south, Yangcun to the north, and Yangfen gang to the west of Tianjin.

9. This census, published in 1846 as the *Jinmen baojia tushuo* (Illustrated explication of Tianjin's Mutual Security Organization) was ordered by the Qing government in 1842 as part of an effort to tighten local *baojia* security arrangements after the Opium War. On *Jinmen baojia tushuo*, see Momose Hiro, "Guanyu Jinmen baojia tushuo," trans. Pu Wenqi, *Tianjinshi yanjiu* 1 (1985): 58–63; Lewis Bernstein, "A History of Tientsin in Early Modern Times, 1800–1910" (Ph.D. diss., University of Kansas, 1988), 79–94.

10. O. D. Rasmussen, *Tientsin: An Illustrated Outline History* (Tianjin: Tientsin Press, 1925), 9.

11. According to the *Jinmen baojia tushuo* survey. This number, although large, is dwarfed in comparison to the hundreds of temples in Qing Beijing: see Susan Naquin, *Peking: Temples and City Life, 1400–1900* (Berkeley: University of California Press, 2001), 20.

12. Rasmussen, *Tientsin*, 34.

13. Ibid.

14. On officials, see Wang Shouxun. *Tianjin zhengsu yan'ge ji* (Record of the evolution of Tianjin's government and customs) (Tianjin: n.p., 1938), 1:19a–b; Zhang Tao, *Jinmen zaji* (1884; reprint, Tianjin: Tianjin guji chubanshe, 1986). On the Eight Great Families, see Tianjinshi zhengxie mishuchu, ed., *Tianjin badajia ji qi houyi* (Tianjin: Tianjinshi zhengxie, 1974); also Kwan, "Merchant World of Tianjin" and *Salt Merchants of Tianjin;* and articles on individual families in the *Tianjin wenshi ziliao* (Tianjin historical materials, hereafter *TJWSZL*), such as Jin Dayang, "Tianjin Li Shanren," *TJWSZL* 7 (1980): 71–85, and Yao Xiyun, "Tianjin Gulaodong Yaojia yishi," *TJWSZL* 47 (1989): 204–42.

15. Chen Yong's analysis of Tianjin's urban structure has shown that each sector of the city was possessed of at least three basic temples—a Sanguan temple, a Guandi temple, and Yaowang temple—that served as the focal point for the neighborhood. On number and location of temples, see Chen Yong, "Mingqing Tianjin chengshi jigou de chu bu kaocha" (Preliminary investigations on Tianjin's urban structure in the Ming-Qing period), *Chengshi shi yanjiu* (Urban history project) 10 (1995): 25–63.

16. The raucous high-low participation in Tianjin's *Huanghui* is a frequent theme in the works of contemporary Tianjin author Feng Jicai. See especially

his prize-winning novella, *Shenbian* (The miraculous pigtail) (Beijing: Zhongguo minjian chubanshe, 1988).

17. On Tianjin's gardens, see Zhang Chunze, "Chengshi yuanlin gaimao," in *Tianjin—yige chengshi de jueqi* (Tianjin: Tianjin renmin chuban she, 1990), 52–63; see also painting of salt merchant Zha Riqian's garden in "Village West of the Waters," in Tianjin lishi bowuguan et al., eds., *Jindai Tianjin tuzhi* (Tianjin: Tianjin guji chubanshe, 1992), 9.

18. A note on medical sources: Tianjin did not produce many famous doctors or medical texts. For this section I extrapolate from Tianjin physician Hong Tianxi's eighteenth-century commentary to Wu Youxing's *Wenyilun, Buzhu wenyi lun* (Supplementary notes to the *Treatise on Epidemic Disease*) (c. 1750; reprint, Beijing: Zhongguo shudian, 1993) and a large compilation of drug formulas by Tianjin native Xu Shiluan, *Yifang conghua* (Tianjin: Tianjin xushi dieyuan, 1889). For additional insights into etiologies and treatments I have also turned to Liu Kui, *Song feng shuo yi* (Beijing: Renmin weisheng chubanshe, 1987). Although not specific to Tianjin, it does describe Liu's experience treating disease in north China around Shandong and Hebei in the early nineteenth century.

19. Charles E. Rosenberg, "Explaining Epidemics," in *Explaining Epidemics and Other Studies in the History of Medicine* (Cambridge: Cambridge University Press, 1992), 295–96.

20. My discussion follows Marta Hanson, "Inventing a Tradition in Chinese Medicine" (Ph.D. diss., University of Pennsylvania, 1997).

21. Ibid., 144.

22. On indeterminacy, see ibid., 146–49. On the decline of cosmological thinking, see John Henderson, *The Development and Decline of Chinese Cosmology* (New York: Columbia University Press, 1984). On regional variation in constitution and disease, see Marta Hanson, "Robust Northerners and Delicate Southerners: The Nineteenth-Century Invention of a Southern Medical Tradition," *positions* 6, no. 3 (1998): 515–50.

23. For Hong Tianxi's biography, see *Tianjin xin xianzhi* (A new gazetteer of Tianjin County, hereafter *TJXXZ*) juan 21: 12a–b.

24. Hong Tianxi, *Buzhu wenyi lun.*

25. Gu Daosheng, "Tianjin chengqu maishui he mai shui jiu su" (Old customs of buying and selling water in the Tianjin area), *Tianjin shizhi* 2 (1990): 49–50.

26. The bean water-treatment technique is mentioned in Xu Shiluan, *Yifang conghua.*

27. Culinary observations below are based on a collection of poems written by Jiang Shi, a Jiangnan scholar touring Tianjin on his way home from taking the capital exams. See Jiang Shi, "Guhe zayong," in *Zili lianzhu ji*, ed. Hua Dingyuan (1879; reprint, Tianjin: Tianjin guji chuban she, 1986), 94.

28. Hua Dingyuan, ed., *Zili lianzhu ji* (1879; reprint, Tianjin: Tianjin guji chubanshe, 1986).

29. This portrait of Tianjin's pleasure quarters derived from Fan, "Jinmen xiaoling," 126–28.

30. Pan Wei, *Yishenji*, 45.

31. Fan, "Jinmen xiaoling," 111.

32. Judith Farquhar, " 'Medicine and the Changes Are One': An Essay on Divination Healing with Commentary," *Chinese Science* 13 (1996): 107–34.

33. Liu Huapu and Bian Xueyue, "Guoyao laodian: Longshunrong" (A venerable purveyor of Chinese medicine), in *Jinmen laozi hao* (Old business of Tianjin), ed. Wenshi ziliao yanjiu weiyuan hui (Tianjin: Baihua wenyi chubanshe, 1992), 64–69.

34. Tianjinshi zhengxie hui—wenshi ziliao yanjiu weiyuanhui, ed., *Tianjin jindai renwu lu* (Biographical dictionary of modern Tianjin) (Tianjin: Tianjinshi difang shizhi bianxiu weiyuan hui zong bianji shi, 1987), 46–49.

35. Robert Hymes, "Not Quite Gentlemen? Doctors in Song and Yuan," *Chinese Science* 8 (Jan. 1987): 9–76.

36. For examples of such families, see Hanson, "Inventing a Tradition"; and Wu Yi-Li, "Transmitted Secrets: The Doctors of the Lower Yangzi Region and Popular Gynecology in Late Imperial China" (Ph.D. diss., Yale University, 1998).

37. Arthur Smith, *Proverbs and Common Sayings from the Chinese* (Shanghai: American Presbyterian Mission Press, 1902), 272.

38. Although it may be argued that Warm Factor and Cold Damage approaches to diagnosis and treatment were not mutually antagonistic, evidence from late-nineteenth-century Tianjin indicates that there were real divisions between the two groups and doctors possessed very clear solidarities with one group or the other.

39. On the Medicine King, Sun Simiao, see Nathan Sivin, *Chinese Alchemy: Preliminary Studies* (Cambridge, Mass.: Harvard University Press, 1968), 81–144. See also Paul Unschuld, *Medicine in China: Historical Artifacts and Images* (Munich and New York: Prestel, 2000).

40. On Fengwo, see Zhang Tao, *Jimen zaji* (Miscellaneous records of Tianjin) 81; Liu Yanchen, *Jinmen zatan* (Miscellaneous discussions on Tianjin) (Tianjin: Sanyou meishu she, 1943). On water guilds, see Chen Ke, "Nongovernmental Organizations and the Urban Control and Management System in Tianjin at the End of the Nineteenth Century," *Social Sciences in China* 11, no. 4 (1990): 61. On Beijing's Medicine King Temples, see Naquin, *Peking: Temples.*

41. Liu Yanchen, *Jinmen zatan*, 19–21; Zhang Tao, *Jinmen zaji*, 76–81; Frederick Brown, *Religion in Tientsin* (Shanghai: Methodist Publishing House, 1908), 15, 33–34.

42. Zhang Tao, *Jinmen zaji*, 86. On such healers in Beijing, see Naquin, *Peking: Temples*, 527, 545.

43. Naquin, *Peking: Temples*, 214, 622–678.

44. Kwan, "The Merchant World of Tianjin," appendix 1b.

45. See Ho Ping-ti, "The Salt Merchants of Yangchou: A Study of Com-

mercial Capitalism in Eighteenth-Century China," *Harvard Journal of Asiatic Studies* 17, nos. 1–2 (1954): 130–68; William Rowe, *Hankow: Commerce and Society in a Chinese City, 1796–1889* (Stanford: Stanford University Press, 1984), 90–121.

46. Ruth Rogaski, "Beyond Benevolence: A Confucian Women's Shelter in Treaty-Port China," *Journal of Women's History* 8, no. 4 (1997): 54–90.

47. Shen Jiaben et al., ed., *Chongxiu Tianjin fuzhi* (Revised gazeteer of Tianjin prefecture, hereafter *CXTJFZ*), 1899, 7: 25b. For the burial regulations of the Yan'ge hui, see Susan Naquin, "Funerals in North China," in *Death Ritual in Late Imperial and Modern China*, ed. James Watson and Evelyn Rawski (Berkeley and Los Angeles: University of California Press, 1988), 47.

48. On the importance of *li* in death rituals, see Evelyn Rawski, "A Historian's Approach to Death Ritual," in Watson and Rawski, *Death Ritual*, 27.

49. On funerals as controlling the spirits of the dead, see James Watson, "Funeral Specialists in Cantonese Society: Pollution, Performance, and Social Hierarchy," in Watson and Rawski, *Death Ritual*, 122–24.

50. Paul Bohr, *Famine in China and the Missionary* (Cambridge, Mass.: Harvard University Press, 1972), 22–23; Angela Ki Che Leung, "Organized Medicine in Ming-Qing China: State and Private Medical Institutions in the Lower Yangzi Region," *Late Imperial China* 8, no. 1 (1987): 163–66; and Pierre-Etienne Will, *Famine and Bureaucracy in Eighteenth-Century China* (Stanford: Stanford University Press, 1990), 36–37.

51. Zhang Tao, *Jinmen zaji*, 49.

52. For nineteenth-century American charitable hospitals, see Charles E. Rosenberg, *The Care of Strangers: The Rise of America's Hospital System* (New York: Basic Books, 1987), 15–46.

53. Wang Shouxun, *Tianjin zhengsu yan'ge ji*, 12:3b–4a. On smallpox inoculation in China before the nineteenth century, see Joseph Needham, *China and the Origins of Immunology* (Hong Kong: Centre of Asian Studies, University of Hong Kong, 1980).

54. Zhu Chungu, *Douzhen dinglun* (Principles of smallpox) (1713; reprint, Tianjin: Wang Xilun, 1898), 78a–b.

55. Yan Renzeng, *Yan xiu xiansheng nianpu* (Chronological biography of Mr. Yan Xiu) (Jinan: Jilu shushe, 1990), 17.

56. Angela Leung, "Variolisation et vaccination dans la Chine prémoderne, 1570–1911" in *L'Aventure de la vaccination*, ed. Anne-Marie Moulin (Paris: Fayard, 1996).

57. Compare with David Arnold, *Colonizing the Body: State, Medicine, and Epidemic Disease in Nineteenth-Century India* (Berkeley and Los Angeles: University of California Press, 1993), 117.

58. Hanson, "Robust Northerners and Delicate Southerners."

59. "Tianjin yiwu shiji," in *Di'er ci yapian zhanzhen* (The second opium war, hereafter *DECYPZZ*), ed. Qi Shihe. Shanghai: Renmin chubanshe, 1978, 2:473.

60. Samuel Wells Williams, *The Journal of S. Wells Williams* (Shanghai: Kelly

and Walsh, 1911), 38. Wells was told by a Chinese elite who had remained that "9/10ths of the good families had run away."

61. *DECYPZZ*, 2: 474. This episode was perhaps recorded as a way of questioning the loyalties of Tianjiners.

62. Hao Purong, "Jinmen shiji quedui" (A record of events in Tianjin, written in couplets), in *DECYPZZ*, 2: 577.

63. Ibid., 2: 571.

CHAPTER 3

1. Kenneth Pomeranz, *The Great Divergence: Europe, China, and the Making of the Modern World Economy* (Princeton, N.J.: Princeton University Press, 2000).

2. On laboratories of modernity, see Ann Laura Stoler, *Race and the Education of Desire: Foucault's History of Sexuality and the Colonial Order of Things* (Durham, N.C.: Duke University Press, 1995), 13–26.

3. Actions and opinions of Dr. Dickson taken from his medical log, "Journal of HM Ship *Chesapeake*, Dr. Walter Dickson, Surgeon, from July 1, 1858, to June 30, 1859, Containing the Cases of the Killed and Wounded in the Attack on the Peiho forts," PRO, Adm., 101/169.

4. Douglas Hurd, *The Arrow War* (London: Collins Press, 1967), 111–12.

5. Richard Gabriel and Karen Metz, *A History of Military Medicine* (New York: Greenwood Press, 1992), 165. The figures in Victor Bonham-Carter, *Surgeon in the Crimea: The Experiences of George Lawson Recorded in the Letters to His Family, 1854–55* (London: Constable, 1968), differ slightly, giving 2,755 killed in action and 16,297 deaths from disease (115). See also the official figures in Royal Army Medical Corps, *Medical and Surgical History of the British Army which Served in Turkey and the Crimea During the War Against Russia in the Years 1854–55–56* (London: Harrison, 1858).

6. C. E. Vulliamy. *Crimea, The Campaign of 1854–56* (London: Jonathan Cape, 1939), 216.

7. Ibid., 219.

8. For an overview of these reforms, see Redmond McLaughlin, *The Royal Army Medical Corps* (London: Leo Cooper Ltd., 1972), 15–20.

9. Warwick Anderson, "Disease, Race, and Empire," *Bulletin of the History of Medicine* 70, no. 1 (1996): 62–67; Mark Harrison, " 'The Tender Frame of Man': Disease, Climate, and Racial Difference in India and the West Indies, 1760–1860," *Bulletin of the History of Medicine* 70, no. 1 (1996): 68–93; Mark Harrison, *Climates and Constitutions: Health, Race, Environment and British Imperialism in India, 1600–1850* (Oxford and New York: Oxford University Press, 1999).

10. Ann Marie Moulin, " 'Tropical Without the Tropics': The Turning Point of Pastorian Medicine in North Africa," in *Warm Climates and Western Medicine: The Emergence of Tropical Medicine, 1500–1900*, ed. David Arnold (Amsterdam and Atlanta, Ga.: Rodopi, 1996), 160–80.

11. An expression that "echoed around the world thrilling the hearts of peoples as perhaps like no expression has ever done," according to Tianjin chronicler O. D. Rasmussen. See Rasmussen, *Tientsin: An Illustrated Outline History* (Tianjin: Tientsin Press, 1925) 21.

12. Ibid., 8.

13. Joseph Lister published his findings about antisepsis in the *Lancet* in 1867. As late as 1882, The American Surgical Association rejected Lister's findings. Gabriel and Metz, *History of Military Medicine*, 164.

14. For a discussion of drugs, medical theory and practice in nineteenth-century United States, see John Harley Warner, *The Therapeutic Perspective: Medical Practice, Knowledge, and Identity in America, 1820–1885* (Cambridge, Mass.: Harvard University Press, 1986), esp. 83–161; Morris J. Vogel and Charles E. Rosenberg, eds., *The Therapeutic Revolution: Essays in the Social History of American Medicine* (Philadelphia: University of Pennsylvania Press, 1979).

15. The list of medicines supplied to navy surgeons included at least a dozen cathartics, emetics, or irritants. See Christopher Lloyd and Jack Coulter, *Medicine and the Navy, 1200–1900*, vol. 4 (Edinburgh: E. and S. Livingstone, 1963), appendix.

16. Lloyd and Coulter, *Medicine and the Navy*, 273. This was particularly true in comparison with the military medicine of the early nineteenth century. The surgeons at Waterloo, according to one author, were "obsessed with the idea of wholesale and immediate amputation." McLaughlin, *Royal Army Medical Corps*, 8.

17. For a view of what these environs were like, see John Bold, *Greenwich: An Architectural History of the Royal Hospital for Seamen and the Queen's House* (New Haven: Yale University Press, 2000).

18. G. J. Wolseley, *Narrative of the War with China in 1860* (London: Longman, Green, Longman and Roberts, 1862), 321.

19. Hao Fusen, "Jinmen wenjian lu" (Memoir of Tianjin), in *Di'er ci yapian zhanzhen* (The second opium war, hereafter *DECYPZZ*), ed. Qi Shihe et al. (Shanghai: Renmin chubanshe, 1978), 2: 590–94.

20. Alain Corbin, *The Foul and the Fragrant: Odor and the French Social Imagination* (Cambridge, Mass.: Harvard Univeristy Press, 1986).

21. Wolseley, journal, WO 147, War Office: Filed Marshall Viscount Garnet Joseph Wolseley Papers, 1860–89, 64 vols., 1: 117.

22. Wolseley, *Narrative of the War with China*, 29.

23. Ibid., 65.

24. Ibid., 53.

25. Ibid., 54.

26. Hao Fusen, "Jinmen wenjianlu," in *DECYPZZ*, 2: 590–94.

27. Quoted in Willam Coleman, "Health and Hygiene in the *Encyclopédie*," *Bulletin of the History of Medicine* 414 (Oct. 1974), 402.

28. For the former, see Samuel E. Finer, *The Life and Times of Sir Edwin Chadwick* (London: Methuen, 1952); for the latter, see Christopher Hamlin, "Ed-

win Chadwick, 'Mutton Medicine,' and the Fever Question," *Bulletin of the History of Medicine* 70 (1996): 233–65; and Hamlin, *Public Health and Social Justice in the Age of Chadwick* (Cambridge: Cambridge University Press, 1998). Margaret Pelling expresses both of these positions well, stating "The rigid moral imperative of the new [Poor] law would have been balanced by action taken upon the concession that the poor were subjected to debilitating physical conditions which were outside their control and responsibility." See Margaret Pelling, *Cholera, Fever, and English Medicine, 1825–1865* (Oxford and New York: Oxford University Press, 1978), 11.

29. Hamlin, "Edwin Chadwick," 233–65; Hamlin, *Public Health and Social Justice.*

30. Dorothy Porter, "Public Health," in *Companion Encyclopedia of the History of Medicine,* ed. W. F. Bynum and Roy Porter (London: Routledge, 1993), 2: 1243.

31. Anthony S. Wohl, *Endangered Lives: Public Health in Victorian Britain* (London: J. M. Dent and Sons, 1983).

32. Kerrie MacPherson, *A Wilderness of Marshes: The Origins of Public Health in Shanghai, 1843–1893* (Hong Kong: Oxford University Press, 1987).

33. John Pickstone, "Dearth, Dirt, and Fever Epidemics: Rewriting the History of British 'Public Health,' 1780–1850," in *Epidemics and Ideas: Essays on the Historical Perception of Pestilence,* ed. Terence Ranger and Paul Slack (New York: Cambridge University Press, 1992), 125–48.

34. Wolseley, *Narrative of the War with China,* 98.

35. Review of "Report on a Hospital at Tientsin for the Treatment of Sick Chinese: Established by the British Army of Occupation, January 11, 1861," *North China Herald* hereafter *NCH*), 19 August 1861.

36. The most influential analysis of the role of the hospital in European medicine remains Michel Foucault, *The Birth of the Clinic,* trans. A. M. Sheridan (New York: Pantheon Books, 1975).

37. *NCH,* 21 June 1862. Dr. Rennie's discovery was lauded in a series of articles that appeared once a week in the *NCH* from 10 May 1862 to 21 June 1862.

38. Ibid., 10 May 1862.

39. Ibid.

40. Ibid., 7 June 1862.

41. Ibid., 21 June 1862.

42. Ibid., 28 June 1862.

43. Christopher Hamlin, *A Science of Impurity: Water Analysis in Nineteenth-Century Britain* (Berkeley: University of California Press, 1990), 129–40.

44. For an overview, see Donald Hopkins, *Princes and Peasants: Smallpox in History* (Chicago: University of Chicago Press, 1983), 9–10.

45. For an overview of European theories of fever before the nineteenth century, see W. F. Bynum and Vivian Nutton, eds., *Theories of Fever from Antiquity to the Enlightenment, Medical History,* supplement no. 1 (1981).

46. Sewers and indoor plumbing did have their detractors, however, who ar-

gued that the introduction of "sewer gasses" into homes was more harmful than the presence of miasmas dissipated into the general atmosphere. See Wohl, *Endangered Lives*, 102–4.

47. On etiology, see Pelling, *Cholera, Fever, and English Medicine*. On the significance of locating lesions, see Foucault, *Birth of the Clinic*.

48. On inconsistencies in early smallpox vaccination, see Francis Barrymore Smith, *The People's Health, 1830–1910* (New York: Holmes and Meier, 1979), 156–70.

49. *NCH*, 28 June 1862.

50. Ibid.

51. Letter from British Consulate at Tientsin to the Medical Officer of H. M. Forces at Tientsin, 8 April 1862, PRO, FO, 674/5.

52. It would spread to Europe in 1865 and then to the Western hemisphere in 1866. See Charles E. Rosenberg, *The Cholera Years: The United States in 1832, 1849, and 1866* (Chicago: University of Chicago Press, 1962).

53. Hao Fusen, *Jinmen wenjian lu* (hand-copied version in Tianjin Academy of Social Sciences, n.d.), 18b.

54. "Journal of Surgeon W. E. O'Brien of H. M. S. *Acorn*," Nov. 1858–Dec. 1860. Includes a "treatise" entitled, "Practical Remarks on Periodic Fevers, Dysentery and Diarrhoea As They Occur on the China Station." PRO, Adm., 101/171.

55. Ibid.

56. For examples of treatment in nineteenth-century Europe and America, see Rosenberg, *The Cholera Years*; Richard J. Evans, *Death in Hamburg: Society and Politics in the Cholera Years, 1830–1910* (New York: Oxford University Press, 1987). For specific examples of cholera treatments used by British army doctors in the mid-nineteenth century, see the medical journals of the HMS *Acorn* (PRO, Adm., 101/174) and the HMS *Euryalus* (PRO, Adm., 101/171).

57. Wang Shixiong, *Huoluan lun* (Treatise on cholera), in *Wang shi qian zhai yi shu shi zhong* (Ten medical books from the subtle studio) (1838; reprint, Taibei: Changjiang chubanshe, 1970).

58. Part of the second world pandemic that had hit Europe and the United States in 1832. See Rosenberg, *The Cholera Years*.

59. Wang Shixiong, "Huoluan lun," 3b (482).

60. Ibid.

61. Ibid., 8b (492)

62. Hao Fusen, *Jinmen wenjian lu* (hand-copied version in Tianjin Academy of Social Sciences, n.d.), 19a.

63. Ibid., 19a–20b.

64. Tianjin zongjiao zhi bianxiu weiyuanhui, ed., *Tianjin zongjiao ziliao xuan* (Historical materials on religion in Tianjin) (Tianjin: Tianjin renmin chubanshe, 1986), 14. Translations from Xavier Sackebant, *Les Premiers martyrs de l' oeuvre de la Sainte Enfance* (Paris: n.p., 1895).

65. Ibid., 17.

66. For discussion of the Tianjin Massacre, see Paul Cohen, *China and Christianity: The Missionary Movement and the Growth of Chinese Antiforeignism, 1860–1870* (Cambridge, Mass.: Harvard University Press, 1963). For a reinterpretation of the massacre from the perspective of the social setting of healing, see Ruth Rogaski, "From Protecting Life to Defending the Nation: The Emergence of Public Health in Tianjin, 1859–1953" (Ph.D. diss., Yale University, 1996).

67. John Dudgeon, *The Diseases of China: Their Causes, Conditions, and Prevalence, Contrasted with Those of Europe* (Glasgow: Dunn and Wright, 1877), 24, 60.

68. Ibid., 53.

69. Ibid., 63.

70. Ibid., 5.

71. Ibid., 60.

72. Ibid., 8.

73. Mark Harrison, " 'The Tender Frame of Man,' " 68–93.

74. Warwick Anderson, "Immunities of Empire: Race, Disease, and the New Tropical Medicine, 1900–1920," *Bulletin of the History of Medicine* 70, no. 1 (1996): 101.

75. On similar British appraisals of Indian medical traditions, see Mark Harrison, "Medicine and Orientalism: Perspectives on Europe's Encounter with Indian Medical Systems," in *Health, Medicine, and Empire*, ed. Biswamoy Pati and Mark Harrison (Hyderabad, India: Orient Longman, 2001).

CHAPTER 4

1. Gyan Prakash, *Another Reason: Science and the Imagination of Modern India* (Princeton, N.J.: Princeton University Press, 1999).

2. Lydia Liu, *Translingual Practice: Literature, National Culture, and Translated Modernity—China, 1900–1937* (Stanford: Stanford University Press, 1995), 40.

3. For a similar sentiment about the importance of the Chinese language as a site of indigenous agency in China, see Shu-mei Shih, *The Lure of the Modern: Writing Modernism in Semicolonial China, 1917–1937* (Berkeley: University of California Press, 2001).

4. Bryna Goodman, *Native Place, City, and Nation: Regional Networks and Identities in Shanghai, 1853–1937* (Berkeley and Los Angeles: University of California Press, 1995).

5. O. D. Rasmussen, *Tientsin: An Illustrated Outline History* (Tianjin: Tientsin Press, 1925), 63.

6. Paul Bohr, *Famine in China and the Missionary* (Cambridge, Mass.: Harvard University Press, 1972); Ruth Rogaski, "Beyond Benevolence: A Confucian Women's Shelter in Treaty-Port China," *Journal of Women's History* 8, no. 4 (1997): 54–90.

7. Goodman, *Native Place*, 41–46, 158–68.

8. Adrian Bennett, *John Fryer: The Introduction of Western Science and Technology into Nineteenth-Century China* (Cambridge, Mass.: East Asian Research Center, Harvard University, 1967); David Wright, *Translating Science: The Transmission of Western Chemistry into Late Imperial China, 1840–1900* (Leiden and Boston: Brill, 2000); James Reardon-Anderson, *The Study of Change: Chemistry in China, 1840–1949* (Cambridge and New York: Cambridge University Press, 1991); Xiong Yuezhi, *Xi xue dong jian yu wan Qing she hui* (The dissemination of Western learning and late Qing society) (Shanghai: Shanghai renmin chubanshe, 1994); Meng Yue, "Hybrid Science Versus Modernity: The Practice of the Jiangnan Arsenal, 1864–1897," *East Asian Science, Technology, and Medicine* 16 (1999): 13–52.

9. Wright, *Translating Science*, 31–71; Wang Guangren, *Zhongguo jindai kexue xianqu Xu Shou fu-zi yanjiu* (Pioneers of modern Chinese science: Xu Shou and son) (Beijing: Qinghua daxue chubanshe, 1998).

10. Wright, *Translating Science*, 232–33. Some scholars now believe that many of Fryer's texts from the 1880s and 1890s, including everything in the *Gezhi huibian* and most of Fryer's missionary textbooks, were in fact cotranslated and coedited by Shandong native Luan Xueqian. See Wang Yangzong, "Gezhi huibian zhi Zhongguo bianjizhe zhi kao" (Investigations into the Chinese editor of the Gezhi huiban), *Wen xian* 63 (Jan. 1995): 237–43. My thanks to Benjamin Elman for pointing out this reference. On Luan, see David Wright, "John Fryer and the Shanghai Polytechnic: Making Space for Science in Nineteenth-Century China," *British Journal of the History of Science* 29, no. 100 (1996): 1–16.

11. David Knight, "Communicating Chemistry," in *Communicating Chemistry: Textbooks and Their Audiences, 1789–1939*, ed. Anders Lundgren and Bernadette Bensaude-Vincent (Canton, Mass.: Science History Publications, 2000), 187–206.

12. *Huaxue weisheng lun* was published in eighty-eight installments in Fryer's *Gezhi huibian*, beginning in 1878. It can be found in *Gezhi huibian* (Nanjing: Nanjing gu jiu shu dian, 1992), beginning in vol. 2, 224.

13. Christopher Hamlin has called this outlook "Chemico-Theology." See his "Providence and Putrefaction: Victorian Sanitarians and the Natural Theology of Health and Disease," *Victorian Studies* 28 (1984–85): 381–411; and Hamlin, "Robert Warington and the Moral Economy of the Aquarium," *Journal of the History of Biology* 1 (1986): 134–41.

14. James F. W. Johnston studied chemistry under Berzelius in Sweden's Uppsala University in the 1830s. He is implicated in the "professional geneology" of several scientists at Yale University, including the renowned chemist Russell Chittenden. See Vera Mainz, Chemical Geneology Database, University of Indiana at Urbana-Champaign, http://www.scs.uiuc.edu/~mainzv/Web_Genealogy/Info/Johnsonjfw.pdf (accessed July 17, 2002).

15. Somnath Ghosh and Pradip Baksi, "The Natural Science Note-Books of Marx and Engels: Middle of 1877 to Early 1883," Hartford Web Publishing World History Archives, http://www.hartford-hwp.com/archives/26/173.html (accessed June 6, 2002).

16. Justus von Liebig, *Familiar Letters on Chemistry: In Its Relations to Physiology, Dietetics, Agriculture, Commerce, and Political Economy* (London: Walton and Maberly, 1859), letter 6.

17. Between 1871 and 1888, Fryer translated or compiled nine texts on chemistry, most with his primary collaborator, Xu Shou. His first important translation, *Huaxue jianyuan* (Mirror of the origins of chemistry) was a translation of the American David Ames Wells's introductory college textbook, *Wells' Principles and Applications of Chemistry* (New York and Chicago: Ivison, Blakeman, Taylor, and Co., 1858). This work, published in 1871, introduced basic concepts of chemistry and began Fryer's long endeavor to produce a unified vocabulary for translating the names of the elements. Wright, *Translating Science*, 50.

18. Qiong Zhang, "Demystifying Qi: The Politics of Cultural Translation and Interpretation in the Early Jesuit Mission to China," in *Tokens of Exchange: The Problem of Translation in Global Circulations*, ed. Lydia H. Liu (Durham, N.C.: Duke University Press, 1999), 74–106.

19. James F. W. Johnston, *The Chemistry of Common Life* (New York: Appleton, 1855), 1: 20; *Huaxue weisheng lun* (installment 5) in Fryer, *Gezhi huibian*, 2: 251.

20. Johnston, *Chemistry of Common Life*, 2: 257.

21. *Huaxue weisheng lun* (installment 76) in Fryer, *Gezhi huibian*, 2: 496.

22. On missionaries' "powers," see Paul Cohen, *China and Christianity: The Missionary Movement and the Growth of Chinese Antiforeignism, 1860–1870* (Cambridge, Mass.: Harvard University Press, 1963). On foreign alchemy, see Wright, *Translating Science*, 9n22, quoting Karl Gutzlaff, *Chinese Repository* 1, no. 4 (1832): 129. My thanks to Benjamin Elman for tracking down this source.

23. On brewing, see Johnston, *Chemistry of Common Life*, 2: 239–45.

24. Ibid., 2: 26.

25. Ibid.

26. Such observations about opium use were decidedly a minority opinion among British missionaries. On missionary anti-opium efforts, see Paul Howard, "Opium Smoking in Qing China: Responses to a Social Problem, 1729–1906" (Ph.D. diss., University of Pennsylvania, 1998).

27. Johnston, *Chemistry of Common Life*, 2.

28. On "racial immunity" and acclimitization, see Mark Harrison, *Climates and Constitutions: Health, Race, Environment, and British Imperialism in India, 1600–1850* (Oxford and New York: Oxford University Press, 1999); and Michael Osborne, "Resurrecting Hippocrates: Hygienic Sciences and the French Scientific Expeditions to Egypt, Morea, and Algeria," in *Warm Climates and Western Medicine: The Emergence of Tropical Medicine, 1500–1900*, ed. David Arnold (Amsterdam and Atlanta, Ga.: Rodopi, 1996), 80–98.

29. Marta Hanson, "Robust Northerners and Delicate Southerners: The Nineteenth-Century Invention of a Southern Medical Tradition," *positions* 6, no. 3 (1998): 515–50; Frank Dikötter, *The Discourse of Race in Modern China* (Stanford: Stanford University Press, 1992); Laura Hotstatler, *Qing Colonial En-*

terprise: Ethnography and Cartography in Early Modern China (Chicago: University of Chicago Press, 2001).

30. *Huaxue weisheng lun* (installment 53, 8b), in Fryer, *Gezhi huibian*, 3: 310.

31. Ibid.

32. Fryer produced these and numerous other texts for the School and Textbook Committee of the General Missionary Conference. By the time the *Weisheng bian* series was published, the committee had changed its name to the more comprehensive Educational Association of China. Xiong, *Xi xue dong jian*, 484.

33. Mary Hannah Hanchett Hunt, *Health for Little Folks* (New York, Cincinnati, and Chicago: American Book Company, 1890); John Harvey Kellogg, *First Book in Physiology and Hygiene* (New York: Harper and Brothers, 1888); James Johonnot and Eugene Bouton, *Lessons in Hygiene, or The Human Body and How to Take Care of It* (New York, Cincinnati, and Chicago: American Book Company, 1889).

34. Ruth Bordin, *Woman and Temperance: The Quest for Power and Liberty, 1873–1900* (Philadelphia: Temple University Press, 1981); Carol Mattingly, *Well-Tempered Women: Nineteenth-Century Temperance Rhetoric* (Carbondale: Southern Illinois University Press, 1998); Ian Tyrrell, *Woman's World/ Woman's Empire: The Woman's Christian Temperance Union in International Perspective, 1800–1930* (Chapel Hill: University of North Carolina Press, 1991).

35. On STI, see Jonathan Zimmerman, *Distilling Democracy: Alcohol Education in America's Public Schools, 1880–1925* (Lawrence: University of Kansas Press, 1999).

36. Ibid., 5.

37. Tyrrell, *Woman's World/ Woman's Empire*, 70.

38. Ibid., 109. On the WCTU's influence in Japan, see Sheldon Garon, "The World's Oldest Debate? Prostitution and the State in Imperial Japan, 1900–1945," *American Historical Review* 98, no. 3 (1993): 710–32; and Garon, *Molding Japanese Minds: The State in Everyday Life* (Princeton, N.J.: Princeton University Press, 1997).

39. On Kellogg, see John Money, *The Destroying Angel: Sex, Fitness, and Food in the Legacy of Degeneracy Theory: Graham Crackers, Kellogg's Corn Flakes, and American History* (Buffalo, N.Y.: Prometheus Books, 1985).

40. Zimmerman, *Distilling Democracy*.

41. *Juzhai weisheng lun* appears in seventeen installments in Fryer's *Gezhi huibian*, beginning in 1879.

42. *Juzhai weisheng lun* (installment 1, 37b) in Fryer, *Gezhi huibian*, 79.

43. Xiong, *Xi xue dong jian*, 492.

44. On Zheng Guanying, see Albert Feuerwerker, *China's Early Industrialization: Shen Hsuan-huai (1844–1916) and Mandarin Enterprise* (Cambridge, Mass.: Harvard University Press, 1958). See also his collected writings, *Zheng Guanying ji*, ed. Xia Dongyuan (Shanghai: Shanghai renmin chuban she, 1982–88).

45. Zheng Guanying, *Zhongwai weisheng yaozhi* (n.p.), Shanghai Munic-

ipal Library. There are two editions: an 1890 edition with 4 juan, and a punctuated 1895 edition with 5 juan. The content of the two editions is essentially the same, with the exception of the addition in the 1895 edition of a translation (in juan 5) of Charles DeLacy's 1885 work, *How to Prolong Life* (translated in 1892 by John Fryer as *Yan nian yishou lun,* see below).

46. Charles de Lacy, *How to Prolong Life: An Inquiry into the Cause of Old Age and Natural Decay, Showing the Diet and Agents Best Adapted for the Lengthened Prolongation of Existence* (London: Balliere, Tindall, and Cox, 1885).

47. Zheng, *Zhongwai weisheng yaozhi* (1895): on public health, 4: 40a–b; on magnetism, 4: 45a; on clitoridectomy, 4: 44b.

48. Zheng, *Zhongwai weisheng yaozhi* (1895), juan 3: 94a–b.

49. Ibid., 3: 16b.

50. Zheng, *Zheng Guanying ji,* 2: 150.

51. Partha Chatterjee, *The Nation and Its Fragments: Colonial and Postcolonial Histories* (Princeton, N.J.: Princeton University Press, 1993).

52. David Arnold, *Colonizing the Body: State, Medicine, and Epidemic Disease in Nineteenth-Century India* (Berkeley and Los Angeles: University of California Press, 1993).

53. Kerrie MacPherson, *A Wilderness of Marshes: The Origins of Public Health in Shanghai, 1843–1893* (Hong Kong: Oxford University Press, 1987).

54. Philip Curtin, "Medical Knowledge and Urban Planning in Tropical Africa," *American Historical Review* 90, no. 3 (1985): 594–613.

55. Robert Bickers and Jeffrey Wasserstrom, "Shanghai's 'Dogs and Chinese Not Admitted' Sign: Legend, History, and Contemporary Symbol," *China Quarterly* 142 (1995):444–66.

56. Zhang Tao, *Jinmen zaji* (Miscellaneous records of Tianjin) (1884; reprint, Tianjin: Tianjin guji chubanshe, 1986), 124–25.

57. Details of interview from Tianjin consul Buslow's confidential report to Peking Embassy, 19 June 1894, PRO, FO, 674/60, 45, emphasis in original. In Hong Kong, plague patients were placed in ice baths in order to reduce high fevers. Brandy and wine were liberally used as pain killers in hospitals of the time. Neither Western nor Chinese medicine of the nineteenth century had any effective treatments for bubonic plague. For Chinese reaction to British public health policy and medical treatments during the 1894 outbreak of bubonic plague in Hong Kong, see Elizabeth Sinn, *Power and Charity: The Early Years of the Tung Wah Hospital* (Hong Kong: Oxford University Press, 1989); Carol Benedict, *Bubonic Plague in Nineteenth-Century China* (Stanford: Stanford University Press, 1996.); Iijima Wataru, *Pesuto to kindai Chûgoku* (Tokyo: Kenbun Shuppan, 2000).

CHAPTER 5

Epigraph: Ban Tadayasu, *Tekijuku to Nagayo Sensai: Eiseigaku to Shôkô shishi* (Osaka: Sogensha, 1987), 156.

1. Frederico Massini, *The Formation of the Modern Chinese Lexicon and Its*

Evolution toward a National Language: The Period from 1840 to 1898 (Berkeley: Journal of Chinese Linguistics, 1993), 202.

2. Ibid.

3. See studies in Lydia H. Liu, ed., *Tokens of Exchange: The Problem of Translation in Global Circulations* (Durham, N.C.: Duke University Press, 1999); and Michael Lackner, Iwo Amelung, and Joachim Kurtz , eds., *New Terms for New Ideas: Western Knowledge and Lexical Change in Late Imperial China* (Leiden: Brill, 2001).

4. James Bartholomew, *The Formation of Science in Japan* (New Haven: Yale University Press, 1989), remains the standard chronicle of the emergence of a modern scientific community. John Bowers described the careers of Western medical teachers and their Japanese students in the waning years of the Tokugawa shogunate in *Western Medical Pioneers in Feudal Japan* (Baltimore: Johns Hopkins University Press, 1970); and *When the Twain Meet: The Rise of Western Medicine in Japan* (Baltimore: Johns Hopkins University Press, 1980). William Johnston, in his magisterial study of tuberculosis in Japan, *The Modern Epidemic: Tuberculosis in Japan* (Cambridge, Mass.: Harvard University Press, 1995), has an excellent introduction to the structures of the Meiji public health system. For recent studies on *eisei*, see Thomas Lamarre, "Bacterial Cultures and Linguistic Colonies: Mori Rintaro's Experiments with History, Science, and Languages," *positions* 6, no. 3 (1998): 597–635; and Susan Burns, "Constructing the National Body: Public Health and the Nation in Nineteenth-Century Japan," in *Nation Work: Asian Elites and National Identities*, ed. Timothy Brook and Andre Schmid (Ann Arbor: University of Michigan Press, 2000).

5. Ban, *Tekijuku to Nagayo Sensai*, 143–47.

6. For an introduction to Nagayo Sensai's early career, see Ann Jannetta, "From Physician to Bureaucrat: The Case of Nagayo Sensai," in *New Directions in the Study of Meiji Japan*, ed. Helen Hardacre (Leiden: Brill, 1997).

7. For an introduction to Dutch Learning, see Donald Keene, *The Japanese Discovery of Europe* (Stanford: Stanford University Press, 1969).

8. On Ogata's translation of Hufeland, see Sugimoto Tsutomu, *Edo Ranpôi kara no messēji* (Tokyo: Perikansha, 1992).

9. For the early years of Western medicine in Japan, see Bowers, *Western Medical Pioneers*; and Bowers, *When the Twain Meet*.

10. Burns, "Constructing the National Body," 22–23.

11. Bowers, *Western Medical Pioneers*, 56.

12. Ban, *Tekijuku to Nagayo Sensai*, 139.

13. Jannetta, "From Physician to Bureaucrat," 158–59.

14. On the rise of German medical education, see Thomas Broman, *The Transformation of German Academic Medicine, 1750–1820* (Cambridge: Cambridge University Press, 1996); and Thomas N. Bonner, *American Doctors and German Universities: A Chapter in International Relations* (Lincoln: University of Nebraska Press, 1963).

15. Anthony S. Wohl, *Endangered Lives: Public Health in Victorian Britain* (London: J. M. Dent and Sons, 1983), 7.

16. Jannetta, "From Physician to Bureaucrat," 160.

17. Rudolf Virchow, *Collected Essays on Public Health and Epidemiology,* ed. L. J. Rather, vol. 2 (Cambridge, Mass.: Science History Publications, 1985).

18. On Pettenkofer's approach, see Erwin Ackerknecht, "Anticontagionism between 1821 and 1867," *Bulletin of the History of Medicine* 22 (1948), 562–93; Wolfgang Locher, "Max von Pettenkofer—Life Stations of a Genius: On the 100th Anniversary of His Death," *International Journal of Hygiene and Environmental Health* 203 (2001): 379–91.

19. For an overview of the influence of Frank on Japanese public health, see Johnston, *The Modern Epidemic.*

20. Quoted in George Rosen, *A History of Public Health* (1958; reprint, Baltimore: Johns Hopkins University Press, 1993).

21. Ban, *Tekijuku to Nagayo Sensai,* 133–34; Burns, "Constructing the National Body," 25.

22. Johnston, *The Modern Epidemic,* 179.

23. Ibid., 179.

24. Ono Yoshirô, *Seiketsu no kindai* (Tokyo: Kôdansha, 1997), 127.

25. Ban, *Tekijuku to Nagayo Sensai,* 47.

26. Sugimoto, *Edo Ranpôi kara no messēji,* 96.

27. C. W. Hufeland, *Enchiridion medicum: Oder Anleitung zur medizinischen Praxis* (Berlin: Jonas Verlagsbuchhandlung, 1836), 709–31.

28. Ogata Koreyoshi, *Eisei shinron* (Osaka: Inada, [1872]), copy in the National Library of Medicine, Washington, D.C. Nagayo Sensai would certainly have known of Ogata's work. The two had studied Dutch medicine together under Pompe and then taught together with Pompe's successor, Antonius Francis Bauduin. After the Meiji Restoration, Nagayo remained in Nagasaki, while Ogata established Osaka's first Western-style hospital and medical school.

29. Ernst Tiegel, *Esei hanron,* trans. Ôi Gendô (Tokyo: Hasunuma, [1880–81]), copy in the National Library of Medicine, Washington, D.C.

30. The authority of Tiegel's lectures received confirmation from none other than Nagayo Sensai, who penned with his own bold calligraphy the text's colophon: "Second to None in Its Comprehensiveness."

31. Ernst Tiegel, *Ifukuryô shikensetsu* (Report on comparative hygienic value of native and foreign clothing, including footwear), trans. Katayama Kuniyoshi (Tokyo: Naimushô, Eiseikyoku, [1881]), copy in the National Library of Medicine, Washington, D.C.

32. Johnston, *The Modern Epidemic,* 168.

33. For police actions, see Yamamoto Shun'ichi, *Nihon korera shi* (Tokyo: Tokyo Daigaku Shuppankai, 1982), 31–40.

34. Tatsukawa Shôji, *Meiji iji ôrai* (Tokyo: Shinchôsha, 1986), 67–73.

35. Johnston, *The Modern Epidemic,* 176.

36. Susan Burns, "Between National Policy and Local Practice: Cholera, Gotô Shimpei, and the Formation of the 'Hygienic Nation,' " (paper presented at the annual meeting of the Association of Asian Studies, Washington, D.C., Apr. 2002).

37. Burns "Constructing the National Body," 17.

38. Kitaoka Shin'ichi, *Gotô Shinpei: gaikô to bijon* (Gotô Shinpei: Diplomacy and vision) (Tokyo: Chûô Kôronsha, 1988), 18–20.

39. Ono, *Seiketsu no kindai*, 111–12.

40. Because Mori went on to become a well-known literary figure, there are many works on his life, including several that focus on his contributions to military medicine and hygiene. See Date Kazuo, *Isei toshite no Mori Ôgai*, 2 vols. (Tokyo: Sekibundô Shuppan, 1981); Maruyama Hiroshi, *Mori Ôgai to Eiseigaku* (Tokyo: Keiso shobo, 1984); Matsui Toshihiko, *Gun-i Mori Ôgai* (Tokyo: Ofusha, 1989); and Miyamoto Shinobu, *Mori Ôgai no igaku shisô* (Tokyo: Keiso Shobo, 1979).

41. On Mori's time in Germany, see his Berlin diary in Mori Ôgai, *Ôgai zenshû*, vol. 38 (Tokyo: Iwanami Shoten, 1971–75).

42. Stefan Tanaka, *Japan's Orient: Rendering Pasts into History* (Berkeley: University of California Press, 1993).

43. The following discussion draws from Mori Ôgai, *Eiseigaku tai-i*, in Mori Ôgai, *Ôgai zenshû*, 30:156–87.

44. On Kitasato, see Bartholemew, *Formation of Science in Japan*, 72–82, 191–92, 205–7.

45. Yasuzumi Saneyoshi, *The Surgical and Medical History of the Naval War Between Japan and China during 1894–1895* (Tokyo: Tokio Printing Co. 1900), 13.

46. Ibid., 256.

47. Date, *Isei toshite no Mori Ôgai*, 2:80. For Mori Ôgai's extensive writings on *kakke*, see Matsui, *Gun-i Mori Ôgai*, 225–80. Beriberi is caused by lack of vitamin B1 (thiamin) and among Asian populations is mostly caused by reliance on thiamin-deficient polished rice for the bulk of calories in the diet. Initial symptoms include fatigue, poor memory, sleep disturbances, abdominal discomfort, and constipation, followed by a burning sensation in feet, cramps in the legs, and a loss of leg muscle control. If left untreated it can result in heart failure and death.

48. Date, *Isei toshite no Mori Ôgai*, 2: 370.

49. Mori Rintarô, *Eisei shinhen*, in Mori Ôgai, *Ôgai zenshû*, vols. 31 and 32.

50. For a discussion of this approach to etiology and diagnosis, see Farquhar, *Knowing Practice*, 119–31.

51. *Zhibao* (The Zhili gazzette), 8 July 1895, 2.

52. Ibid., 27 July 1895, 3.

53. Ibid., 5 October 1895, 3.

54. Ono, *Seiketsu no kindai*, 5–10.

CHAPTER 6

Epigraphs: James Ricalton, *China Through the Stereoscope: A Journey Through the Dragon Empire at the Time of the Boxer Uprising*, ed. Jim Zwick (New York: Underwood and Underwood, 1901; revised and enlarged edition, BoondocksNet, http://www.boondocksnet.com/china, 2000). Lyautey quoted in

Roy Porter, *The Greatest Benefit to Mankind: A Medical History of Humanity from Antiquity to the Present* (London: HarperCollins, 1997), 463.

1. See James L. Hevia, "Leaving a Brand on China: Missionary Discourse in the Wake of the Boxer Movement," *Modern China* 18, no. 3 (1992), 304–32; Paul Cohen, *History in Three Keys: The Bowers as Event, Experience, and Myth* (New York: Columbia University Press, 1997); Lydia Liu, *Translingual Practice: Literature, National Culture, and Translated Modernity — China, 1900–1937* (Stanford: Stanford University Press, 1995), 28; Prasenjit Duara, *Rescuing History from the Nation: Questioning Narratives of Modern China* (Chicago: University of Chicago Press, 1995); Feng Jicai, *Shenbian* (The miraculous pigtail) (Beijing: Zhonguo minjian chubanshe, 1988); Wang Shuo, *Please Don't Call Me Human (Qianwang bie ba wo dang ren)*, trans. Howard Goldblatt (New York: Hyperion, 2000).

2. Shu-mei Shih, *The Lure of the Modern: Writing Modernism in Semicolonial China, 1917–1937* (Berkeley: University of California Press, 2001), 373.

3. Gail Hershatter, *The Workers of Tianjin, 1900–1949* (Stanford: Stanford University Press, 1986).

4. Shang Keqiang and Liu Haiyan, eds., *Tianjin zujie shehui yanjiu* (Tianjin: Tianjin renmin chuban she, 1994), 11–12.

5. British Consul, 2 December 1884, PRO, FO, 674/8, letter no. 44. The foreign population increased substantially after the Boxer Uprising. By the first formal census in 1906, a total of 6,341 foreigners lived in the concessions of Tianjin. Li Jingneng, ed., *Tianjin renkoushi* (Tianjin: Nankai daxue chubanshe, 1990), 307.

6. Liu Mengyang, "Tianjin quanfei bianluan jishi," in *Yihetuan* (The Boxers), ed. Jian Bozan, Zhongguo shixue hui (Shanghai: Shen zhou guo guang she, 1951), 9: 8.

7. Joseph Esherick, *The Origins of the Boxer Uprising* (Berkeley and Los Angeles: Univesity of California Press, 1987).

8. O. D. Rasmussen, *Tientsin: An Illustrated Outline History* (Tianjin: Tientsin Press, 1925) 131–33.

9. Rasmussen, *Tientsin*, 114. See Mori Etsuko, "Tenshinto tôgamon no tsuite" (On the Tianjin Provincial Government), *Tôyôshi kenkyû* 67, no. 2 (1988): 318.

10. Cohen, *History in Three Keys*.

11. James L. Hevia, "Looting Beijing: 1860, 1900," in *Tokens of Exchange: The Problem of Translation in Global Circulations*, ed. Lydia H. Liu (Durham, N.C.: Duke University Press, 1999), 192–213.

12. See Zhu Renxun, *Wenjian lu* (Recollections) (hand-copied manuscript, Tianjin: Tianjin Academy of Social Sciences, n.d.), entries GX 26/11/9 (30 Dec. 1900), GX 26/11/17 (7 Jan, 1901).

13. Liu Xizi, "Jinxi piji" (Anxious record from west of Tianjin), in *Yihetuan* (The Boxers), ed. Jian Bozan, Zhongguo shixue hui (Shanghai: Shen zhou guo guang she, 1951).

14. Liu Mengyang, "Tianjin quanfei bianluan jishi," 9: 11.

15. Ibid., 9: 12. See also the memoirs of Hua Xuelan, "Gengzi riji," in *Gengzi jishi* (Memoirs of 1900), ed. Zhongguo shehui kexue yuan jindaiyanjiu suo (Beijing: n.p., 1978), 102.

16. Zhu Renxun, *Wenjian lu*, entry GX 26/6/18 (12 July 1900).

17. See Rasmussen, *Tientsin*, 224.

18. Gunji jôhô (Military information) Web site, Okiraku gunji kinkyû kai, http://www51.tok2.com/home/okigunnji/akiyamakouko.htm.

19. Mori Etsuko, " 'Tenshinto tôgamon no tsuite,' " 316.

20. Ôta Azan, *Fukushima shôgun iseki: denki Fukushima Yasumasa* (Tokyo: Ôzorasha, 1997).

21. Warwick Anderson, "Excremental Colonialism,"*Critical Inquiry* 21, no. 3 (spring 1995): 640–69; Bruno Latour, *The Pasteurization of France* (Cambridge, Mass.: Harvard University Press, 1988).

22. John Farley, *Bilharzia: A History of Imperial Tropical Medicine* (New York and Cambridge: Cambridge University Press, 1991); Douglas Haynes, *Imperial Medicine: Patrick Manson and the Conquest of Tropical Disease* (Philadelphia: University of Pennsylvania Press, 2001).

23. Philip Curtin "Medical Knowledge and Urban Planning in Tropical Africa," *American Historical Review* 90, no. 3 (1985): 594–613.

24. Roger Cooter, Mark Harrison, and Steve Sturdy, eds., *War, Medicine, and Modernity* (Stroud: Sutton, 1998).

25. See illustration of mass burials in Liu Mengyang, "Tianjin quanfei bianluan jishi."

26. Lewis Bernstein, "A History of Tientsin in Early Modern Times, 1800–1910" (Ph.D. diss., University of Kansas, 1988), 236.

27. Zhu Renxun, *Wenjian lu*, entries GX 26/8/23 (16 Sept. 1900), GX 26/run8/20 (13 Oct, 1900). For Chinese burial practices as a point of contention between Chinese and foreigners, see Bryna Goodman, *Native Place, City, and Nation: Regional Networks and Identities in Shanghai, 1853–1937* (Berkeley and Los Angeles: University of California Press, 1995), 154–55.

28. Bernstein, *History of Tientsin*, 235.

29. Ibid., 250. On incarceration and modernity in China, see Michael Dutton, *Policing and Punishment in China: From Patriarchy to "The People"* (Cambridge and New York: Cambridge University Press, 1992); Frank Dikötter, *Crime, Punishment, and the Prison in Modern China* (New York: Columbia University Press, 2002).

30. Zhu Renxun, *Wenjian lu*, entry GX 26/6/23 (19 July 1900).

31. Ibid., entry GX 28/5/19 (24 June 1902).

32. Ibid., entry GX 26/9/3 (25 Oct. 1900).

33. On the remarkably indiscriminate excretory habits of Europeans before the arrival of "civilization," see Norbert Elias, *The Civilizing Process* (London: Blackwell, 1993).

34. Dipesh Chakrabarty, "Open Space, Public Place: Garbage, Modernity, and India," *South Asia: Journal of South Asian Studies* 14, no. 1 (1991): 15–31.

35. Anderson, "Excremental Colonialism."

36. Zhu Renxun, *Wenjian lu,* entries GX 28/4/24 (10 May 1902), GX 28/5/22 (27 June 1902). This privatized system continued throughout the Republican period and into the PRC.

37. On Beijing's walls, see Susan Naquin, *Peking: Temples and City Life, 1400–1900* (Berkeley: University of California Press, 2001), 4–10.

38. Mori Etsuko, " 'Tenshinto tôgamon no tsuite,' " 321.

39. *Dutong yamen huiyi jiyao* (Minutes of the meetings of the Tianjin provisional government, hereafter *DTYMHYJY*), translation of *Procès-verbaux des séance du conseil du gouvernement provisoire de Tientsin* (handwritten manuscript, Tianjin: Tianjin Academy of Social Sciences, n.d.). Segments of this translation have been published as "Tianjin dutong yamen huiyiji yaoxuan," ed. Liu Haiyan and Hao Kelu, *Jindai shi ziliao* 79 (1991): 34–75. On the establishment of brothels, see entries for meetings on 10 Aug. 1900 and 27 Aug. 1900.

40. On lock hospitals and brothels in Japan, see Sheldon Garon, "The World's Oldest Debate? Prostitution and the State in Imperial Japan, 1900–1945," *American Historical Review* 98, no. 3 (1993): 710–33. On debates on lock hospitals in the British empire, see Antoinette Burton, *Burdens of History: British Feminists, Indian Women, and Imperial Culture, 1865–1915* (Chapel Hill: University of North Carolina Press, 1994).

41. Zhu Renxun, *Wenjian lu,* entry GX 26/11/17 (7 Jan. 1901).

42. For report and directives, see *DTYMHYJY* for 2 and 6 June 1902.

43. Zhu Renxun, *Wenjian lu,* entry GX 28/5/11 (16 June 1902).

44. *Peking and Tientsin Times,* editorial, 7 June 1902.

45. Ibid., editorial, 14 June 1902.

46. Tezuka Akira, *Bakumatsu, Meiji kaigai tokôsha sôran* (Tokyo: Kashiwa Shobô, 1992), 2: 82. My thanks to Professor Yoshizawa Seiichirô of Tokyo University for tracking down the identity of Dr. Tsuzuki.

47. All information on Dr. Tsuzuki from J. Tsuzuki, "Bericht uber meine epidemioligischen Beobachtungen und Forschundgen wahrend der Choleraepedemie im Nordchina im Jahre 1902" (Report on my epidemiological observations and researches during the cholera epidemic of 1902 in north China), in *Archiv für Schiffs und Tropen-Hygiene* (Archives for naval and tropical hygiene) (Leipzig, 1904).

48. Tenshin kyoryûmindan, *Tenshin kyoryû mindan nijû shûnen kinenshi* (Tianjin: n.p., 1930), 543.

49. On Japanese formation of nationality/ethnicity vis-à-vis the West, see Stefan Tanaka, *Japan' s Orient: Rendering Pasts into History* (Berkeley: University of California Press, 1993); Louise Young, *Japan' s Total Empire: Manchuria and the Culture of Wartime Imperialism* (Berkeley: University of California Press, 1998); Frank Dikötter, ed., *The Construction of Racial Identities in China and Japan: Historical and Contemporary Perspectives* (London: Hurst and Co., 1997). On the impact that the varied class background of Japanese sojourners had on Japanese identity formation in the colonies, see Barbara Brooks, "Colonial Power and Public Health in Japanese-Held Korea" (paper presented at the annual meeting of the Association of Asian Studies, Washington, D.C., Mar. 2002).

50. *DTYMHYJY*, 96.

51. Yan Xiu, *Yan Xiu xiansheng nian pu* (The chronological biography of Mr. Yan Xiu) (Jinan: Jilu Press, 1990), 130.

52. Hua Xuelan, *Xinchou riji* (1901 diary) (Shanghai: Shangwu yinshu guan, 1936), 1–17. Hua was an 1886 *jinshi* degree holder and was related by marriage to other powerful salt merchant families, including the Yans. He went on to become active in education reform and published books on mathematics and chemistry.

53. Ibid., x.

54. Susan Naquin, *Millenarian Rebellion in China: The Eight Trigrams Uprising of 1813* (New Haven: Yale University Press, 1976).

55. Ranajit Guha, *Dominance Without Hegemony: History and Power in Colonial India* (Cambridge, Mass.: Harvard University Press, 1997).

56. Hershatter, *Workers of Tianjin*, 25.

57. The relationship between sanitary policing and territorial claims is addressed in Goodman, *Native Place*, 154–57. Also see Bridie Andrews, *The Making of Modern Chinese Medicine* (Cambridge: Cambridge University Press, 2004).

58. For an overview of these reforms, see Stephen R. MacKinnon, *Power and Politics in Late Imperial China: Yuan Shikai in Beijing and Tianjin, 1901–1908* (Berkeley and Los Angeles: University of California Press, 1980), chaps. 4 and 5.

59. Gan Houci, ed., *Beiyang gongdu leizuan* (Classified collection of public documents of the commissioner of trade for the northern ports, hereafter *BYGDLZ*) (1907; reprint, Taibei: Wenhai chuban she, 1966), 25, 1836.

60. The most detailed description of the Tianjin Army Medical School is in *Ershi shiji chu de Tianjin gaikuang* (Conditions in early-twentieth-century Tianjin), a translation of Shinkoku chûtongun shireibu, ed., *Tenshinshi* (Tianjin gazetteer) (Tokyo: Hakubunkan, 1909), trans. Hou Zhentong (Tianjin: Tianjin difang shizhi bianxiu weiyuanhui zongbianjishi chuban, 1986), 318–19. My thanks to Professor Yoshizawa Seiichirô for providing the citation for the original source.

61. On the Dôjinkai, see Ming-Cheng M. Lo, *Doctors Within Borders: Profession, Ethnicity, and Modernity in Colonial Taiwan* (Berkeley: University of California Press, 2002) 151–79.

62. Gan Houci, *BYGDLZ*, 1825.

63. Ibid., 1828–30.

64. The following discussion on the duties of Tianjin police comes from the police regulations, *Tianjin nanduan xuncha zongju zhangcheng*, 1907, Tianjin Academy of Social Sciences, History Research Library copy. Also see Gan Houci, *BYGDLZ*, juan 8.

65. On the Japanese influence in the Beijing and Baoding Police Academies, see Douglas Reynolds, *China: 1898–1912* (Cambridge, Mass.: Harvard University Press, 1993), 161–74; and David Strand, *Rickshaw Beijing: City People and Politics in the 1920s* (Berkeley and Los Angeles: University of California Press, 1989), 67–69. According to Reynolds, Kawashima spent a brief ten days in Baod-

ing laying the groundwork for the Zhili Police Academy, which trained police for Tianjin. On the development of modern police systems throughout China, see Frederic Wakeman, *Policing Shanghai, 1927–1937* (Berkeley and Los Angeles: University of California Press, 1995). On Tianjin's police, see Yoshizawa Seiichirô, *Tenshin no kindai* (Nagoya: Nagoya University Press, 2002).

66. Dipesh Chakrabarty, "Postcoloniality and the Artifice of History: Who Speaks for 'Indian' Pasts?" in *A Subaltern Studies Reader, 1986–1995*, ed. Ranajit Guha (Minneapolis: University of Minnesota Press, 1997), 263–93 (288).

CHAPTER 7

1. On the physical transformation of Chinese cities in the first decades of the twentieth century, see the studies included in Joseph Esherick, ed., *Remaking the Chinese City: Modernity and National Identity, 1900–1950* (Honolulu: University of Hawaii Press, 2000). Monographs on individual cities include Michael Tsin, *Nation, Governance, and Modernity in China: Canton, 1900–1927* (Stanford: Stanford University Press, 1999); Kristen Stapleton, *Civilizing Chengdu: Chinese Urban Reform, 1895–1937* (Cambridge: Harvard University Press, 2000); David Strand, *Rickshaw Beijing: City People and Politics in the 1920s* (Berkeley: University of California Press, 1989).

2. On sewers, water pipes, and the city, see Lewis Mumford, *The City in History: Its Origins, Its Transformations, and Its Prospects* (New York: Harcourt Brace, 1961); Richard Sennet, *Flesh and Stone: The Body and the City in Western Civilization* (New York: W. W. Norton, 1994); David Jordon, *Transforming Paris: The Life and Labors of Baron Haussmann* (New York: The Free Press, 1995); Donald Reid, *Paris Sewers and Sewermen: Realities and Representations* (Cambridge: Harvard University Press, 1991); Jean-Pierre Goubert, *The Conquest of Water: The Advent of Health in the Industrial Age* (Cambridge: Polity Press, 1986); Christopher Hamlin, *A Science of Impurity: Water Analysis in Nineteenth Century Britain* (Berkeley: University of California Press, 1991).

3. Lai Xinxia, ed., *Tianjin jindaishi* (Modern Tianjin history). (Tianjin: Nankai Daxue chubanshe, 1987) chart between pages 196 and 197.

4. Timothy Mitchell, *Colonising Egypt* (Cambridge: Cambridge University Press, 1991), 12.

5. For photographs of Tianjin's foreign architecture in the 1920s, see O. D. Rasmussen, *Tientsin: An Illustrated Outline History* (Tianjin: Tientsin Press, 1925); see also Tianjin jindai jianzhu bianxie zu, *Tianjin jindai jianzhu* (Tianjin's modern architecture) (Tianjin: Tianjin kexue jishu chuban she, 1990).

6. Gail Hershatter, *The Workers of Tianjin, 1900–1949* (Stanford: Stanford University Press, 1986), 17.

7. *Tianjin renkou shi*, 6. See also chart in Luo Shuwei et al., ed., *Jindai Tianjin chengshi shi* (The modern history of Tianjin) (Beijing: Zhongguo shehui kexue chubanshe, 1993), 455.

8. With its flourishing drug trade, the Japanese concession became known

as the "heart of north China's heroin belt." On the Japanese concession under-world, see Marcus Mervine, "The Japanese Concession in Tientsin and the Nar-cotics Trade," *Information Bulletin of the Council on International Affairs* 3, no. 4 (1937): 83–95; Sun Limin and Xin Gongxian, "Tianjin ri zujie gaikuang" (The Japanese concession in Tianjin), *Tianjin wenshi ziliao xuanji*, 18 (1982): 11–151; and Motohiro Kobayashi, "Drug Operations by Resident Japanese in Tianjin," in Timothy Brook and Bob Tadashi Wakabayashi, ed., *Opium Regimes* (Berkeley: University of California Press, 2000).

9. Luo Shuwei, *Jindai Tianjin chengshi shi*, 335.

10. Sun Xuelian, *Tianjin zhinan* (A guide to Tianjin) (Tianjin: Zhonghua shuju, 1923), 6.

11. For photographs of the "New City," see Tianjin, ed., *Jindai Tianjin tuzhi*, 141.

12. For a list of police stations housed in temples, see Song Yunpu, ed., *Tianjin zhilue* (A brief gazetteer of Tianjin) (1931, reprint, Taibei: Chengwen chuban-she, 1969), 41. On co-opting of Daoist temples by modern government concerns, see Prasenjit Duara, *Culture, Power, and the State: Rural North China, 1900–1942* (Stanford: Stanford University Press, 1988); *Rescuing History from the Nation: Questioning Narratives of Modern China* (Chicago: University of Chicago Press, 1995). By 1904, the number of active temples in Tianjin had de-creased from 324 (c. 1870) to 169. *Ershi shiji chu de Tianjin gaikuan*, 130.

13. Doctors of Chinese medicine who had their offices in the French con-cession include the prolific medical writer Ding Zilang (see chapter 8).

14. Gan Minyang, ed., *Xin Tianjin zhinan* (New guide to Tianjin) (Tianjin: Jiangxue zhai shuju, 1927), 8.

15. Daniel Headrick, *The Tentacles of Progress: Technology Transfer in the Age of Imperialism, 1850–1940* (New York: Oxford University Press, 1988), 166–67.

16. British Municipal Area, Tientsin, "Municipal Bye-laws [sic], 1919" (Tianjin: Tientsin Press, n.d.).

17. Tianjin jindai jianzhu bianxie zu, *Tianjin jindai jianzhu.*

18. British Municipal Council, Tientsin, "Municipal Bye-Laws [sic]": Sani-tary Section (Tianjin: Tientsin Press, 1929).

19. British Municipal Council, Tientsin, "1929 Annual Report," 72.

20. Ibid., 32.

21. On Tianjin's workshops, see Hershatter, *The Workers of Tianjin.*

22. Tianjin health department to the Tianjin Chamber of Commerce, GX 32/2/4 (24 Feb. 1906), in Tianjinshi dang'an guan, ed., *Tianjin shanghui dang' an huibian* (Tianjin Chamber of Commerce Archives), vol. 2 (Tianjin: Tianjin Chamber of Commerce, 1903–11), 2275.

23. Ibid., 2276.

24. Ibid., 2277–78.

25. *Da gongbao* (Tianjin), 9 Feb. 1907.

26. On Tianjin's transport workers, see Hershatter, *The Workers of Tianjin.*

27. For a marvelously detailed description of the skills of the night-soil car-

rier, see Hanchao Lu, *Beyond the Neon Lights: Everyday Shanghai in the Early Twentieth Century* (Berkeley: University of California Press, 1999), 189–98.

28. For examples of water-carrier organization, see William Rowe, *Hankow: Conflict and Community in a Chinese City, 1796–1895* (Stanford: Stanford University Press, 1986); Lu, *Beyond the Neon Lights.*

29. Gu Daosheng, "Tianjin chengqu mai shui he mai shui jiu su," *Tianjin shizhi* 2 (1990): 49–50.

30. Hershatter, *The Workers of Tianjin,* 125–28; Man-bun Kwan, "Order in Chaos: Tianjin's *Hunhunr* and Urban Identity in Modern China," *Journal of Urban History* 27, no. 1 (2000): 75–91.

31. Ke Chen, "Nongovernmental Organizations and the Urban Control and Management System in Tianjin at the End of the Nineteenth Century," *Social Sciences in China* 11, no. 4 (1990): 54–77.

32. *The Chinese Times,* 12 Oct. 1889.

33. *The Peking and Tientsin Times,* 14 Sept. 1895.

34. Ibid., 21 Sept. 1895.

35. Ibid., 26 Feb.1898.

36. Ibid., 31 Dec. 1898.

37. Ibid., 26 Aug. 1899.

38. British Municipal Council, Tientsin, "Annual Report, 1939" (Tianjin: Tientsin Press, 1940).

39. Shang Keqiang and Liu Haiyan, ed., *Tianjin zujie shehui yanjiu* (Tianjin: Tianjin renmin chuban she, 1994), 126–27; Katsuragawa Mitsumasa, "Sokai zaijû Nihonjin no Chûgoku ninshiki, Tenshin o ichirei to shite" (The perception of China by Japanese residents in the concessions: The case of Tianjin), *Kindai Nihon no Ajia ninshiki* (Modern Japanese perceptions of China), ed. Furuya Tetsuo (Kyoto: Kyoto daigaku jinbun kagaku kenkyûjo, 1994).

40. Tenshin kyoryû mindan, *Tenshin kyoryû mindan nijisshûnen kinenshi* (Tianjin Japanese Residents' Association Twentieth Anniversary Report), (Tianjin: n.p., 1930), 648.

41. Ibid., 649.

42. Ibid., 650.

43. Like the British settlement, several streets in the Japanese concession recalled the names of military men involved in the "conquests" of China, including Fukushima Yasumasa and Akiyama Yoshifuru.

44. Tenshin kyoryûmindan, *Tenshin kyoryûmindan jimu hôkoku* (Tianjin Japanese Settlement Corporation Annual Report) (Tianjin: n.p., 1928), 293, 511.

45. Ibid., 294.

46. On the founding of the Tientsin Native City Waterworks Company, see Li Shaobi and Ni Pujun, "Tianjin zilaishui shiye jianshi" (A brief history of water supply in Tianjin), *Tianjin wenshi ziliao xuanji* 21 (Aug. 1982): 36–37.

47. On the Zha family garden, see Wang Huachang, ed., *Tianjin—yige chengshi de jueqi* (Tianjin—The rise of a city) (Tianjin: Renmin chuban she, 1990), 54; and Tianjin lishi bowuguan et al., eds., *Jindai Tianjin tuzhi,* 9.

48. Li Shaobi and Ni Pujun, "Tianjin zilaishui shiye jianshi," 37.

49. See photograph in Tianjin lishi bowuguan et al., eds., *Jindai Tianjin tuzhi* (Illustrated history of modern Tianjin), (Tianjin: Tianjin guji chubanshe, 1992), 8.

50. See list of streets laid in bills from the waterworks to the public works department, dated 5 May 1910 and 29 Jan. 1912, *Ji' an zilaishui* archive (hereafter JA), file 23, TMA.

51. From the public works department, per Tsaolong Lee, to the Native City Waterworks, 5 July 1904, JA 23.

52. Expressed by the company as one thousand gallons per yuan, a rate understood by the Chinese as 140 *dan* per yuan. This price seems to have remained relatively consistent throughout the company's history. Although I do not attempt in this chapter to discuss the profitability of the water company, it is worthwhile to note that an internal communication from 1931 placed production cost at .08 yuan per one thousand gallons, thus revealing the company's considerable profit margin.

53. Report from Chief Engineer Hansen to Board of Directors, 27 Jan. 1931, JA 36. The 78-percent figure also included water supplied to public bath houses. The main point of this figure is to show that the proportion of private household meter installations was relatively small in the Chinese city.

54. See communication from Engineer in Chief, Native City Waterworks, to the French Municipal Council Secretary, 7 April 1926, JA 28.

55. See report from Engineer in Chief to Board of Directors, "The Effect of Artesian Wells upon the Sale of Water in the Hopei District," 26 Feb. 1931, JA 36.

56. Waterworks to Dr. K. Y. Kwan, Director of the Sanitary Department, 29 July 1907, JA 23.

57. Tientsin Police Taotai to the Tientsin Native City Waterworks, 22 Feb. 1910, company translation of Chinese original, JA 23 (emphasis added).

58. Waterworks to the Director of the Tientsin Police, 22 Feb. 1910, JA 23.

59. For these insights, see Erland Mårald, "Everything Circulates: Agricultural Chemistry and Re-cycling Theories in the Second Half of the Nineteenth Century," (paper presented at the conference of IFF Social Ecology, Nature, Society, History: Long Term Dynamics of Social Metabolism, Vienna, Austria, Sept. 1999). http://www.univie.ac.at/iffsocec/conference99/pdf/poMarald.pdf.

CHAPTER 8

1. Liu Na'ou, "Etiquette and Hygiene" (Liyi he weisheng), quoted in Shumei Shih, *The Lure of the Modern: Writing Modernism in Semicolonial China, 1917–1937* (Berkeley: University of California Press, 2001), 291.

2. On the creator of Pink Pills, see L. Loeb, "George Fulford and Victorian Patent Medicine Men: Quack Mercenaries or Smilesian Entrepreneurs?" *Canadian Bulletin of Medical History* 16, no. 1 (1999): 125–45. On similar patent medicines, see Sarah Stage, *Female Complaints: Lydia Pinkham and the Business of Women' s Medicine* (New York: W. W. Norton, 1979).

3. *Da gong bao* (Tianjin), 9 Sept. 1920, 1.

4. The ability of Chinese marketers to tailor advertisements for foreign products to the tastes of a Chinese audience can be understood through Sherman Cochran's work on business in China. See *Big Business in China: Sino-Foreign Rivalry in the Cigarette Industry, 1890–1930* (Cambridge, Mass.: Harvard University Press, 1980); and *Encountering Chinese Networks: Western, Japanese, and Chinese Corporations in China, 1880–1937* (Berkeley: University of California Press, 2000). On the culture of Chinese medicine advertisements in the republican era, see Sherman Cochran, "Medicine and Advertising Dreams in China, 1900–1950," in *Becoming Chinese: Passages to Modernity and Beyond,* ed. Wen-hsin Yeh (Berkeley: University of California Press, 2000); Huang Ke-wu, "Cong *Shenbao* yiyao guangao kan Min chu Shanghai de yiliao wenhua yu shehui shenghuo, 1912–1926" (The Medical Culture and Social Life of Early Republican Shanghai as Seen Through Medicine Advertisements in the *Shenbao),* *Zhongyang yaunjiu yuan jindai shi yanjiu suo jikan* 17 (Dec. 1989), 141–94.

5. *Da gong bao,* 28 Sept. 1920, 1.

6. *Da gong bao,* 14 June 1920, 1; 8 Aug. 1920, 1.

7. Charlotte Furth, *A Flourishing Yin: Gender in China's Medical History, 950–1665* (Berkeley: University of California Press, 1998).

8. *Da gong bao,* 14 July 1920, 1

9. Shigehisa Kuriyama, "Interpreting the History of Bloodletting," *Journal of the History of Medicine and the Allied Sciences* 50 (1995): 11–46.

10. Jintan was developed in 1905 by the Morishita Company in Osaka. It went on to become one of the most well-known patent medicines in Japan.

11. *Da gong bao,* 28 Oct. 1920, 1 Mar. 1920.

12. *Da gong bao,* 20 Sept. 1920. On the association of lower back pain with male sexual deficiency, see Hugh Shapiro, "The Puzzle of Spermatorrhea in Republican China" in *positions* 6, no. 3 (1998): 551–96.

13. *Da gong bao,* 9 June 1932, 23 May 1932, 14 July 1937.

14. *Da gong bao,* 26 July 1937.

15. Nancy Tomes, *The Gospel of Germs: Men, Women, and the Microbe in American Life* (Cambridge, Mass.: Harvard University Press, 1998).

16. Frank Dikötter, *Sex, Culture, and Modernity in China: Medical Science and the Construction of Sexual Identities in the Early Republican Period* (London: Hurst and Co., 1995).

17. Gail Hershatter, *Dangerous Pleasures* (Berkeley: University of California Press, 1997), 226, 324.

18. Christian Henriot, *Shanghai, 1927–1937: Municipal Power, Locality, and Modernization* (Berkeley: University of California Press, 1993); Gail Hershatter *Dangerous Pleasures* (Berkeley: University of California Press, 1997); Frederic Wakeman, *Policing Shanghai, 1927–1937* (Berkeley: University of California Press, 1995); William Kirby, "Engineering China: Birth of the Developmental State,' in *Becoming Chinese: Passages to Modernity and Beyond,* ed. Wen-hsin Yeh (Berkeley: University of California Press, 2000), 137–60.

19. Ralph Croizier, *Traditional Medicine in Modern China: Science, Na-*

tionalism, and the Tensions of Cultural Change. (Cambridge, Mass.: Harvard University Press, 1968); Sean Hsiang-lin Lei, "When Chinese Medicine Encountered the State: 1910–1949" (Ph.D. diss., University of Chicago, 1999).

20. For an overview of warlord conflicts in Tianjin during the Guomindang period, see Tianjin shehui kexueyuan lishi yanjiu suo, ed., *Tianjin jian shi* (Tianjin: Tianjin renmin chubanshe, 1987), 302–3.

21. For information on Quan, see *Weisheng zazhi* (Hygiene magazine), vol. 2 (1929), 1–2.

22. On Li, see Diyi yiyuan zhi bian hui, ed., *Diyi yiyuan zhi* (Chronicle of the Number One Hospital) (Tianjin: n.p., 1990).

23. Ibid.

24. See various cases in Tianjin shili diyi yiyuan (Tianjin Number One Municipal Hospital, hereafter DYYY), record group 123, File 22, TMA.

25. Ibid.

26. For an overview of the YMCA in China, see Shirley Garret, *Social Reformers in Urban China: The Chinese Y.M.C.A., 1895–1926* (Cambridge, Mass.: Harvard University Press, 1970).

27. On Nankai Middle School and Tianjin education reformers Yan Xiu and Zhang Boling, see Sarah Coles-McElroy, "Transforming China through Education: Yan Xiu, Zhang Boling, and the Effort to Build a New School System, 1901–1927" (Ph.D. diss., Yale University, 1997). On the experience of Nankai Middle School's most famous alumnus, see Chae-Jin Lee, *Zhou En-lai: The Early Years* (Stanford: Stanford University Press, 1994).

28. For examples of such public lectures, see *Tianjin tebieshi weisheng ju yuekan* (Monthly journal of the Tianjin Special Municipality Public Health Department), vol. 3, 55.

29. For an overview of the New Life Movement, see Lloyd Eastman, *The Abortive Revolution: China under Nationalist Rule, 1927–1937* (Cambridge, Mass.: Harvard University Press, 1974); Arif Dirlik, "The Ideological Foundations of the New Life Movement: A Study in Counterrevolution," *Journal of Asian Studies* 34, no. 4 (1975): 945–80.

30. Pei-kai Cheng, Michael Lestz, with Jonathan D. Spence, *The Search for Modern China: A Documentary Collection* (New York: W. W. Norton, 1999).

31. *Tianjin weisheng ziliao* (Tianjin public health historical materials), vol. 8 (1988): 106.

32. Tianjin shili diyi yiyuan (The Tianjin Number One Municipal Hospital, hereafter DYYY), record group 123, File 13, TMA.

33. *Weisheng zazhi*, vol. 7 (1930): 1–2.

34. See, for example, Feng Jishun, "Lun mianyi chuanran fa" (On methods of preventing infectious diseases), which includes glosses such as "The number of bacteria" (for the simple phrase *xi jun de shu mu*) and "The is non-Pathogenic bacteria" [sic] (for *fei bingyuan jun*), *Weisheng zazhi* vol. 8, 16.

35. Zhong Huilan, "Lun zhongguo ji yi fazhan gonggong weisheng" (China should immediately develop public health), *Weisheng zazhi*, vol. 22: 1–4.

36. *Weisheng zazhi*, vol. 7 (1930): 1–2.

37. On Pan Guangdan, see Frank Dikötter, *The Discourse of Race in Modern China*, 174–82. For the text of Pan's Tianjin lecture, "Yousheng yu minzu jiankang" (Eugenics and racial health), see Pan Guangdan, *Minzu texing yu minzu weisheng* (Racial characteristics and racial hygiene) (Shanghai, 1937), 31–44.

38. Pan, *Minzu texing yu minzu weisheng*, 34.

39. Ibid., 43.

40. On Pan's life, see Dikötter, *The Discourse of Race in Modern China;* Howard L. Boorman, ed., *Biographical Dictionary of Republican China* (New York: Columbia University Press, 1967–79).

41. On Japanese and Korean involvement in opium trade, see Timothy Brook and Bob Wakabayashi, *Opium Regimes: China, Britain, and Japan, 1839–1952* (Berkeley, Los Angeles, and London: University of California Press, 2000); Kathryn Meyer and Terry Parssinen, *Webs of Smoke: Smugglers, Warlords, Spies, and the History of the International Drug Trade* (Lanham, Md.: Rowman and Littlefield, 1998); Wataru Masuda, *Japan and China: Mutual Representations in the Modern Era*, trans. Joshua Fogel (Richmond and Surrey: Curzon, 2000); Edward Slack, *Opium, State, and Society: China's Narco-Economy and the Guomindang, 1924–1937* (Honolulu: University of Hawaii Press, 2001).

42. The largest incident before 1937 was the "Tianjin Outbreak" of November 1931. On the situation in Shanghai, see Frederic Wakeman, *The Shanghai Badlands: Wartime Terrorism and Urban Crime, 1937–1941* (New York: Cambridge University Press, 1996).

43. Pan, *Minzu texing yu minzu weisheng*, 35.

44. Huntington went on to become one of American academia's foremost advocates of eugenics. The year Pan gave his eugenics lecture in Tianjin (1935), Huntington published his well-known eugenics manifesto *Tomorrow's Children: The Goal of Eugenics* (New York: J. Wiley and Sons, Inc.; London: Chapman and Hall, Ltd., 1935).

45. Arthur Smith, *Chinese Characteristics* (New York: Revell, 1894). For a history of the translations of Arthur Smith available in China in the twentieth century, see Lydia Liu, *Translingual Practice: Literature, National Culture, and Translated Modernity — China, 1900–1937* (Stanford: Stanford University Press, 1995), 28.

46. Ibid., 29–35.

47. Pan, *Minzu texing yu minzu weisheng*, 313–54.

48. Li Jinghan in Ibid., 1.

49. Pan, *Minzu texing yu minzu weisheng*, 317–18.

50. For a brief biography of Ding, see Zhongguo renmin zhengzhi xieshang huiyi Tianjin shi weiyuanhui, wen shi ziliao yanjiu weiyuan hui, ed., *Jindai Tianjin renwu lu* (Biographical dictionary of modern Tianjin) (Tianjin: Tianjinshi difang shizhi bianxiu weiyuan hui zong bianji shi, 1987), 1.

51. On the founding of the Medical Research Association, see Ding Zilang, ed., *Zhu yuan cong hua* (Collected talks from the Bamboo Garden), 1923–26, vol. 18, 112–15. For the content of association meetings, see example report of

monthly meeting held GX 32/9/24 (10 Nov. 1906), in vol. 12, 122–125. Copies in the Tianjin Municipal Library.

52. In Ding Zilang, *Zhu yuan cong hua*, vol. 10, 71.

53. On Ding Fubao, see Bridie Andrews, *The Making of Modern Chinese Medicine* (Cambridge and New York: Cambridge University Press, 2004).

54. Ding Zilang, "Zai shuo huoluan bing," *Zhu yuan cong hua*, vol. 6, 125.

55. Preface to *Shuo yi*, reprinted in Ding Zilang, *Zhu yuan cong hua*, vol. 10, 113–116.

56. Ding Zilang, "Duiyu wairen fangyi fanhe zhi ganyan," *Zhu yuan cong hua*, vol. 11, 42–50

57. Ding Zilang, *Zhu yuan cong hua*, vol. 1, 114.

58. Ibid., vol 17, 106.

59. Ibid., vol. 2, 128

60. Ibid., 129.

61. *Guoyi zhen yan* (True words on the national medicine), Vol. 8, 3–6. Tianjin History Museum collection.

62. Shu-mei Shih, *The Lure of the Modern: Writing Modernism in Semicolonial China, 1917–1937* (Berkeley: University of California Press, 2001), 304.

63. Partha Chatterjee, *Nationalist Thought and the Colonial World: A Derivative Discourse* (Minneapolis: University of Minnesota Press, 1986).

64. Ashis Nandy, "Modern Medicine and Its Non-Modern Critics," in *The Savage Freud and Other Essays on Possible and Retrievable Selves* (Princeton: Princeton University Press, 1995), 159.

65. Ibid.

66. Gyan Prakash, *Another Reason: Science and the Imagination of Modern India* (Princeton, N.J.: Princeton University Press), 1999.

67. Bridie Andrews, "Tuberculosis and the Assimilation of Germ Theory in China, 1895–1937," *Journal of the History of Medicine and Allied Sciences* 52, no. 1 (1997): 114–57.

68. Prakash, *Another Reason*, 158.

CHAPTER 9

1. Ramon H. Myers and Mark R. Peattie, ed., *The Japanese Colonial Empire, 1895–1945* (Princeton, N.J.: Princeton University Press, 1984); Peter Duus, Ramon H. Myers, and Mark R. Peattie, ed., *The Japanese Informal Empire in China, 1895–1973* (Princeton, N.J.: Princeton University Press, 1989); and Duus, Myers, and Peattie, ed., *The Japanese Wartime Emprie, 1931–1945* (Princeton, N.J.: Princeton University Press, 1996).

2. Ann Laura Stoler and Frederick Cooper, ed., *Tensions of Empire: Colonial Cultures in a Bourgeois World* (Berkeley: University of California Press, 1997); Ann Laura Stoler, *Race and the Education of Desire: Foucault's History of Sexuality and the Colonial Order of Things* (Durham, N.C.: Duke University Press, 1995).

3. Stefan Tanaka, *Japan' s Orient: Rendering Pasts into History* (Berkeley: University of California Press, 1993).

4. Barbara Brooks, "Reading the Japanese Colonial Archive: Gender and Bourgeois Civility in Korea and Manchuria to 1932," in *Gendering Modern Japanese History*, ed. Kathleen Uno and Barbara Molony, eds. (Cambridge, Mass.: Harvard East Asian Monographs, forthcoming); also Barbara Brooks, "Colonial Power and Public Health in Japanese-Held Korea" (paper presented at the annual meeting of the Association of Asian Studies, Washington, D.C., Apr. 2002). See also Louise Young, *Japan' s Total Empire: Manchuria and the Culture of Wartime Imperialism* (Berkeley: University of California Press, 1998).

5. Leo T. S. Ching, *Becoming "Japanese": Colonial Taiwan and the Politics of Identity Formation* (Berkeley: University of California Press, 2001).

6. Barbara Brooks, "Colonial Power and Public Health in Japanese-Held Korea."

7. Barbara Brooks, "Japanese Colonial Citizenship in Treaty-Port China: The Location of Koreans and Taiwanese in the Imperial Order," in *New Frontiers: Imperialism' s New Communities in East Asia, 1843–1953*, ed. Robert Bickers and Christian Henriot (Manchester and New York: Manchester University Press, 2000), 109–24.

8. Joshua Fogel, "Akutakaga Ryûnosuke in China," *Chinese Studies in History* 30, no. 4 (1997): 6–55; Inger Sigrun Brodey and Ikuo Tsunematsu, ed., *Rediscovering Natsume Soseki* (Folkestone: Global Oriental, 2000).

9. Peter Duus, *The Abacus and the Sword* (Berkeley: University of California Press, 1995), 399–406; Barbara Brooks, "Reading the Japanese Colonial Archive."

10. Paul Katz, "Germs of Disaster—The Impact of Epidemics on Japanese Military Campaigns in Taiwan, 1874 and 1895," *Annales de Demographie Historique* (1996): 195–220.

11. Iijima Wataru and Wakamura Kohei, "Eisei to teikoku: Nichi-Ei shokuminchishugi no hikakushi teki kôsatsu ni mukete" (Hygiene and empire: Toward a comparative history of Japanese and British colonialism), *Nihon shi kenkyu* (Research in Japanese history) 462 (Feb. 2001); Liu Shiyong, "Qingjie, weisheng, yu baojian: Rizhi shiqi Taiwan shehui gonggong weisheng guannian zhi zhuanbian" (Cleanliness, hygiene, and health: Transformations of concepts of public health in Taiwan society during the Japanese colonial period), *Taiwan shi yanjiu* (Research in the history of Taiwan) 8, no. 1 (2000): 41–88.

12. Iijima and Wakamura, "Eisei to teikoku," 7–8.

13. Gyan Prakash, *Another Reason*, 123–158.

14. Iijima and Wakamura, "Eisei to teikoku," 9.

15. Barbara Brooks, "Colonial Power and Public Health in Japanese-Held Korea." On Japanese-trained doctors in Taiwan, see Ming-cheng M. Lo, *Doctors Within Borders: Profession, Ethnicity, and Modernity in Colonial Taiwan* (Berkeley: University of California Press, 2002).

16. Barbara Brooks, "Reading the Japanese Colonial Archive."

17. Liu Shiyong, "Qingjie, weisheng, yu baojian."

18. Iijima Wataru, *Pesuto to kindai Chûgoku* (Tokyo: Kenbun Shuppan, 2000).

19. Ibid.; Robert Perrins, "Combating Illness and Constructing Public Health: Disease and Hospitals in Japanese-Controlled Southern Manchuria" (paper presented at the annual meeting of the Association for Asian Studies, Washington, D.C., Apr. 2002).

20. Iijima, *Pesuto to kindai Chûgoku.*

21. Mark R. Peattie, "Japanese Treaty-Port Settlements in China, 1895–1937," *The Japanese Informal Empire in China, 1895–1937* (Princeton, N.J.: Princeton University Press, 1989), 166–209.

22. Tenshin kyoryû mindan, *Tenshin kyoryû mindan nijisshûnen kinenshi* (Tianjin: n.p., 1930), 618.

23. Peattie, "Japanese Treaty Ports Settlements in China, 1895–1937," 178.

24. Tenshin kyoryû mindan, *Tenshin kyoryû mindan jimu hôkoku* (Tianjin Japanese settlement corporation annual report), (Tianjin,: n.p., 1928), 120–21.

25. Sun Xuelian, *Tianjin zhinan* (A guide to Tianjin) (Tianjin: Zhonghua shuju, 1923).

26. Barbara Brooks, *Japan's Imperial Diplomacy: Consuls, Treaty Ports, and War in China, 1895–1938* (Honolulu: University of Hawaii Press, 2000). On consuls, see 79–116.

27. On Japanese residents' associations in China, see Joshua Fogel, "Shanghai-Japan": The Japanese Residents' Association of Shanghai," *Journal of Asian Studies* 59, 4 (2000):927–950.

28. On the Tianjin garrison, see Furuno Naoya, *Tenshin Gunshireibu: 1901–1937* (Tokyo: Kokusho Kankôkai, 1989).

29. Tenshin kyoryû mindan, *Tenshin kyoryû mindan jimu hôkoku*, 1928, 285.

30. From 1927 to 1933, mortality rates dropped from 16.5 to 14.4 in Tokyo, while Osaka dropped from 18.8 to 16.3. Government of Japan, Ministry of Health, Labour, and Welfare, "Trends in Vital Statistics by Prefecture in Japan, 1899–1998" http://www.mhlw.go.jp/english/database/db-hw/ vs_8/index.html.

31. Tenshin kyoryû mindan, *Tenshin kyoryû mindan jimu hôkoku*, 1928, 262; ibid., 1933, 185.

32. For general studies of the Manchurian plague crisis of 1911, see Carl Nathan, *Plague Prevention and Politics in Manchuria, 1910–1931* (Cambridge: East Asian Research Center, Harvard University, 1967); Lien-teh Wu, *Plague Fighter: The Autobiography of a Modern Chinese Physician* (Cambridge: Heffer and Sons, 1959); and Carol Benedict *Bubonic Plague in Nineteenth-Century China* (Stanford: Stanford University Press, 1996), 155–63.

33. Tenshin kyoryû mindan, *Tenshin kyoryû mindan nijisshûnen kinenshi* (Tianjin: n.p., 1930), 559.

34. On radical plague prevention measures in the Shanghai International Settlement and the resulting Chinese riots, see Bryna Goodman, *Native Place, City, and Nation: Regional Networks and Identities in Shanghai, 1853–1937* (Berkeley and Los Angeles: University of California Press, 1995), 154–55.

35. These Japanese techniques closely resembled the plague control policy

enacted in India by British authorities, a policy that the British settlers in Tianjin had been reluctant to undertake. See David Arnold, *Colonizing the Body: State, Medicine, and Epidemic Disease in Nineteenth-Century India* (Berkeley and Los Angeles: University of California Press, 1993), 203–30.

36. *Tenshin kyoryû mindan nijisshûnen kinenshi* (Tianjin Japanese Residents' Association Twentieth Anniversary Report), (Tianjin: n.p., 1930), 559.

37. Tenshin kyoryû mindan, *Tenshin kyoryû mindan jimu hôkoku*, 1911.

38. Ibid., 1928, 284.

39. Based on comparisons between populations statistics for 1933 (Tenshin kyoryû mindan, *Tenshin kyoryû mindan jimu hôkoku*, 98) and prostitute inspection statistics (130). For mainland Japan, Sheldon Garon estimates that in 1925, one out of every thirty-one young women worked as a prostitute. Garon, *Molding Japanese Minds: The State and Everyday Life* (Princeton, N.J.: Princeton University Press, 1997), 94.

40. On the emergence of a modern licensed prostitution system in Japan, see , *Molding Japanese Minds*, 90–94.

41. Tenshin kyoryû mindan, *Tenshin kyoryû mindan jimu hôkoku*, 1933. For the incidence of venereal disease among prostitutes in Shanghai, see Hershatter, *Dangerous Pleasures*, 230, 319.

42. On treatments available before World War II, see Hershatter, *Dangerous Pleasures*, 231.

43. Frederic Wakeman, *The Shanghai Badlands: Wartime Terrorism and Urban Crime, 1937–1941* (New York: Cambridge University Press, 1996); Brian Martin, *The Shanghai Green Gang: Politics and Organized Crime, 1919–1937* (Berkeley: University of California Press, 1996).

44. On the battle for Tianjin, see Liu Jingyue, "Tianjin lunxian qian de zuihou yi zhan" (The last battle for Tianjin), in Tianjinshi zhengxie hui—wenshi ziliao yanjiu weiyuanhui, ed., *Lunxian shiqi de Tianjin* (Tianjin during the occupation) (Tianjin: Jinghai xian yinshuachang, 1992), 1–8. In an irony of modernization and militarization, the Japanese airfield that launched the planes that bombed Nankai was located just east of Tianjin at Dong Juzi, the site of Li Hongzhang's original Beiyang Arsenal.

45. The Japanese population would increase beyond seventy thousand as the war dragged on; see Li Jingneng, ed., *Tianjin renkoushi* (Tianjin: Nankai daxue chuban she, 1990), 273.

46. On Tianjin's Security Preservation Committee, see Tianjinshi zhengxie hui—wenshi ziliao yanjiu weiyuanhui, ed., *Lunxian shiqi de Tianjin*. On Peace (Security) Preservation Committees as a wartime phenomenon, see Lo Jiu-jung, "Survival as Justification for Collaboration, 1937–1945" in David Barrett and Larry Shyu, ed., *Chinese Collaboration: The Limits of Accommodation* (Stanford: Stanford University Press, 2001), 116–32.

47. Communication from Tianjinshi zhi'an weichi weiyuanhui weisheng ju (hereafter ZAWSJ) to Weisheng ju units, 8 Aug. 1937, Tianjin shi Weisheng chu (hereafter WSC) 115-1-2, Tianjin Municipal Archives (hereafter TMA).

48. Personnel list, n.d., WSC 115–1-2, TMA.

49. Communication from ZAWSJ to Weisheng ju units, 7 and 12 Aug. 1937, WSC 115–1-12, TMA.

50. See reports from Chuanran bing yiyuan to ZAWSJ, July–Aug. 1937, WSC 115–1-28, TMA.

51. Photographs in Tianjin tebie shi weishengchu, *Tianjin tebieshi fangyi gongzuo baogao* (Tianjin Special Municipality Epidemic Prevention Work Report) 1938, Tianjin Municipal Library.

52. For reports filled out by Chinese personnel, see "Qu jianyi gongzuo baogao," 28 Sept. to 10 Oct. 1937, WSC 115–1-1948, 115–1-1950, TMA.

53. For reports from Japanese military see file "Hokushi jimusho bôeki jôhô," 28 Sept. to 10 Oct. 1937, WSC 115–1-1974, TMA.

54. For Fu zhi hui participation and the text of the lectures, see WSC 115–1-340, TMA.

55. Tenshin kyoryû mindan, *Tenshin kyoryû mindan jimu hôkoku*, 1939, 1943.

56. Ibid., 1943.

57. R. Keith Schoppa, "Patterns and Dynamics of Elite Collaboration in Occupied Shaoxing County," in David Barrett and Larry Shyu, ed., *Chinese Collaboration: The Limits of Accommodation* (Stanford: Stanford University Press, 2001), 156–79; Lo Jiu-jung, "Survival as Justification for Collaboration, 1937–1945" in Barrett and Shyu, *Chinese Collaboration*, 116–32.

58. Prasenjit Duara, "Transnationalism and the Predicament of Sovereignty: China 1900–1945, *American Historical Review* 102, no. 4 (1997): 1030–51; Poshek Fu, *Passivity, Resistance, and Collaboration: Intellectual Choices in Occupied Shanghai, 1937–1945* (Stanford: Stanford University Press, 1993). See also Rana Mitter, *The Manchurian Myth* (Berkeley: University of California Press, 2000).

59. Ming-cheng M. Lo, *Doctors Within Borders: Profession, Ethnicity, and Modernity in Colonial Taiwan* (Berkeley: University of California Press, 2002).

60. For doctors' registration records, see WSC 115–1-237 through 115–1-242, TMA.

61. Hou had a Chinese surname, but this does not rule out the possibility that he may have had a Japanese mother.

62. On the Weisheng ju's management of the epidemic, see WSC 115–1-567 and 115–1-605, TMA.

63. Report from Hou Fusang, director, Chuanranbing yiyuan (Contagious disease hospital), to Weisheng chu (Health Department) director Fu Ruqin, 1 July 1938, WSC 115–1-561, TMA.

64. For a discussion of the textile factories and the lives of workers, see Hershatter, *Workers of Tianjin*, 140–80.

65. All of the application materials of all physicians (Chinese and Western medicine) who registered during the Japanese occupation are available in the TMA, WSC 115–1-196 through 115–1-237.

66. On government examinations for physicians of Chinese medicine, see

Sean Hsiang-lin Lei, "When Chinese Medicine Encountered the State: 1910–1949" (Ph.D. diss., University of Chicago, 1999).

67. Minutes of health department meeting, 18 July 1938, WSC 115-1-583, TMA.

68. Letter from the Zhongguo huijiao hui (Chinese Islamic Association) to the Weisheng chu (Health Department), 7 Aug.1938, WSC 115-1-583, TMA.

69. Report from Chuanranbing yiyuan (Contagious disease hospital) to Weisheng chu (Health Department), 5 Sept. 1938, WSC 115-1-583, TMA.

70. On Japanese biological warfare in China, see Sheldon Harris, *Factories of Death: Japanese Biological Warfare, 1932–1945, and the American Cover-up* (London and New York: Routledge, 1994); and Peter Williams and David Wallace, *Unit 731: The Japanese Army' s Secret of Secrets* (London: Hodder and Stoughton, 1989).

71. Williams and Wallace, *Unit 731,* 9.

72. Sheldon Harris, *Factories of Death,* 111.

73. Zhongyang danganguan, Zhongguo dier lishi danganguan, Jilinshen shehui kexueyuan, *Xijunzhan yu duqi zhan* (Beijing: Zhonghua shuju, 1989), 192.

74. Luise White, *Speaking with Vampires: Rumor and History in Colonial Africa* (Berkeley: University of California Press, 2000); and Nancy Rose Hunt, *A Colonial Lexicon of Birth Ritual, Medicalization, and Mobility in the Congo* (Durham, N.C.: Duke University Press, 1999).

CHAPTER 10

1. Several works have been published recently on the Korean War germ warfare allegations. Katherine Weathersby argues that the allegations were nothing but a hoax. See her "Deceiving the Deceivers: Moscow, Beijing, Pyongyang, and the Allegations of Bacteriological Weapons Use in Korea," *Cold War International History Project Bulletin,* 11 (winter 1998): 176–84. Stephen Endicott and Edward Hagerman, *The United States and Biological Warfare: Secrets from the Early Cold War and Korea* (Bloomington: Indiana University Press, 1998), argue that the United States did use biological weapons in the Korean War.

2. For the fighting leading up to the surrender, see Chen Changjie, "Tianjin zhanyi gaishu," in *Pingjin zhanyi qin liji* (General description of the battle for Tianjin) (Beijing: Zhonghua wenshi chuban she, 1989), 170–84.

3. For the general situation in Tianjin in the first few weeks after liberation, see Zhong gong Tianjinshi wei et al., *Tianjin jieguan shilu* (Beijing: Zhong gong dang shi shubanshe, 1991), 1–30. See also Kenneth Lieberthal, *Revolution and Tradition in Tientsin, 1949–1952* (Stanford: Stanford University Press, 1980), 28–35.

4. On the arrest of GMD spies, see Lieberthal, *Revolution and Tradition in Tientsin,* 57–60.

5. Zhong gong Tianjinshi wei et al., *Tianjin jieguan shilu,* 145.

6. Lieberthal, *Revolution and Tradition in Tientsin.*

7. Han Feng, "Qudi jiu Tianjin changye jishi," in Ma Weigang, ed., *Jin chang jin du* (Beijing: Jing guan jiaoyu chuban she, 1993), 50.

8. On the Three- and Five-Anti Campaigns and Thought Reform, see Lieberthal, *Revolution and Tradition in Tientsin.*

9. Zhang Rongqing, "Fangyi gongzuo yu mianyi zhidu" (Epidemic prevention work and vaccination system) *Tianjin weisheng shiliao* 2 and 3 (1987): 47.

10. Xin Zhongguo yufang yixue lishi jingyan bian weiyuanhui, ed., *Xin Zhongguo yufang yixue lishi jingyan* (The historical experiences of preventive medicine in New China) (Beijing: Renmin weisheng chubanshe, 1991).

11. Cai Gongqi, "Tianjin shi weisheng ju 1951 nian gongzuo jihua" (Tianjin Public Health Bureau work report for 1951 [27 Jan. 1951]). Tianjin: Tianjin Public Health Bureau Archives.

12. "1950 nian yinshui jihua" (1950 Drinking Water Plan), Tianjin Health Bureau Archives.

13. Ibid.

14. Tianjin shi fangyi weiyuanhui (Tianjin municipal epidemic prevention committee), 1949. "Heji ge qu fangyi fenhui huiyi jilu" (Minutes of the joint meeting of all district epidemic prevention committees), Nov. 15, Tianjin: Tianjin Public Health Bureau Archives.

15. "Report on the Condition in Hospitals Founded by Foreigners" (c. 1950), Tianjin Communist Party internal document.

16. I did not find any information on the fates of physicians who had served under the Japanese occupation government.

17. Tsao Yu, *Bright Skies* (Beijing: Foreign Language Press, 1960), 112–13.

18. See for example "Democratic Parties Protest US Shocking Crime," 25 Feb. 1952; "European Press Condemn New U.S. Atrocities," 29 Feb. 1952; "WFTU Urges UN to Halt Germ War," 6 Mar. 1952; "Tientsin, Shanghai Catholics Protest U.S. Germ Warfare," 7 Mar. 1952; "National Minorities Denounce U.S. Germ Warfare," 15 Apr. 1952, all cited in *Hsinhua News Agency Daily News* (hereafter *Hsinhua*).

19. Weisheng ju bangongshi (Public health bureau office), "Tianjin shi weisheng weiyuanhui 1952 aiguo weisheng yundong zongjie baogao" (Final report of the Tianjin public health committee 1952 patriotic hygiene campaign), 31 Oct. 1952. Tianjin: Tianjin Public Health Bureau Archives.

20. *Renmin ribao,* 5 Mar. 1952.

21. Chinese People's Committee for World Peace, *Exhibition on Bacteriological War Crimes Committed By the Government of the United States of America* (Beijing 1952).

22. For a general overview of the Patriotic Hygiene Campaign, see Albert E. Cowdrey, " 'Germ Warfare' and Public Health in the Korean Conflict," *Journal of the History of Medicine and Allied Sciences* 39 (1984): 153–72.

23. The Five Annihilations were a precursor to the better-known Four Pest Eradications (Chu si hai) Campaigns of the 1950s and 1960s, when the hapless sparrow was added to the usual suspects of flies, rats, and mosquitoes. Judith Shapiro, *Mao's War Against Nature: Politics and the Environment in Rev-*

olutionary China (Cambridge and New York: Cambridge University Press, 2001).

24. Tianjin shehui kexue yuan yuqing zhongxin (Tianjin academy of social science public opinion center). 1999. *Survey on China's Patriotic Hygiene Campaign*. 200 respondents.

25. Weisheng ju bangongshi (Public health bureau office), "Tianjin shi weisheng weiyuanhui 1952 aiguo weisheng yundong zongjie baogao" (Final report of the Tianjin public health committee 1952 patriotic hygiene campaign), 31 Oct. 1952. Tianjin: Tianjin Public Health Bureau Archives.

26. Tianjin shi hezuoshe xitong (Tianjin cooperative society system), "Tianjin shi hezuoshe xitong aiguo weisheng yundong zongjie baogao" (Tianjin cooperative society system patriotic hygiene campaign final report), 1953. Municipal Government File, Folder 1929. Tianjin: Tianjin Municipal Archives.

27. Ibid.

28. Dangdai Zhongguo congshu bianjibu, *Dangdai Zhongguode weisheng shiye* (Contemporary China's public health) (Beijing: Zhongguo shehui kexue chubanshe, 1986), 1: 51, 53.

29. Frank Dikötter, *Imperfect Conceptions: Medical Knowledge, Birth Defects, and Eugenics in China* (New York: Columbia University Press, 1998).

CONCLUSION

1. Frantz Fanon, *Black Skin, White Masks* (London: Granada, 1970); Ashis Nandy, *The Intimate Enemy: Loss and Recovery of Self under Colonialism* (New Delhi: Oxford University Press, 1984); John Fitzgerald, "Chinese, Dogs, and the State that Stands on Two Legs," in *Bulletin of Concerned Asian Scholars* 29, no. 4 (1997): 54–61.

2. John Fitzgerald, *Awakening China: Politics, Culture and Class in the Nationalist Revolution* (Stanford: Stanford University Press, 1996).

3. Shu-mei Shih, *The Lure of the Modern: Writing Modernism in Semicolonial China, 1917–1937* (Berkeley: University of California Press, 2001), 291.

4. Fitzgerald, "Chinese, Dogs, and the State that Stands on Two Legs," 60. As Prasenjit Duara has pointed out, any comparison between Gandhi and Mao as revolutionaries "must break down with respect to Mao's ultimate adherence to the Enlightenment project and his violent rejection of the past." *Rescuing History from the Nation: Questioning Narratives of Modern China* (Chicago: University of Chicago Press, 1995), 216.

5. Duara, *Rescuing History from the Nation*, 221; also *Culture, Power, and the State: Rural North China, 1900–1942* (Stanford: Stanford University Press, 1988).

6. Shih, *The Lure of the Modern*.

7. Prasenjit Duara, "Transnationalism and the Predicament of Sovereignty: China 1900–1945," *American Historical Review* 102, no. 4 (1997): 1030–51.

8. Paul Unschuld, "Epistemological Issues and Changing Legitimation: Traditional Chinese Medicine in the Twentieth Century," in *Paths to Asian Med-*

ical Knowledge, ed. Charles Leslie and Allan Young (Berkeley: University of California Press, 1992).

9. Nancy Chen, "Urban Spaces and Experiences of Qigong," in *Urban Spaces: Autonomy and Community in Post-Mao China,* ed. D. Davis (New York and Cambridge: Cambridge University Press, 1995).

10. Elisabeth Hsu, *The Transmission of Chinese Medicine* (Cambridge: Cambridge University Press, 1999).

11. Judith Farquhar, *Knowing Practice: The Clinical Encounter of Chinese Medicine.* (Boulder, Colo.: Westview Press, 1994); Bridie Andrews, *The Making of Modern Chinese Medicine* (Cambridge: Cambridge University Press, 2004); Elisabeth Hsu, *The Transmission of Chinese Medicine* (Cambridge: Cambridge University Press, 1999); Volker Schied, *Chinese Medicine in Contemporary China: Plurality and Synthesis* (Durham, N.C.: Duke University Press 2002); Marta Hanson, "Inventing a Tradition in Chinese Medicine" (Ph.D. diss., University of Pennsylvania, 1997); Yi-Li Wu, "Transmitted Secrets: The Doctors of the Lower Yangzi Region and Popular Gynecology in Late Imperial China" (Ph.D. diss., Yale University, 1998); Vivienne Lo, "The Influence of Western Han Nurturing Life Literature on the Development of Acumoxa Therapy" (Ph.D. diss., London University, 1998); T. J. Hinrichs, "New Geographies of Chinese Medicine," in "Beyond Joseph Needham: Science, Technology, and Medicine in East and Southeast Asia" *Osiris* 13 (1998).

Bibliography

Ackerknecht, Erwin. "Anticontagionism between 1821 and 1867." *Bulletin of the History of Medicine* 22 (1948): 562–93.

Anderson, Warwick. "Disease, Race, and Empire." *Bulletin of the History of Medicine* 70, no. 1 (1996): 62–67.

———. "Excremental Colonialism." *Critical Inquiry* 21, no. 3 (spring 1995): 640–69.

———. "Immunities of Empire: Race, Disease, and the New Tropical Medicine, 1900–1920." *Bulletin of the History of Medicine* 70, no. 1 (1996): 94–118.

———. "Where is the Postcolonial History of Medicine?" *Bulletin of the History of Medicine* 79, no. 3 (1998): 522–30.

Andrews, Bridie. "Tuberculosis and the Assimilation of Germ Theory in China, 1895–1937." *Journal of the History of Medicine and Allied Sciences* 52, no. 1 (1997): 114–57.

———. *The Making of Modern Chinese Medicine.* Cambridge: Cambridge University Press, 2004.

———. "The Making of Modern Chinese Medicine, 1895–1937." Ph.D. diss., Cambridge University, 1996.

Andrews, Bridie, and Chris Cunningham, eds. *Western Medicine as Contested Knowledge.* Manchester and New York: Manchester University Press, 1997.

Arnold, David. *Colonizing the Body: State, Medicine, and Epidemic Disease in Nineteenth-Century India.* Berkeley and Los Angeles: University of California Press, 1993.

———, ed. *Imperial Medicine and Indigenous Societies.* Manchester: Manchester University Press, 1988.

———, ed. *Warm Climates and Western Medicine: The Emergence of Tropical Medicine, 1500–1900.* Amsterdam and Atlanta, Ga.: Rodopi, 1996.

Ban Tadayasu. *Tekijuku to Nagayo Sensai: eiseigaku to Shôkô shishi* (The Tekijuku and Nagayo Sensai: Hygienics and the fragrant pine memoirs). Osaka: Sogensha, 1987.

Bartholomew, James. *The Formation of Science in Japan.* New Haven: Yale University Press, 1989.

Bederman, Gail. *Manliness and Civilization*. Chicago: University of Chicago Press.

"Beiyang lujun weisheng fangyi zhangcheng" (Beiyang army's regulations concerning sanitation and the prevention of contagious disease). *Dongfang zazhi* 2, no. 9 (1905).

"Beiyang yiyuan yuni sheli zhandi yiyuan" (The Beiyang hospital's plans for the establishment of a battlefield hospital). *Dongfang zazhi* 2, no. 9 (1905).

Benedict, Carol. *Bubonic Plague in Nineteenth-Century China*. Stanford: Stanford University Press, 1996.

———. "Policing the Sick: Plague and the Origins of State Medicine in Late Imperial China." *Late Imperial China* 14, no. 2 (1993): 60–77.

Bennett, Adrian. *John Fryer: The Introduction of Western Science and Technology into Nineteenth-Century China*. Cambridge, Mass.: East Asian Research Center, Harvard University, 1967.

Bernstein, Lewis. "A History of Tientsin in Early Modern Times, 1800–1910." Ph.D. diss., University of Kansas, 1988.

Bickers, Robert, and Jeffrey Wasserstrom. "Shanghai's 'Dogs and Chinese Not Admitted' Sign: Legend, History, and Contemporary Symbol." *China Quarterly* 142 (1995): 444–66.

Bohr, Paul. *Famine in China and the Missionary*. Cambridge, Mass.: Harvard University Press, 1972.

Bold, John. *Greenwich: An Architectural History of the Royal Hospital for Seamen and the Queen's House*. New Haven: Yale University Press, 2000.

Bonham-Carter, Victor. *Surgeon in the Crimea: The Experiences of George Lawson Recorded in the Letters to His Family, 1854–55*. London: Constable, 1968.

Bonner, Thomas N. *American Doctors and German Universities: A Chapter in International Relations*. Lincoln: University of Nebraska Press, 1963.

Boorman, Howard L., ed. *Biographical Dictionary of Republican China*. 5 vols. New York: Columbia University Press, 1967–79.

Bordin, Ruth. *Woman and Temperance: The Quest for Power and Liberty, 1873–1900*. Philadelphia: Temple University Press, 1981.

Bowers, John Z. *Western Medical Pioneers in Feudal Japan*. Baltimore: Johns Hopkins University Press, 1970.

———. *Western Medicine in a Chinese Palace: Peking Union Medical College, 1917–1951*. Philadelphia: Josiah Macy Jr. Foundation, 1972.

———. *When the Twain Meet: The Rise of Western Medicine in Japan*. Baltimore: Johns Hopkins University Press, 1980.

Bowers, John Z., and Elizabeth F. Purcell, eds. *Medicine and Society in China*. New York: Josiah Macy Jr. Foundation, 1974.

Brodey, Inger Sigrun, and Ikuo Tsunematsu, eds. *Rediscovering Natsume Soseki* (Folkestone: Global Oriental, 2000).

Brokaw, Cynthia. "Commercial Publishing in Late Imperial China: The Zou and Ma Family Businesses of Sibao, Fujian." *Late Imperial China* 17, no. 1 (1996): 49–92.

———. "Field Work on the Social and Economic History of the Chinese Book."

Paper presented at the annual meeting of the Association for Asian Studies, Chicago, Ill., Mar. 2001.

Broman, Thomas. *The Transformation of German Academic Medicine, 1750–1820*. Cambridge: Cambridge University Press, 1996.

Brooks, Barbara. "Colonial Power and Public Health in Japanese-Held Korea." Paper presented at the annual meeting of the Association of Asian Studies, Washington, D.C., Apr. 2002.

———. "Japanese Colonial Citizenship in Treaty-Port China: The Location of Koreans and Taiwanese in the Imperial Order." In *New Frontiers: Imperialism's New Communities in East Asia, 1843–1953*, ed. Robert Bickers and Christian Henriot. Manchester and New York: Manchester University Press, 2000.

———. *Japan's Imperial Diplomacy: Consuls, Treaty Ports, and War in China, 1895–1938*. Honolulu: University of Hawaii Press, 2000.

———. "Reading the Japanese Colonial Archive: Gender and Bourgeois Civility in Korea and Manchuria to 1932." In *Gendering Modern Japanese History*, in Kathleen Uno and Barbara Molony. Cambridge, Mass.: Harvard East Asian Monographs, forthcoming.

Brook, Timothy. *Confusions of Pleasure: Commerce and Culture in Ming China*. Berkeley: University of California Press, 1998.

Brook, Timothy, and Bob Tadashi Wakabayashi. *Opium Regimes: China, Britain, and Japan, 1839–1952*. Berkeley: University of California Press, 2000.

Brown, Frederick. *Religion in Tientsin*. Shanghai: Methodist Publishing House, 1908.

Buell, Paul D., and Eugene N. Anderson. *A Soup for the Qan: Chinese Dietary Medicine of the Mongol Era as Seen in Hu Szu-Hui's Yin-shan cheng yao*. London and New York: Kegan Paul International, 2000.

Bullock, Mary. *An American Transplant: The Rockefeller Foundation and the Peking Union Medical College*. Berkeley and Los Angeles: University of California Press, 1980.

Burns, Susan. "Between National Policy and Local Practice: Cholera, Gotô Shimpei, and the Formation of the 'Hygienic Nation.'" Paper presented at the annual meeting of the Association of Asian Studies, Washington, D.C., Apr. 2002.

———. "Constructing the National Body: Public Health and the Nation in Nineteenth-Century Japan." In *Nation Work: Asian Elites and National Identities*, ed. Timothy Brook and Andre Schmid. Ann Arbor: University of Michigan Press, 2000.

Burton, Antoinette. *Burdens of History: British Feminists, Indian Women, and Imperial Culture, 1865–1915*. Chapel Hill: University of North Carolina Press, 1994.

Bynum, W. F., and Vivian Nutton, eds. *Theories of Fever from Antiquity to the Enlightenment. Medical History*, supplement no. 1 (1981).

Bynum, W. F., and Roy Porter, eds. *Medical Fringe and Medical Orthodoxy*. London: Croom Helm, 1987.

Cai Gongqi. "Tianjin shi weisheng ju 1951 nian gongzuo jihua" (Tianjin Public Health Bureau Work report for 1951 [27 Jan. 1951]). Tianjin: Tianjin Public Health Bureau Archives.

Carroll, Peter. "Between Heaven and Modernity: The Late Qing and Early Republic (Re)Construction of Suzhou Urban Space." Ph.D. diss., Yale University, 1998.

Chadwick, Edwin. *Report on an Inquiry into the Sanitary Conditions of the Labouring Population of Great Britain.* London, 1842.

Chakrabarty, Dipesh. "Open Space, Public Place: Garbage, Modernity, and India." *South Asia: Journal of South Asian Studies* 14, no. 1 (1991): 15–31.

———. "Postcoloniality and the Artifice of History: Who Speaks for 'Indian' Pasts?" In *A Subaltern Studies Reader, 1986–1995,* ed. Ranajit Guha. Minneapolis: University of Minnesota Press, 1997.

Chang, Che-chia. "The Therapeutic Tug of War: The Imperial Physician-Patient Relationship in the Era of Empress Dowager Cixi, 1874–1908." Ph.D. diss., University of Pennsylvania, 1998.

Chang, Chia-feng. "Aspects of Smallpox and Its Significance in Chinese History." Ph.D. diss., University of London, 1996.

Chang, K. C. *Food in Chinese Culture.* New Haven: Yale University Press, 1977.

Chatterjee, Partha. *The Nation and Its Fragments: Colonial and Postcolonial Histories.* Princeton, N.J.: Princeton University Press, 1993.

———. *Nationalist Thought and the Colonial World: A Derivative Discourse.* Minneapolis: University of Minnesota Press, 1986.

Chemical Genealogy Database. Available from http://www.scs.uiuc.edu/~mainzv/Web_Geneology/Info?Johnsonjfw.pdf (accessed July 17, 2002).

Chen, Ke. "Nongovernmental Organizations and the Urban Control and Management System in Tianjin at the End of the Nineteenth Century." *Social Sciences in China* 11, no. 4 (1990): 54–77.

Chen, Nancy. "Urban Spaces and Experiences of Qigong." In *Urban Spaces: Autonomy and Community in Post-Mao China,* ed. D. Davis. New York and Cambridge, England: Cambridge University Press, 1995.

Chen Yong. "Mingqing Tianjin chengshi jigou de chu bu kaocha" (Preliminary investigations on Tianjin's urban structure in the Ming-Qing period). *Chengshi shi yanjiu* (Urban history project) 10 (1995): 25–63.

Chen, Yuan-peng. "Food and Healing in the Tang and Sung: The Shih-chih Chapter in Sun Szu-miao's Ch'ien-chin Yao-fang." *Bulletin of the Institute of History and Philology: Academia Sinica* 69, no. 4 (1998): 765–825.

Chen Zhengjiang, ed. *Yihetuan wenxian jizhu yu yanjiu* (Annotation and analysis of the historical materials on the Boxer movement). Tianjin: Tianjin renmin chubanshe, 1985.

Cheng, Pei-kai, and Michael Lestz, with Jonathan D. Spence. *The Search for Modern China: A Documentary Collection.* New York: W. W. Norton, 1999.

Chinese Times (Tientsin), 1886–91.

Cochran, Sherman. *Big Business in China: Sino-Foreign Rivalry in the Cigarette Industry, 1890–1930.* Cambridge, Mass.: Harvard University Press, 1980.

————. *Encountering Chinese Networks: Western, Japanese, and Chinese Corporations in China, 1880–1937.* Berkeley: University of California Press, 2000.

————. "Medicine and Advertising Dreams in China, 1900–1950," in *Becoming Chinese: Passages to Modernity and Beyond,* ed. Wen-hsin Yeh. Berkeley: University of California Press, 2000.

Cohen, Paul. *History in Three Keys: The Boxers as Event, Experience, and Myth.* New York: Columbia University Press, 1997.

————. *China and Christianity: The Missionary Movement and the Growth of Chinese Antiforeignism, 1860–1870.* Cambridge, Mass.: Harvard University Press, 1963.

Coleman, William. *Death Is a Social Disease: Public Health and Political Economy in Early Industrial France.* Madison, Wisc.: University of Wisconsin, 1982.

————. "Health and Hygiene in the *Encyclopédie.*" *Bulletin of the History of Medicine* 414 (Oct. 1974): 399–421.

Coles-McElroy, Sarah. "Transforming China through Education: Yan Xiu, Zhang Boling, and the Effort to Build a New School System, 1901–1927." Ph.D. diss., Yale University, 1997.

Confucius. *The Analects.* Trans. D. C. Lau. New York: Penguin, 1979.

Cooter, Roger. *Studies in the History of Alternative Medicine.* Basingstoke: Macmillan in association with St. Antony's College Oxford, 1988.

Cooter, Roger, Mark Harrison, and Steve Sturdy, eds. *War, Medicine, and Modernity.* Stroud: Sutton, 1998.

Corbin, Alain. *The Foul and the Fragrant: Odor and the French Social Imagination.* Cambridge, Mass.: Harvard University Press, 1986.

Cowdrey, Albert E. " 'Germ Warfare' and Public Health in the Korean Conflict." *Journal of the History of Medicine and Allied Sciences* 39 (1984): 153–72.

Croizier, Ralph. *Traditional Medicine in Modern China: Science, Nationalism, and the Tensions of Cultural Change.* Cambridge, Mass.: Harvard University Press, 1968.

Cumings, Bruce, and Jon Halliday. *Korea, the Unknown War.* London: Viking/Penguin Press, 1988.

Curtin, Philip. "Medical Knowledge and Urban Planning in Tropical Africa." *American Historical Review* 90, no. 3 (1985): 594–613.

Da gong bao (L'Impartial; Tianjin), 1902–38.

Dai Yuyan. *Gushui jiuwen* (Old things heard about Tianjin). 1936. Reprint, Tianjin: Tianjin guji chubanshe, 1986.

Dangdai Zhongguo congshu bianjibu, ed. *Dangdai Zhongguode weisheng shiye* (Contemporary China's public health). Beijing: Zhongguo shehui kexue chubanshe, 1986.

————. *Kang Mei yuan Chao zhanzheng* (The Korean War). Beijing: Zhongguo shehuikexue chubanshe, 1990.

————. *Dangdai Zhongguo de Tianjin* (Contemporary Tianjin). Beijing: Zhongguo shehui kexue chubanshe, 1989.

Date Kazuo. *Isei toshite no Mori Ôgai* (Mori Ôgai as military doctor). 2 vols. Tokyo: Sekibundô Shuppan, 1981.

De Bevoise, Ken. *Agents of Apocalypse: Epidemic Disease in the Colonial Philippines.* Princeton, N.J.: Princeton University Press, 1995.

de Lacy, Charles. *How to Prolong Life: An Inquiry into the Cause of Old Age and Natural Decay, Showing the Diet and Agents Best Adapted for the Lengthened Prolongation of Existence.* London: Balliere, Tindall, and Cox, 1885.

Despeux, Catherine. *La Moelle du Phénix Rouge: Santé et longue vie dans la Chine du XVIe siècle.* Paris: Guy Tredaniel, 1988.

Deutsche Niederlassunger Gemeinde in Tientsin: Abchluss und Jahresbericht (Annual report and budget of the German settlement in Tianjin). Tianjin: n.p., 1916.

Dickson, Walter. "Journal of HM Ship *Chesapeake,* Dr. Walter Dickson, Surgeon, from 1 July 1958 to 30 June 1959, Containing the Cases of the Killed and Wounded in the Attack on the Peiho forts." PRO, Adm., 101/169.

Ding Zilang, ed. *Zhu yuan cong hua* (Collected talks from the Bamboo Garden). Tianjin. 1923–26.

Diyi yiyuan zhi bian hui, ed. *Diyi yiyuan zhi.* (Chronicle of the Number One Hospital). Tianjin: n.p., 1990.

Dongbei ribao (Northeast daily; Shenyang), 1952–53.

Dikötter, Frank, ed. *The Construction of Racial Identities in China and Japan: Historical and Contemporary Perspectives.* London: Hurst and Co., 1997.

———. *The Discourse of Race in Modern China.* Stanford: Stanford University Press, 1992.

———. *Imperfect Conceptions: Medical Knowledge, Birth Defects, and Eugenics in China.* New York: Columbia University Press, 1998.

———. *Crime, Punishment, and the Prison in Modern China.* New York: Columbia University Press, 2002.

———. *Sex, Culture, and Modernity in China: Medical Science and the Construction of Sexual Identities in the Early Republican Period.* London: Hurst and Co., 1995.

Dirlik, Arif. "The Ideological Foundations of the New Life Movement: A Study in Counterrevolution." *Journal of Asian Studies* 34, no. 4 (1975): 945–80.

Duara, Prasenjit. *Culture, Power, and the State: Rural North China, 1900–1942.* Stanford: Stanford University Press, 1988.

———. *Rescuing History from the Nation: Questioning Narratives of Modern China.* Chicago: University of Chicago Press, 1995.

———. "Transnationalism and the Predicament of Sovereignty: China 1900–1945." *American Historical Review* 102, no. 4 (1997): 1030–51.

Dudgeon, John. *The Diseases of China: Their Causes, Conditions, and Prevalence, Contrasted with Those of Europe.* Glasgow: Dunn and Wright. 1877.

Duffy, John. *The Sanitarians: A History of American Public Health.* Champaign-Urbana: University of Illinois Press, 1990.

Dunstan, Helen. "Late Ming Epidemics: A Preliminary Survey." *Ch'ing-shih wen-t'i* 3, no. 3 (1975): 1–75.

Dutong yamen huiyi jiyao (Minutes of the meetings of the Tianjin Provisional Government, *DTYMHYJY*), translation of *Procès-verbaux des séance du conseil du gouvernement provisoire de Tientsin*. Handwritten manuscript, Tianjin Academy of Social Sciences, n.d.

Dutton, Michael. *Policing and Punishment in China: From Patriarchy to "The People."* Cambridge and New York: Cambridge University Press, 1992.

Duus, Peter, Ramon H. Myers, and Mark R. Peattie, eds. *The Japanese Informal Empire in China, 1895–1973*. Princeton, N.J.: Princeton University Press, 1989.

———. *The Japanese Wartime Empire, 1931–1945*. Princeton, N.J.: Princeton University Press, 1996.

Eastman, Lloyd. *The Abortive Revolution: China under Nationalist Rule, 1927–1937*. Cambridge, Mass.: Harvard University Press, 1974.

Elias, Norbert. *The Civilizing Process*. London: Blackwell, 1993.

Elman, Benjamin. *A Cultural History of Civil Examinations in Late Imperial China*. Berkeley: University of California Press, 2000.

———. *From Philosophy to Philology: Intellectual and Social Aspects of Change in Late Imperial China*. Cambridge, Mass.: Harvard University Press, 1984.

Endicott, Stephen, and Edward Hagerman. *The United States and Biological Warfare: Secrets from the Early Cold War and Korea*. Bloomington: Indiana University Press, 1998.

Engels, Dagmar, and Shula Marks, eds. *Contesting Colonial Hegemony: State and Society in Africa and India*. London: I. B. Taurus, 1994.

Ershi shiji chu de Tianjin gaikuang (Conditions in early twentieth-century Tianjin). Chinese translation of *Tenshinshi* (Tianjin gazetteer), ed. Shinkoku chûtongun shireibu. Tokyo: Hakubunkan, 1909. Trans. Hou Zhentong. Tianjin: Tianjin difang shizhi bianxiu weiyuanhui zongbianjishi chuban, 1986.

Esherick, Joseph. *The Origins of the Boxer Uprising*. Berkeley and Los Angeles: University of California Press, 1987.

———, ed. *Remaking the Chinese City: Modernity and National Identity, 1900–1950*. Honolulu: University of Hawaii Press, 2000.

Evans, Richard J. *Death in Hamburg: Society and Politics in the Cholera Years, 1830–1910*. New York: Oxford University Press, 1987.

Fan Bin. "Jinmen xiaoling" (Poems in praise of Tianjin). 1819. In *Zili lianzhu ji* (String of pearls from my home), ed. Hua Dingyuan. 1879. Reprint, Tianjin: Tianjin guji chubanshe, 1986.

Fanon, Frantz. *Black Skin, White Masks*. London: Granada, 1970.

Farley, John. *Bilharzia: A History of Imperial Tropical Medicine*. New York and Cambridge: Cambridge University Press, 1991.

Farquhar, Judith. *Knowing Practice: The Clinical Encounter of Chinese Medicine*. Boulder, Colo.: Westview Press, 1994.

———. " 'Medicine and the Changes Are One': An Essay on Divination Healing with Commentary." *Chinese Science* 13 (1996): 107–34.

———. "Multiplicity, Point of View, and Responsibility in Traditional Chinese Healing." In *Body, Subject, and Power in China*, ed. Angela Zito and Tani Barlow. Chicago: University of Chicago Press, 1994.

Feng Jicai. *Shenbian* (The miraculous pigtail). Beijing: Zhongguo minjian chubanshe, 1988.

Feng Zhaozhan. *Douzhen quanji* (Complete book of smallpox). 1702. Reprint, Taibei: Zhengwen shuju, 1975.

Feuerwerker, Albert. *China's Early Industrialization: Shen Hsuan-huai (1844–1916) and Mandarin Enterprise.* Cambridge, Mass.: Harvard University Press, 1958.

Fileti, Vincenzo. *La Concessione Italiana di Tien-tsin.* Genova: Barabina e Graeve, 1921.

Finer, Samuel E. *The Life and Times of Sir Edwin Chadwick.* London: Methuen, 1952.

Fitzgerald, John. *Awakening China: Politics, Culture, and Class in the Nationalist Revolution.* Stanford: Stanford University Press, 1996.

———. "Chinese, Dogs, and the State that Stands on Two Legs." *Bulletin of Concerned Asian Scholars* 29, no. 4 (1997): 54–61.

Fogel, Joshua. "Akutakaga Ryûnosuke in China." *Chinese Studies in History* 30, no. 4 (1997): 6–55.

———. "Shanghai-Japan": The Japanese Residents' Association of Shanghai." *Journal of Asian Studies* 59, no. 4 (2000): 927–50.

Foucault, Michel. *The Birth of the Clinic.* Trans. A. M. Sheridan. New York: Pantheon Books, 1975.

———. *Discipline and Punish: The Birth of the Prison.* New York: Vintage 1979.

———. *The History of Sexuality.* New York: Vintage, 1985.

———. *Power/Knowledge: Selected Interviews and Other Writings, 1972–1977.* Ed. Colin Gordon. New York: Pantheon Books, 1980.

Frank, Johann Peter. *System einer vollstandigen medicinischen Polizey.* Frankenthal: Verlag der Gegelischen Buchdruckerey und Buchhandlung, 1791.

Fryer, John, ed. *Gezhi huibian* (The Chinese scientific magazine). Nanjing: Nanjing gu jiu shu dian, 1992.

Fu, Poshek. *Passivity, Resistance, and Collaboration: Intellectual Choices in Occupied Shanghai, 1937–1945.* Stanford: Stanford University Press, 1993.

Furth, Charlotte. "Blood, Body, and Gender: Medical Images of the Female Condition in China 1600–1850." *Chinese Science* 7 (1986): 43–66.

———. "Concepts of Pregnancy, Childbirth, and Infancy." *Journal of Asian Studies* 46, no. 1 (1987): 7–31.

———. *A Flourishing Yin: Gender in China's Medical History, 950–1665.* Berkeley: University of California Press, 1999.

Furuno Naoya. *Tenshin Gunshireibu: 1901–1937.* Tokyo: Kokusho Kankôkai, 1989.

Gabriel, Richard, and Karen Metz. *A History of Military Medicine.* New York: Greenwood Press, 1992.

Gan Houci, ed. *Beiyang gongdu leizuan* (Classified collection of public documents of the commissioner of trade for the northern ports, *BYGDLZ*). 1907. Reprint, Taibei: Wenhai chubanshe, 1966.

Gan Minyang, ed. *Xin Tianjin zhinan* (New guide to Tianjin). Tianjin: Jiangxue zhai shuju, 1927.

Gao Lingwen, ed. *Tianjin xian xin zhi* (A new gazetteer of Tianjin county). Tianjin: Jinyue, 1930.

Garon, Sheldon. *Molding Japanese Minds: The State in Everyday Life.* Princeton, N.J.: Princeton University Press, 1997.

———. "The World's Oldest Debate? Prostitution and the State in Imperial Japan, 1900–1945." *American Historical Review* 98, no. 3 (1993): 710–33.

Garret, Shirley. *Social Reformers in Urban China: The Chinese Y.M.C.A., 1895–1926.* Cambridge, Mass.: Harvard University Press, 1970.

Geison, Gerald L. ed. *Physiology in the American Context, 1850–1940.* Baltimore, Md.: American Physiological Society, 1987; distributed by Williams and Wilkins.

Ghosh, Somnath, and Pradip Baksi. "The Natural Science Note-Books of Marx and Engels: Middle of 1877 to Early 1883." Hartford Web Publishing World History Archives, http://www.hartford-hwp.com/archives/26/173.html.

Glosser, Susan. "'The Truths I Have Learned': Nationalism, Family Reform, and Male Identity in China's New Culture Movement, 1915–1923." In *Chinese Feminities, Chinese Masculinities,* ed. Susan Brownell and Jeffrey Wasserstrom. Berkeley: University of California Press, 2002.

Gongzhongdang Guanxu chao zouzhe (Secret palace memorials of the Guangxu period). 26 vols. Taibei: National Palace Museum, 1974.

Goodman, Bryna. "Improvisations on a Semicolonial Theme, or, How to Read a Celebration of Transnational Urban Community." *Journal of Asian Studies* 59, no. 4 (2000): 889–926.

———. *Native Place, City, and Nation: Regional Networks and Identities in Shanghai, 1853–1937.* Berkeley and Los Angeles: University of California Press, 1995.

Goodrich, L. Carrington, ed. *Dictionary of Ming Biography, 1368–1644.* New York: Columbia University Press, 1976.

Gordon, C. A. *An Epitome of the Reports of the Medical Officers to the Imperial Maritime Customs Service, from 1871 to 1882.* Shanghai: Kelly and Walsh, 1884.

Goubert, Jean-Pierre. *The Conquest of Water: The Advent of Health in the Industrial Age.* Cambridge: Polity Press, 1986.

Graham, A. C. *Chuang-tzu: The Seven Inner Chapters and Other Writings from the Book Chuang-tzu.* London and Boston: Allen and Unwin, 1981.

Graham, Gerald. *The China Station: War and Diplomacy, 1830–1860.* New York: Oxford University Press, 1978.

Gu Daosheng, "Tianjin chengqu maishui he mai shui jiu su" (Old customs of buying and selling water in the Tianjin area). *Tianjin shizhi* 2 (1990): 49–50.

Guha, Ranajit. *Dominance Without Hegemony: History and Power in Colonial India.* Cambridge, Mass.: Harvard University Press, 1997.

Guo Aichun, ed., *Huangdi neijin suwen jiaozhu yuyi* (Basic questions from the Inner Canon of the Yellow Emperor: Annotated with explanations in modern Chinese). Beijing: Renmin weisheng chubanshe, 1992.

Guo Zuyuan, ed. *Tianjin shangxiashuidao gongcheng* (Construction of Tianjin's sewers and water system). Tianjin: Tianjin diliushiyiqu nonghui, 1947.

Guoyi zhen yan (True words on the national medicine) (Tianjin), 1934. Tianjin History Museum collection.

Hamlin, Christopher. "Edwin Chadwick, 'Mutton Medicine,' and the Fever Question." *Bulletin of the History of Medicine* 70 (1996): 233–65.

———. "Providence and Putrefaction: Victorian Sanitarians and the Natural Theology of Health and Disease." *Victorian Studies* 28 (1984–85): 381–411.

———. *Public Health and Social Justice in the Age of Chadwick.* Cambridge: Cambridge University Press, 1998.

———. "Robert Warington and the Moral Economy of the Aquarium." *Journal of the History of Biology* 1 (1986): 134–41.

———. *A Science of Impurity: Water Analysis in Nineteenth-Century Britain.* Berkeley: University of California Press, 1990.

Han Feng. "Qudi jiu Tianjin changye jishi" (Events in the elimination of Old Tianjin's prostitution industry). In *Jin chang jin du* (The crackdown on prostitution and drugs), ed. Ma Weigang. Beijing: Jing guan jiaoyu chubanshe, 1993.

Hanson, Marta. "Inventing a Tradition in Chinese Medicine." Ph.D. diss., University of Pennsylvania, 1997.

———. "Robust Northerners and Delicate Southerners: The Nineteenth-Century Invention of a Southern Medical Tradition." *positions* 6, no.3 (1998): 515–50.

Harper, Donald. *Early Chinese Medical Literature: The Mawangdui Medical Manuscripts.* London and New York: Kegan Paul International, 1998.

Hao Fusen. *Jinmen wenjian lu* (Memoir of Tianjin). Hand-copied version in Tianjin Academy of Social Sciences, Tianjin, n.d.

———. "Jinmen wenjian lu" (Memoir of Tianjin). In *Di'er ci yapian zhanzhen* (The second opium war, *DECYPZZ*), ed. Qi Shihe et al. Shanghai: Renmin chubanshe, 1978.

Hao Purong. "Jinmen shiji quedui" (A record of events in Tianjin, written in couplets). In *Di'er ci yapian zhanzhen* (The second opium war, *DECYPZZ*), ed. Qi Shihe et al. Vol. 2. Shanghai: Renmin chubanshe, 1978.

Harris, Sheldon. *Factories of Death: Japanese Biological Warfare, 1932–1945, and the American Cover-up.* London and New York: Routledge, 1994.

Harrison, Mark. *Climates and Constitutions: Health, Race, Environment, and British Imperialism in India, 1600–1850.* Oxford and New York: Oxford University Press, 1999.

———. "The Identity of Cholera in British India, 1860–1890." In *Warm Cli-*

mates and Western Medicine: The Emergence of Tropical Medicine, 1500–1900, ed. David Arnold. Amsterdam and Atlanta, Ga.: Rodopi, 1996.

———. "Medicine and Orientalism: Perspectives on Europe's Encounter with Indian Medical Systems." In *Health, Medicine, and Empire*, ed. Biswamoy Pati and Mark Harrison. Hyderabad, India: Orient Longman, 2001.

———. *Public Health in British India: Anglo-Indian Preventive Medicine, 1859–1914*. Cambridge: Cambridge University Press, 1994.

———. " 'The Tender Frame of Man': Disease, Climate, and Racial Difference in India and the West Indies, 1760–1860." *Bulletin of the History of Medicine* 70, no. 1 (1996): 68–93.

Hart, Roger. "Translating the Untranslatable: From Copula to Incommensurable Worlds." In *Tokens of Exchange: The Problem of Translation in Global Circulations*, ed. Lydia H. Liu. Durham, N.C.: Duke University Press, 1999.

Hayes, Douglas. *Imperial Medicine: Patrick Manson and the Conquest of Tropical Disease*. Philadelphia: University of Pennsylvania Press, 2001.

Headrick, Daniel. *The Tentacles of Progress: Technology Transfer in the Age of Imperialism, 1850–1940*. New York: Oxford University Press, 1988.

Henderson, John. *The Development and Decline of Chinese Cosmology*. New York: Columbia University Press, 1984.

Henriot, Christian. "Medicine, V.D., and Prostitution in Pre-Revolutionary China." *Social History of Medicine* 5, no. 1 (1992): 95–120.

———. *Shanghai, 1927–1937: Municipal Power, Locality, and Modernization*. Berkeley and Los Angeles: University of California Press, 1993.

Hershatter, Gail. *Dangerous Pleasures*. Berkeley: University of California Press, 1997.

———. *The Workers of Tianjin, 1900–1949*. Stanford: Stanford University Press, 1986.

Hevia, James L. "Leaving a Brand on China: Missionary Discourse in the Wake of the Boxer Movement." *Modern China* 18, no. 3 (1992), 304–32.

———. "Looting Beijing: 1860, 1900." In *Tokens of Exchange: The Problem of Translation in Global Circulations*, ed. Lydia H. Liu. Durham, N.C.: Duke University Press, 1999.

Hinrichs, T. J. "New Geographies of Chinese Medicine." In "Beyond Joseph Needham: Science, Technology, and Medicine in East and Southeast Asia." *Osiris* 13 (1998).

Ho, Ping-ti. "The Salt Merchants of Yangchou: A Study of Commercial Capitalism in Eighteenth-Century China." *Harvard Journal of Asiatic Studies* 17, nos. 1–2 (1954): 130–68.

Hong Tianxi. *Buzhu wenyi lun* (Supplementary notes to the treatise on epidemic disease). Circa 1750. Reprint, Beijing: Zhongguo shu dian, 1993.

Honig, Emily. *Sisters and Strangers: Women in the Shanghai Cotton Mills, 1919–1949*. Stanford: Stanford University Press, 1986.

Hopkins, Donald. *Princes and Peasants: Smallpox in History*. Chicago: University of Chicago Press, 1983.

Hotstatler, Laura. *Qing Colonial Enterprise: Ethnography and Cartography in Early Modern China.* Chicago: University of Chicago Press, 2001.

Howard, Paul. "Opium Smoking in Qing China: Responses to a Social Problem, 1729–1906." Ph.D. diss., University of Pennsylvania, 1998.

Hsiung, Ping-chen. "More or Less: Cultural and Medical Factors Behind Marital Fertility in Late Imperial China." In *Abortion, Infanticide, and Reproductive Culture in Asia: Past and Present,* ed. James Z. Lee and Osamu Saito. Oxford: Oxford University Press, forthcoming.

Hsu, Elizabeth. *The Transmission of Chinese Medicine.* Cambridge: Cambridge University Press, 1999.

Hu Wenhuan, ed. *Lei xiu yao jue* (Essential formulas for self-cultivation, divided in categories). 1600. Reprint, Shanghai: Shanghai zhongyi xueyuan chubanshe, 1989.

———, comp. *Shouyang cong shu* (Collected works on cultivating longevity). In *Beijing tushuguan guji zhenben congkan* (Rare books from the Beijing Library). Vol. 82. Beijing: Beijing tushuguan guji chubanshe, 1987.

Hua Dingyuan, ed. *Zili lianzhu ji.* 1879. Reprint, Tianjin: Tianjin guji chubanshe, 1986.

Hua Xuelan. "Gengzi riji." In *Gengzi jishi* (Memoirs of 1900), ed. Zhongguo shehui kexue yuan jindaiyanjiu suo. Beijing: n.p., 1978.

———. *Xinchou riji* (1901 diary). Shanghai: Shangwu yinshu guan, 1936.

Huang Ke-wu. "Cong *Shenbao* yiyao guangao kan Min chu Shanghai de yiliao wenhua yu shehui shenghuo, 1912–1926." (The medical culture and social life of early Republican Shanghai as seen through medicine advertisements in the *Shenbao.*) *Zhongyang yaunjiu yuan jindai shi yanjiu suo jikan* 17 (Dec. 1989): 141–94.

Hufeland, C. W. *Enchiridion medicum: Oder Anleitung zur medizinischen Praxis* (Handbook of medicine, or, A code of medical practice). Berlin: Jonas Verlagsbuchhandlung, 1836.

Hunt, Mary Hannah Hanchett. *Haitong weisheng bian.* Trans. John Fryer. Shanghai: The Chinese Scientific Book Depot, 1894.

———. *Health for Little Folks.* New York, Cincinnati, and Chicago: American Book Company, 1890.

Hunt, Nancy Rose. *A Colonial Lexicon of Birth Ritual, Medicalization, and Mobility in the Congo.* Durham, N.C.: Duke University Press, 1999.

Huntington, Ellsworth, in conjunction with the directors of the American Eugenics Society. *Tomorrow's Children: The Goal of Eugenics.* New York: J. Wiley and Sons, Inc.; London: Chapman and Hall, Ltd., 1935.

Hurd, Douglas. *The Arrow War.* London: Collins Press, 1967.

Husihui. *Yinshan zhengyao* (Principles of a Correct Diet). 1330. Reprint, Shanghai: Shanghai guju chubanshe, 1994.

Hymes, Robert. "Not Quite Gentlemen? Doctors in Song and Yuan." *Chinese Science* 8 (Jan. 1987): 9–76.

Iijima Wataru and Wakamura Kohei. "Eisei to teikoku: Nichi-Ei shokumin-chishugi no hikakushi teki kôsatsu ni mukete" (Hygiene and empire: Toward a comparative history of Japanese and British Colonialism). *Nihon shi kenkyu* (Research in Japanese history) 462 (Feb. 2001).

——. "Kindai higashi Ajia ni okeru pesuto no ryûkô ni tsuite" (On the prevalence of the plague in modern East Asia). *Shichô* 29 (1991): 24–39.

——. *Pesuto to kindai Chûgoku.* Tokyo: Kenbun Shuppan, 2000.

Imperial Maritime Customs. *Decennial Reports, 1882–1931.* 5 vols. Shanghai: Kelly and Walsh, 1882–1931.

Inspectorate General of Customs. *Decennial Reports, 1882–91.* Shanghai: Kelly and Walsh, 1892.

——. *Decennial Reports, 1892–1901.* Shanghai: Kelly and Walsh, 1902.

——. *Decennial Reports, 1902–11.* Shanghai: Kelly and Walsh, 1912.

——. *Decennial Reports, 1912–21.* Shanghai: Kelly and Walsh, 1922.

Jannetta, Ann. "From Physician to Bureaucrat: The Case of Nagayo Sensai." In *New Directions in the Study of Meiji Japan,* ed. Helen Hardacre. Leiden: Brill, 1997.

Jiang Shi. "Guhe zayong" (Miscellaneous chants from the ancient river). In *Zili lianzhu ji* (String of pearls from my hometown), ed. Hua Dingyuan. 1879. Reprint, Tianjin: Tianjin guji chubanshe, 1986.

Jin Dayang. "Tianjin Li Shanren" (Tianjin's "Charitable Li"). *Tianjin wenshi ziliao* (Tianjin historical materials, *TJWSZL*) 7 (1980): 71–85.

Jindai Tianjin renwu lu (Biographical dictionary of modern Tianjin). Tianjin: Tianjinshi difang shizhi bianxiu weiyuan hui zong bianji shi, 1987.

Jinmen jinghua shilu (Record of the cultural essence of Tianjin). Tianjin: Zhonghua yutu xue she, 1918.

"Jinmen shiji quedui" (An accurate record of the events at Tianjin, in couplets). In *Di'er ci yapian zhanzhen* (The second opium war, *DECYPZZ*), ed. Qi Shihe. Vol. 2. Shanghai: Renmin chubanshe, 1978.

Johnson, Kay Ann. *Women, the Family and Peasant Revolution in China.* Chicago: University of Chicago Press, 1983.

Johnston, James F. W. *Chemistry of Common Life.* New York: Appleton, 1855.

Johnston, William. *The Modern Epidemic: Tuberculosis in Japan.* Cambridge, Mass.: Harvard University Press, 1995.

Johonnot, James, and Eugene Bouton. *Lessons in Hygiene, or The Human Body and How to Take Care of It.* New York, Cincinnati, and Chicago: American Book Company, 1889.

——. *Youtong weisheng bian.* Trans. John Fryer. Shanghai: The Chinese Scientific Book Depot, 1894.

Jordon, David. *Transforming Paris: The Life and Labors of Baron Haussmann.* New York: The Free Press, 1995.

Katsuragawa Mitsumasa. "Sokai zaijû Nihonjin no Chûgoku ninshiki, Tenshin o ichirei to shite" (The perception of China by Japanese residents in the concessions: The case of Tianjin). *Kindai Nihon no Ajia ninshiki* (Modern Japanese perceptions of China), ed. Furuya Tetsuo. Kyoto: Kyoto daigaku jinbun kagaku kenkyûjo, 1994.

Katz, Paul. *Demon Hordes and Burning Boats: The Cult of Marshal Wen in Late*

Imperial Chekiang. SUNY Series in Chinese Local Studies. Albany: SUNY Press, 1995.

———. "Germs of Disaster—The Impact of Epidemics on Japanese Military Campaigns in Taiwan, 1874 and 1895." *Annales de Demographie Historique* (1996): 195–220.

Kellogg, John Harvey. *First Book in Physiology and Hygiene.* New York: Harper and Brothers, 1888.

———. *Chuxue weisheng bian.* Trans. John Fryer. Shanghai: The Chinese Scientific Book Depot, 1896.

Keene, Donald. *The Japanese Discovery of Europe.* Stanford: Stanford University Press, 1969.

Kirby, William. *Germany and Republican China.* Stanford: Stanford University Press, 1984.

———. "Engineering China: Birth of the Developmental State." In *Becoming Chinese: Passages to Modernity and Beyond,* ed. Wen-hsin Yeh. Berkeley: University of California Press, 2000.

———. "The Internationalization of China: Foreign Relations at Home and Abroad in the Republican Era." *China Quarterly* 150 (1997): 433–58.

Kitaoka Shin'ichi. *Gotô Shinpei: gaikô to bijon* (Gotô Shinpei: diplomacy and vision). Tokyo: Chûô Kôronsha, 1988.

Kleinman, Arthur, ed. *Culture and Healing in Asian Societies: Anthropological, Psychiatric, and Public Health Studies.* Boston: G. K. Hall, 1978.

———. *Patient and Healing in the Context of Culture.* Berkeley and Los Angeles: University of California Press, 1980.

———, et al., eds. *Medicine in Chinese Cultures.* Washington, D.C.: U.S. Department of Health, Education, and Welfare, National Institute of Health, 1975.

Knight, David. "Communicating Chemistry." In *Communicating Chemistry: Textbooks and Their Audiences, 1789–1939,* ed. Anders Lundgren and Bernadette Bensaude-Vincent. Canton, Mass.: Science History Publications, 2000.

Kobayashi, Motohiro. "Drug Operations by Resident Japanese in Tianjin." In *Opium Regimes,* ed. Timothy Brook and Bob Tadashi Wakabayashi. Berkeley: University of California Press, 2000.

Kohn, Livia. *The Taoist Experience: An Anthology.* Albany, N.Y.: SUNY Press, 1993.

———, ed. *Taoist Meditation and Longevity Techniques.* Ann Arbor: University of Michigan, Michigan Monographs in Chinese Studies, vol. 61, 1989.

Kraut, Alan. *Silent Travelers: Germs, Genes, and the "Immigrant Menace."* New York: Basic Books, 1994.

Kuriyama, Shigehisa. *The Expressiveness of the Body and the Divergence of Greek and Chinese Medicine.* New York: Zone Books, 1999.

———. "The Imagination of Winds and the Development of the Chinese Conception of the Body." In *Body, Subject, and Power in China,* ed. Angela Zito and Tani E. Barlow. Chicago: University of Chicago Press, 1994.

———. "Interpreting the History of Bloodletting." *Journal of the History of Medicine and the Allied Sciences* 50 (1995): 11–46.

———. "Visual Knowledge in Classical Chinese Medicine." In *Knowledge and the Scholarly Medical Traditions,* ed. Don Bates. Cambridge and New York: Cambridge University Press, 1995.

Kwan, Man-bun. "The Merchant World of Tianjin: Society and Economy of a Chinese City." Ph.D. diss., Stanford University, 1990.

———. "Order in Chaos: Tianjin's *Hunhunr* and Urban Identity in Modern China." *Journal of Urban History* 27, no. 1 (2000): 75–91.

———. *The Salt Merchants of Tianjin: State-Making and Civil Society in Late Imperial China.* Honolulu: University of Hawaii Press, 2001.

Lackner, Michael, Iwo Amelung, and Joachim Kurtz, eds. *New Terms for New Ideas: Western Knowledge and Lexical Change in Late Imperial China.* Leiden: Brill, 2001.

Lai Xinxia, ed. *Tianjin jindaishi* (Modern Tianjin history). Tianjin: Nankai Daxue chubanshe, 1987.

Lamarre, Thomas. "Bacterial Cultures and Linguistic Colonies: Mori Rintaro's Experiments with History, Science, and Languages." *positions* 6, no. 3 (1998): 597–635.

Lao-tzu. *Tao te ching.* Trans. James Legge. Taipei: Ch'eng-wen Publishing Company, 1969.

Latour, Bruno. *The Pasteurization of France.* Cambridge, Mass.: Harvard University Press, 1988.

Lee, Chae-Jin. *Zhou En-lai: The Early Years.* Stanford: Stanford University Press, 1994.

Lee, James Z., and Wang Feng. *One Quarter of Humanity: Malthusian Mythology and Chinese Realities, 1700–2000.* Cambridge, Mass.: Harvard University Press, 1999.

Lei, Sean Hsiang-lin. "When Chinese Medicine Encountered the State: 1910–1949." Ph.D. diss., University of Chicago, 1999.

Leung, Angela Ki Che. "Organized Medicine in Mid-Qing China: State and Private Medical Institutions in the Lower Yangzi Region." *Late Imperial China* 8, no. 1 (1987): 155–66.

———. "To Chasten Society: The Development of Widow Homes in the Qing, 1773–1911." *Late Imperial China* 14, no. 2 (1993): 1–32.

Li Chih-ch'ang [Li Zhichang]. *The Travels of an Alchemist: The Journey of the Daoist Ch'ang Ch'un from China to the Hindukush at the Summons of Chingiz Khan.* Trans. Arthur Waley. London: George Routledge and Sons, Ltd., 1931.

Li Jingneng, ed. *Tianjin renkoushi* (Population history of Tianjin). Tianjin: Nankai daxue chubanshe, 1990.

——— et al., eds. *Zhongguo renkou: Tianjin fence* (China's population: Tianjin edition). Beijing: Zinhua shudian, 1987.

Li Shaobi and Ni Pujun. "Ji Tianjin zilaishui chuangban wushi nian" (Recollecting fifty years of Tianjin's water system). Unpublished manuscript (Tianjin zhengxiehui, wenshi ziliao guan, Tianjin), 1981.

————. "Tianjin zilaishui shiye jianshi" (A brief history of water supply in Tianjin). *Tianjin wenshi ziliao xuanji* 21 (Aug. 1982): 27–53.

Li Shizhen. *Ben cao gang mu*. 1596, 1885 edition. Reprint, Beijing: Renmin weisheng shuban she, 1957.

Li Wenhai. *Jindai Zhongguo zaihuang jinian* (Chronicle of modern China's natural disasters). Changsha: Hunan jiaoyu chubanshe, 1990.

————. *Zaihuang yu jijin* (Natural disasters and famine). Beijing: Gaodengjiaoyu chubanshe, 1991.

Li Zhichang [Li Chih-ch'ang]. *Chang Chun zhen ren xi you ji* (The journey to the west of the Perfected One Chang Chun). 1228. In *Kuo hsueh chi pen cong shu*, vol. 349, ed. Wang Yunwu. Taibei: Shangwu jin shu guan, 1968.

Liang Qizi [Leung, Angela]. "Minjian cishan huodong di xingqi: yi Jiang Zhe diqu weili" (The rise of private philanthropy in late Ming and early Qing: Examples from Jiangsu and Zhejiang). *Shih-huo* 15, nos. 7–8 (1986): 304–31.

————. *Shishan yu jiaohua: Ming Qin de cishan zuzhi* (Doing good and moral transformation: Ming-Qing philanthropic organizations). Taibei: Lianjing, 1997.

————. "Variolisation et vaccination dans la Chin prémoderne, 1570–1911." In *L'Aventure de la vaccination*, ed. Anne-Marie Moulin. Paris: Fayard, 1996.

Liebig, Justus, Freiherr von. *Familiar Letters on Chemistry: In Its Relations to Physiology, Dietetics, Agriculture, Commerce, and Political Economy*. London: Walton and Maberly, 1859.

Lieberthal, Kenneth. *Revolution and Tradition in Tientsin, 1949–1952*. Stanford: Stanford University Press, 1980.

Liu Haiyan. "Jindai Zhongguo chengshishi yanjiu de huigu yu zhanwang" (Modern Chinese urban history: Its past and future prospects). *Lishi yanjiu* 3 (1992): 14–31.

————. "Youguan Tianjin jiao'an de jige wenti" (Some issues related to the Tianjin massacre). *Jindai Zhongguo jiaoan yanjiu* (Research in modern China's missionary cases). Chengdu: Sichuan sheng shehui kexueyuan chubanshe, 1979.

Liu Haiyan and Hao Kelu, eds. "Tianjin dutong yamen huiyiji yaoxuan" (Excerpts from the minutes of the Tianjin Provisional Government). *Jindai shi ziliao* (Materials for modern history) 79 (1991): 34–75.

Liu Huapu and Bian Xueyue. "Guoyao laodian: Longshunrong" (A venerable purveyor of Chinese medicine: Longshunrong). In *Jinmen laozi hao* (Old business of Tianjin), ed. Wenshi ziliao yanjiu weiyuan hui. Tianjin: Baihua wenyi chubanshe, 1992.

Liu Jiantang and Wei Jiao. *Jinmen tan gu* (Tales of old Tianjin). Tianjin: Beihua wenyi chubanshe, 1991.

Liu Jingyue. "Tianjin lunxian qian de zuihou yi zhan" (The last battle for Tianjin). In *Lunxia shiqi de Tianjin*, ed. Tianjinshi zhengxie hui—wenshi ziliao yanjiu weiyuanhui. (Tianjin during the occupation). Tianjin: Jinghai xian yinshuachang, 1992.

Liu Kui. *Song feng shuo yi* (Discussion on epidemics from Pine Peak). Beijing: Ren min wei sheng chubanshe, 1987.

Liu, Lydia H., ed. *Tokens of Exchange: The Problem of Translation in Global Circulations.* Durham, N.C.: Duke University Press, 1999.

———. *Translingual Practice: Literature, National Culture, and Translated Modernity—China, 1900–1937.* Stanford: Stanford University Press, 1995.

Liu Mengyang. "Tianjin quanfei bianluan jishi" (Record of Tianjin during the Boxer debacle). In *Yihetuan* (The Boxers), ed. Jian Bozan, Zhongguo shixue hui, vol. 9. Shanghai: Shen zhou guo guang she, 1951.

Liu Shiyong. "Qingjie, weisheng, yu baojian: Rizhi shiqi Taiwan shehui gong-gong weisheng guannian zhi zhuanbian" (Cleanliness, hygiene, and health: Transformations of concepts of public health in Taiwan society during the Japanese colonial period). *Taiwan shi yanjiu* (Research in the history of Taiwan) 8, no. 1 (2000).

Liu Xizi. "Jinxi piji" (Anxious record from west of Tianjin). In *Yihetuan* (The Boxers), ed. Jian Bozan, Zhongguo shixuehui. Shanghai: Shen zhou guo guang she, 1951.

Liu Yanchen. *Jinmen zatan* (Miscellaneous discussions of Tianjin). Tianjin: Sanyou meishu she, 1943.

Liu Zaisu, ed. *Tianjin kuailan* (Tianjin at a glance). Shanghai: Shijie shuju, 1926.

Lloyd, Christopher, and Jack Coulter. *Medicine and the Navy, 1200–1900.* Vol. 4. Edinburgh: E. and S. Livingstone, 1963.

Lo, Jiu-jung. "Survival as Justification for Collaboration, 1937–1945." In *Chinese Collaboration: The Limits of Accommodation,* ed. David Barrett and Larry Shyu. Stanford: Stanford University Press, 2001.

Lo, Ming-Cheng M. *Doctors Within Borders: Profession, Ethnicity, and Modernity in Colonial Taiwan.* Berkeley: University of California Press, 2002.

Lo, Vivienne. "The Influence of Western Han Nurturing Life Literature on the Development of Acumoxa Therapy." Ph.D. diss., London University, 1998.

Locher, Wolfgang. "Max von Pettenkofer—Life Stations of a Genius: On the 100th Anniversary of His Death." *International Journal of Hygiene and Environmental Health* 203 (2001): 379–91.

Loeb, L. "George Fulford and Victorian Patent Medicine Men: Quack Mercenaries or Smilesian Entrepreneurs?" *Canadian Bulletin of Medical History* 16, no. 1 (1999): 125–45.

Lu Weicheng. "Shiheng paishui gongcheng jianshe shilue" (A brief history of drainage construction). In *Tianjin: yige cheng de quqi* (Tianjin: The rise of a city), ed. Tianjinshi zhengxie hui—wenshi ziliao yanjiu weiyuanhui. Tianjin: Renmin chubanshe, n.d.

Lucas, AnElissa. *Chinese Medical Modernization: Comparative Policy Continuities, 1930s–1980s.* New York: Praeger, 1982.

Luo Hongxian (attrib.). *Wan shou xian shu* (The book of the everlasting immortals, c. 1560). Daoguang renzhen ed. (1832), comp. Cao Ruoshui. In *Zhongguo yixue dacheng sanbian* (Great compendium of Chinese medicine, in three parts), ed. Qiu Peiran, et al. Vol. 8. Changsha: Yuelu shu she, 1994.

——— (attrib.). *Weisheng zhen jue* (True formulas for guarding life). Circa 1560. Reprint, Beijing: Weisheng chubanshe, 1987.

Luo Shuwei et al., eds. *Jindai Tianjin chengshi shi* (The modern history of Tianjin). Beijing: Zhongguo shehui kexue chubanshe, 1993.

Luo Tianyi (fl. 1246–1283). *Weisheng baojian* (A precious mirror for guarding life). Reprint edition. Beijing: Weisheng chubanshe, 1987.

MacKinnon, Stephen R. *Power and Politics in Late Imperial China: Yuan Shikai in Beijing and Tianjin, 1901–1908.* Berkeley and Los Angeles: University of California Press, 1980.

MacLeod, Roy, ed. *Disease, Medicine, and Empire.* London: Routledge, 1988.

MacPherson, Kerrie. *A Wilderness of Marshes: The Origins of Public Health in Shanghai, 1843–1893.* Hong Kong: Oxford University Press, 1987.

Mair, Victor H. *Wandering on the Way: Early Taoist Tales and Parables of Chuang Tzu.* Honolulu: University of Hawaii Press, 1994.

Mårald, Erland. "Everything Circulates: Agricultural Chemistry and Re-cycling Theories in the Second Half of the Nineteenth Century." Paper presented at the conference of IFF Social Ecology, Nature, Society, History: Long Term Dynamics of Social Metabolism, Vienna, Austria, 1999, http://www.univie.ac.at/iffsocec/conference99/pdf/poMarald.pdf.

Marcovich, Ann. "French Colonial Medicine and Colonial Rule: Algeria and Indochina." In *Disease, Medicine, and Empire,* ed. Roy MacLeod. London: Routledge, 1988.

Marcus, Alan I. *Plague of Strangers: Social Groups and the Origins of City Services in Cincinnati, 1819–1870.* Columbus, Ohio: Ohio State University Press, 1991.

Martin, Brian. *The Shanghai Green Gang: Politics and Organized Crime, 1919–1937.* Berkeley: University of California Press, 1996.

Martin, Emily. *The Woman in the Body: A Cultural Analysis of Reproduction.* Boston: Beacon Press, 1987.

Maruyama Hiroshi. *Mori Ôgai to Eiseigaku* (Mori Ôgai and hygienics). Tokyo: Keiso shobo, 1984.

Maspero, Henri. *Taosim and Chinese Religion.* Amherst, Mass.: University of Amherst Press, 1981.

Masini, Frederico. *The Formation of the Modern Chinese Lexicon and Its Evolution Toward a National Language: The Period from 1840 to 1898.* Berkeley: Journal of Chinese Linguistics, 1993.

Masuda, Wataru. *Japan and China: Mutual Representations in the Modern Era.* Trans. Joshua Fogel. Richmond and Surrey: Curzon, 2000.

Matsui Toshihiko. *Gun-i Mori Ôgai* (Mori Ôgai as military doctor). Tokyo: Ofusha, 1989.

Mattingly, Carol. *Well-Tempered Women: Nineteenth-Century Temperance Rhetoric.* Carbondale: Southern Illinois University Press, 1998.

Mayer, Georg. *Hygienische Studien in China* (Studies of hygiene in China). Leipzig: Johann Ambrosius Barth, 1904.

McLaughlin, Redmond. *The Royal Army Medical Corps.* London: Leo Cooper, 1972.

Meng Xian (c. 621–c. 713). *Shiliao ben cao.* Reprint, Beijing: Zhongguo shangye chubanshe, 1992.

Meng Yue. "Hybrid Science Versus Modernity: The Practice of the Jiangnan Arsenal, 1864–1897." *East Asian Science, Technology, and Medicine* 16 (1999): 13–52.

Mervine, Marcus. "The Japanese Concession in Tientsin and the Narcotics Trade." *Information Bulletin of the Council on International Affairs* 3, no. 4 (1937): 83–95.

Meyer, Kathryn, and Terry Parssinen. *Webs of Smoke: Smugglers, Warlords, Spies, and the History of the International Drug Trade.* Lanham, Md.: Rowman and Littlefield, 1998.

Mikkeli, Heikii. *Hygiene in the Early Modern Medical Tradition.* Helsinki: Academica Scientiarum Fennica, 1999.

Mitchell, Timothy. *Colonising Egypt.* Cambridge: Cambridge University Press, 1991.

Mitter, Rana. *The Manchurian Myth.* Berkeley: University of California Press, 2000.

Miyamoto Shinobu. *Mori Ôgai no igaku shisô* (Mori Ôgai's medical thought). Tokyo: Keiso Shobo, 1979.

Momose Hiro. "Guanyu Jinmen baojia tushuo" (On the "Illustrated Treatise of Tianjin's Baojia System"). Trans. Pu Wenqi. *Tianjinshi yanjiu* 1 (1985).

Money, John. *The Destroying Angel: Sex, Fitness, and Food in the Legacy of Degeneracy Theory: Graham Crackers, Kellogg's Corn Flakes, and American History.* Buffalo, N.Y.: Prometheus Books, 1985.

Morache, Georges. *Pekin et ses habitants: etude d'hygiene* (Peking and its inhabitants: A study of hygiene). Paris: J. B. Balliere et fils, 1869.

Mori Etsuko. "Tenshinto tôgamon no tsuite" (On the Tianjin Provincial Government). *Tôyôshi kenkyû* 67, no. 2 (1988).

Mori Ôgai. *Eiseigaku tai-i.* In *Ôgai zenshû.* Vol. 30. Tokyo: Iwanami Shoten, 1971–75.

———. *Ôgai zenshû.* 38 vols. Tokyo: Iwanami Shoten, 1971–75.

Mori Rintarô. *Eisei shinhen.* In Mori Ôgai, *Ôgai zenshû,* vols. 31 and 32. Tokyo: Iwanami Shoten, 1971–75.

Mote, Frederick W. "Yuan and Ming." In *Food in Chinese Culture,* ed. K. C. Chang. New Haven: Yale University Press, 1977.

Moulin, Ann Marie. " 'Tropical Without the Tropics': The Turning Point of Pastorian Medicine in North Africa." In *Warm Climates and Western Medicine: The Emergence of Tropical Medicine, 1500–1900,* ed. David Arnold. Amsterdam and Atlanta, Ga.: Rodopi, 1996.

Mumford, Lewis. *The City in History: Its Origins, Its Transformations, and Its Prospects.* New York: Harcourt Brace, 1961.

Myers, Ramon H., and Mark R. Peattie, eds. *The Japanese Colonial Empire, 1895–1945.* Princeton: Princeton University Press, 1984.

Naquin, Susan. "Funerals in North China." In *Death Ritual in Late Imperial and Modern China*, ed. James Watson and Evelyn Rawski. Berkeley and Los Angeles: University of California Press, 1988.

―――. *Millenarian Rebellion in China: The Eight Trigrams Uprising of 1813.* New Haven: Yale University Press, 1976.

―――. *Peking: Temples and City Life, 1400–1900.* Berkeley: University of California Press, 2001.

Nandy, Ashis. *The Intimate Enemy: Loss and Recovery of Self under Colonialism.* (New Delhi: Oxford University Press, 1984.

―――. "Modern Medicine and Its Non-modern Critics." In *The Savage Freud and Other Essays on Possible and Retrievable Selves.* Princeton, N.J.: Princeton University Press, 1995.

Nathan, Carl. *Plague Prevention and Politics in Manchuria, 1910–1931.* Cambridge, Mass.: Harvard University, East Asian Research Center, 1967.

Needham, Joseph. *China and the Origins of Immunology.* Hong Kong: Centre of Asian Studies, University of Hong Kong, 1980.

―――, et al. *Science and Civilisation in China.* 7 vols. Cambridge: Cambridge University Press, 1954–.

―――. *Science and Civilisation in China.* Vol. 2, *History of Scientific Thought.* Cambridge: Cambridge University Press, 1991.

―――. *Science and Civilization in China.* Vol. 5, *Chemistry and Chemical Technology,* part 2, *Spagyrical Invention and Discovery: Magisteries of Gold and Immortality.* Cambridge: Cambridge University Press, 1974.

―――. *Science and Civilisation in China.* Vol. 6, *Biology and Biological Technology,* part 6, *Medicine.* Edited and with an introduction by Nathan Sivin. Cambridge: Cambridge University Press, 2000.

Needham, Joseph, and Lu Gwei-djen. "Hygiene and Preventive Medicine in Ancient China." In *Clerks and Craftsmen in China and the West,* ed. Joseph Needham et al., pp. 340–78. Cambridge: Cambridge University Press, 1970.

―――. *Science and Civilisation in China.* Vol. 5, *Chemistry and Chemical Technology,* part 5, *Spagyrical Discovery and Invention: Physiological Alchemy,* 1983.

North China Herald and Supreme Court and Consular Gazette (Shanghai), 1858–95.

Ogata Koreyoshi. *Eisei shinron* (A new treatise on hygiene). Osaka: Inada, [1872].

Ono Yoshirô. *Seiketsu no kindai* (A clean modern). Tokyo: Kôdansha, 1997.

Osborne, Michael. "Resurrecting Hippocrates: Hygienic Sciences and the French Scientific Expeditions to Egypt, Morea, and Algeria." In *Warm Climates and Western Medicine: The Emergence of Tropical Medicine, 1500–1900,* ed. David Arnold. Amsterdam and Atlanta, Ga.: Rodopi, 1996.

Osterhammel, Jürgen. "Semicolonialism and Informal Empire in Twentieth-Century China: Towards a Framework of Analysis." In *Imperialism and After: Continuities and Discontinuities,* ed. Wolfgang Mommsen and Jürgen Osterhammel. London: Allen and Unwin, 1986.

Ôta Azan. *Fukushima shôgun iseki: denki Fukushima Yasumasa* (Traces of General Fukushima: A biography of Fukushima Yasumasa). Tokyo: Ôzorasha, 1997.

Pan Guangdan, *Minzu texing yu minzu weisheng* (Racial characteristics and racial hygiene). Shanghai: Shangwu yinshuguan, 1937.

Pan Wei. *Yishenji: Neigong tushuo* (Illustrated techniques of inner practice). Beijing: Renmin weisheng chubanshe, 1982.

Peattie, Mark. "Japanese Treaty-Port Settlements in China, 1895–1937." In *The Japanese Informal Empire in China, 1895–1937*. Princeton, N.J.: Princeton University Press, 1989.

Peking and Tientsin Times (Tianjin), 1894–1902.

Pelling, Margaret. *Cholera, Fever, and English Medicine, 1825–1865*. Oxford and New York: Oxford University Press, 1978.

Perrins, Robert. "Combating Illness and Constructing Public Health: Disease and Hospitals in Japanese-Controlled Southern Manchuria." Paper presented at the annual meeting of the Association for Asian Studies Annual, Washington, D.C., Apr. 2002.

Pickowicz, Paul G. "The Theme of Spiritual Pollution in Chinese Films of the 1930s." *Modern China* 17, no. 1 (1991): 38–75.

Pickstone, John. "Dearth, Dirt, and Fever Epidemics: Rewriting the History of British 'Public Health,' 1780–1850." In *Epidemics and Ideas: Essays on the Historical Perception of Pestilence*, ed. Terence Ranger and Paul Slack. New York: Cambridge University Press, 2000.

Pomeranz, Kenneth. *The Great Divergence: Europe, China, and the Making of the Modern World Economy*. Princeton, N.J.: Princeton University Press, 2000.

Porkert, Manfred. *The Theoretical Foundations of Chinese Medicine: Systems of Correspondence*. Cambridge, Mass.: MIT Press, 1974.

Porter, Dorothy. *Health, Civilization, and the State: A History of Public Health from Ancient to Modern Times*. London: Routledge, 1999.

———. "Public Health." In *Companion Encyclopedia of the History of Medicine*, ed. W. F. Bynum and Roy Porter. London: Routledge, 1993.

Porter, Roy, ed., *Patients and Practitioners: Lay Perceptions of Medicine in Pre-industrial Society*. Cambridge: Cambridge University Press, 1985.

Porter, Roy, and Dorothy Porter. *In Sickness and in Health: The British Experience, 1650–1850*. London: Fourth Estate, 1988.

Prakash, Gyan. *Another Reason: Science and the Imagination of Modern India*. Princeton, N.J.: Princeton University Press, 1999.

Proctor, Robert. *Racial Hygiene: Medicine Under the Nazis*. Cambridge, Mass.: Harvard University Press, 1988.

Qi Shihe, ed. *Di'erci yapian zhanzheng* (The second opium war, *DECYPZZ*). Vol. 2. Shanghai: Renmin chubanshe, 1978.

Qu Hongjun. "Wo dui kaizhan weisheng fangyi gongzuo de zhuyao jingyan he shiwu" (My estimation of the experiences and mistakes in the beginning of epidemic prevention work in Tianjin). *Tianjin weisheng shiliao* (Historical materials on Tianjin public health) 10 (1992): 1–5.

Rankin, Mary Backus. *Elite Activism and Political Transformation in China: Zhejiang Province, 1865–1911*. Stanford: Stanford University Press, 1986.

Rasmussen, O. D. *Tientsin: An Illustrated Outline History*. Tianjin: Tientsin Press, 1925.

Rawski, Evelyn. "A Historian's Approach to Death Ritual." In *Death Ritual in Late Imperial and Modern China*, ed. James Watson and Evelyn Rawski. Berkeley and Los Angeles: University of California Press, 1988.

Reardon-Anderson, James. *The Study of Change: Chemistry in China, 1840–1949*. Cambridge and New York: Cambridge University Press, 1991.

Reid, Donald. *Paris Sewers and Sewermen: Realities and Representations*. Cambridge: Harvard University Press, 1991.

Renmin ribao (People's daily; Beijing), 1952.

Reynolds, Douglas. *China: 1898–1912*. Cambridge, Mass.: Harvard University Press, 1993.

Ricalton, James. *China Through the Stereoscope: A Journey Through the Dragon Empire at the Time of the Boxer Uprising*. Ed. Jim Zwick. New York: Underwood and Underwood, 1901. Revised and enlarged edition, BoondocksNet, http://www.boondocksnet.com/china, 2000.

Robinet, Isabelle. *Taoist Meditation: The Mao-shan Tradition of Great Purity*. Trans. Julian Pas and Norman Giradot. Albany, N.Y.: SUNY Press, 1993.

Rogaski, Ruth. "Beyond Benevolence: A Confucian Women's Shelter in Treaty-Port China." *Journal of Women's History* 8, no. 4 (1997): 54–90.

———. "From Protecting Life to Defending the Nation: The Emergence of Public Health in Tianjin, 1859–1953." Ph.D. diss., Yale University, 1996.

———. "Germs and the Reach of the Modern State, Tianjin 1949–1952." In *Proceedings of the International Symposium on China and the World in the Twentieth Century*. Taipei: The Institute of Modern History, Academia Sinica, 2001.

———. "Hygienic Modernity in Tianjin." In *Remaking the Chinese City: Modernity and National Identity*, ed. Joseph Esherick. Honolulu: University of Hawaii Press, 2000.

———. "Nature, Annihilation, and Modernity: China's Korean War Germ Warfare Experience Revisited." *Journal of Asian Studies* 61, no. 2 (2002): 381–415.

Rosen, George. *From Medical Police to Social Medicine: Essays on the History of Health Care*. New York: Science Publications, 1974.

———. *A History of Public Health*. 1958. Reprint, Baltimore: Johns Hopkins University Press, 1993.

Rosenberg, Charles E. *The Care of Strangers: The Rise of America's Hospital System*. New York: Basic Books, 1987.

———. *The Cholera Years: The United States in 1832, 1849, and 1866*. Chicago: University of Chicago Press, 1962.

———. "Explaining Epidemics." In *Explaining Epidemics and Other Studies in the History of Medicine*. Cambridge: Cambridge University Press, 1992.

Rowe, William. *Hankow: Commerce and Society in a Chinese City, 1796–1889*. Stanford: Stanford University Press, 1984.

―――. *Hankow: Conflict and Community in a Chinese City, 1796–1895*. Stanford: Stanford University Press, 1986.

Royal Army Medical Corps. *Medical and Surgical History of the British Army which Served in Turkey and the Crimea During the War Against Russia in the Years 1854–55–56*. London: Harrison, 1858.

Ryan, Mark. *Chinese Attitudes Toward Nuclear Weapons: China and the United States During the Korean War*. Armonk, N.Y.: M. E. Sharpe, 1989.

Saneyoshi, Yasuzumi. *The Surgical and Medical History of the Naval War Between Japan and China during 1894–1895*. Tokyo: Tokio Printing Co., 1900.

Schied, Volker. *Chinese Medicine in Contemporary China: Plurality and Synthesis*. Durham, N.C.: Duke University Press 2002.

Schoppa, R. Keith. "Patterns and Dynamics of Elite Collaboration in Occupied Shaoxing County." In *Chinese Collaboration: The Limits of Accommodation*, ed. David Barrett and Larry Shyu. Stanford: Stanford University Press, 2001.

Schwartz, Benjamin. *In Search of Wealth and Power: Yen Fu and the West*. Cambridge, Mass.: Harvard University Press, 1964.

Sennet, Richard. *Flesh and Stone: The Body and the City in Western Civilization*. New York: W. W. Norton, 1994.

Shang Keqiang and Liu Haiyan, eds. *Tianjin zujie shehui yanjiu* (Research in the society of Tianjin's concessions). Tianjin: Tianjin renmin chubanshe, 1994.

Shapiro, Hugh. "The Puzzle of Spermatorrhea in Republican China." *positions* 6, no. 3 (1998): 550–96.

Shapiro, Judith. *Mao's War Against Nature: Politics and the Environment in Revolutionary China*. Cambridge and New York: Cambridge University Press, 2001.

Shen bao (Shanghai), 1872–88.

Shen Jiaben and Zongliang et al., ed. *(Chongxiu) Tianjin fuzhi* (Revised gazetteer of Tianjin prefecture). 1899.

Shi Mingzheng. "Beijing Transforms: Urban Infrastructure, Public Works, and Social Change in the Chinese Capital, 1900–1928." Ph.D. diss., Columbia University, 1993.

Shih, Shu-mei. "Gender, Race, and Semicolonialism: Liu Na'ou's Urban Shanghai Landscape." *Journal of Asian Studies* 55, no. 4 (1996): 934–56.

―――. *The Lure of the Modern: Writing Modernism in Semicolonial China, 1917–1937*. Berkeley: University of California Press, 2001.

Sigerist, Henry. *Landmarks in the History of Hygiene*. Oxford: Oxford University Press, 1956.

Sinn, Elizabeth. *Power and Charity: The Early History of the Tung Wah Hospital*. Hong Kong: Oxford University Press, 1989.

Sivin, Nathan. *Chinese Alchemy: Preliminary Studies*. Cambridge, Mass.: Harvard University Press, 1968.

―――. "Science and Medicine in Imperial China—The State of the Field." *Journal of Asian Studies* 47, no. 1 (1988): 41–90.

―――. "State, Cosmos, and the Body in the Last Three Centuries B.C." *Harvard Journal of Asiatic Studies* 55, no. 1 (1995): 5–38.

———. *Traditional Medicine in Contemporary China*. Ann Arbor: Center for Chinese Studies, University of Michigan, 1987.

Slack, Edward. *Opium, State, and Society: China's Narco-Economy and the Guomindang, 1924–1937*. Honolulu: University of Hawaii Press, 2001.

Smith, Arthur. *Chinese Characteristics*. New York: Revell, 1894.

———. *Proverbs and Common Sayings from the Chinese*. Shanghai: American Presbyterian Mission Press, 1902.

Smith, Francis Barrymore. *The People's Health, 1830–1910*. New York: Holmes and Meier, 1979.

Smith, Virginia. "Prescribing the Rules of Health: Self-Help and Advice in the Late Eighteenth Century." In *Patients and Practitioners: Lay Perceptions of Medicine in Pre-industrial Society*, ed. Roy Porter. Cambridge: Cambridge University Press, 1985.

Song Lianbi. *Yifang xiaopin* (Humble prescriptions). Tianjin: n.p., early nineteenth century.

Song Yunpu, ed. *Tianjin zhilue* (A brief gazetteer of Tianjin). 1931. Reprint, Taibei: Chengwen chubanshe, 1969.

Spence, Jonathan. "Aspects of Western Medical Experience in China, 1850–1910." In *Medicine and Society in China*, ed. John Z. Bowers and Elizabeth F. Purcell. New York: Josiah Macy Jr. Foundation, 1974.

———. "Commentary on Historical Perspectives and Ch'ing Medical Systems." In *Medicine in Chinese Cultures*, ed. Arthur Kleinman et al., Washington, D.C.: U.S. Department of Health, Education, and Welfare, National Institute of Health, 1975.

Stage, Sarah. *Female Complaints: Lydia Pinkham and the Business of Women's Medicine*. New York: W. W. Norton, 1979.

Stapleton, Kristen. *Civilizing Chengdu: Chinese Urban Reform, 1895–1937*. Cambridge: Harvard University Press, 2000.

Stepan, Nancy Leys. *The Hour of Eugenics: Race, Gender, and Nation in Latin America*. Ithaca: Cornell University Press, 1991.

Stoler, Ann Laura. *Race and the Education of Desire: Foucault's History of Sexuality and the Colonial Order of Things*. Durham, N.C.: Duke University Press, 1995.

Stoler, Ann Laura, and Frederick Cooper, eds. *Tensions of Empire: Colonial Cultures in a Bourgeois World*. Berkeley: University of California Press, 1997.

Strand, David. *Rickshaw Beijing: City People and Politics in the 1920s*. Berkeley and Los Angeles: University of California Press, 1989.

Sugimoto Tsutomu, ed. *Edo no hon'yakukatachi* (Edo translators). Tokyo: Waseda Daigaku Shuppanbu, 1995.

———. *Edo Ranpôi kara no messēji* (The message from Edo's physicians of "Dutch Medicine"). Tokyo: Perikansha, 1992.

———. *Zuroku Rangaku jishi* (Illustrated history of Dutch Learning). Tokyo: Waseda Daigaku Shuppanbu, 1985.

Sun Dagan. *Tianjin jingshihua* (Tales of the economic history of Tianjin). Tianjin: Shehuikexueyuan chubanshe, 1989.

Sun Limin and Gongxian Xin. "Tianjin Ri zujie gaikuang" (The Japanese concession in Tianjin). *Tianjin wenshi ziliao xuanji* (Selected cultural and historical materials of Tianjin) 18 (1982): 11–151.

Sun Simiao. *Qian jin fang* (Prescriptions worth a thousand). Circa 652 C.E. Reprint, Beijing: Huaxia chubanshe, 1993.

———. *Qian jin shi zhi* (Dietary cures from presciptios worth a thousand). Circa 652 C.E. Reprint, Beijing: Zhongguo shangye chubanshe, 1985.

Sun Xuelian. *Tianjin zhinan* (A guide to Tianjin). Tianjin: Zhonghua shuju, 1923.

Sun Yat-sen. *Guofu quanji* (Complete writings of the Father of the Nation). Vol. 1, *San-min chu-yi* (Three principles of the people). Lecture 2: 19. Taibei: Chung-yang wen-wu kung-ying she, 1961.

Tanaka, Stefan. *Japan's Orient: Rendering Pasts into History*. Berkeley: University of California Press, 1993.

Tatsukawa Shôji. *Meiji iji ôrai*. (Medical doings in the Meiji period). Tokyo: Shinchôsha, 1986.

Tenshin kyoryû mindan. *Gyôsei gaiyô* (Administration outline). Tianjin, 1942.

———. *Tenshin kyoryû mindan nijisshûnen kinenshi*. (Tianjin Japanese Residents' Association Twentieth Anniversary Report). Tianjin: n.p., 1908–43.

———. *Tenshin kyoryû mindan jimu hôkoku* (Tianjin Japanese Residents' Association Twentieth Anniversary Report). Tianjin, 1930.

———. *Tenshin kyoryû mindan zeikisoku* (Tianjin Japanese Residents' Association tax regulations). Tianjin: n.p., 1942.

Tenshin nihon sokai keibôdan. *Keibôdan jistumu yôryô* (Civilian police business affairs summary). Tianjin, 1941.

Tezuka Akira. *Bakumatsu, Meiji kaigai tokôsha sôran* (Overview of travelers abroad in the Bakumatsu and Meiji periods). Tokyo: Kashiwa Shobô, 1992.

Tientsin British Municipal Area Bye-Laws. Tianjin: Tientsin Press, 1919.

Tientsin British Municipal Council Building Sanitary By-Laws. Tianjin: Tientsin Press, 1925.

Tientsin British Municipal Council Reports. Tianjin: Tientsin Press, 1929–39.

Tianjin difangzhi ziliao lianhe mulu bianji zu. *Tianjin difangshi ziliao lianhe mulu* (Catalogue of Tianjin local history materials). Vols. 1–3. Tianjin: Tianjin tushuguan, 1980–82.

———. *Tianjin shi baokan lunwen ziliao suoyin (1949–1980)* (Index of articles in Tianjin newspapers and journals). Tianjin: Tianjin tushuguan, 1982.

———. *Tianjin shi qikan lunwen ziliao suoyin (1860–1949)* (Index of articles in Tianjin periodicals). Tianjin: Tianjin tushuguan, 1985.

Tianjin hongshizihui pingmin yiyuan bao gao (Tianjin Red Cross commoners' hospital reports). Tianjin: n.p., 1926–30.

Tianjin jiaotongju, ed. *Tianjin gonglu yunshu shi* (A history of roads and transportation in Tianjin). Beijing: Renmin jiaotong chubanshe, 1988.

Tianjin jindai jianzhu bianxie zu. *Tianjin jindai jianzhu* (The modern architecture of Tianjin). Tianjin: Tianjin kexue jishu chubanshe, 1990.

Tianjin lishi bowuguan et al., eds. *Jindai Tianjin tuzhi* (Illustrated history of modern Tianjin). Tianjin: Tianjin guji chubanshe, 1992.

Tianjin nanduan xuncha zongju zhangcheng (Regulations of the southern section police headquarters). Tianjin, 1907. Tianjin Academy of Social Sciences, History Research Library copy.

Tianjin shehui kexueyuan lishi yanjiusuo, ed. *Tianjin shanghui dang'an huibian* (Collected archival documents from the Tianjin Chamber of Commerce). Tianjin: Tianjin renmin chubanshe, 1989–93.

———. Tianjin shehui kexueyuan lishiyanjiu suo, ed. *Tianjin jianshi*. Tianjin: Renmin chubanshe, 1987.

Tianjin shi dang'an guan, ed. *Tianjin zujie dang'an xuanbian* (Collected archival documents from Tianjin concessions). Tianjin: Tianjin renmin chubanshe, 1992.

Tianjin shi zhengfu gongbao (Bulletin of the Tianjin city government). Tianjin: Tianjin tebie shi, 1929–37.

Tianjin shili jiujiyuan sheshi jiyao (Overview of the establishment of the Tianjin Municipal Relief Institute). Tianjin: Tianjinshi shehuiju, 1935.

Tianjin shiyi ji shi wenjian lu (Traces of Tianjin's past). 1879 (?). Reprint, Tianjin: Tianjin guji chubanshe, 1986.

Tianjin shizhi bianxiu weiyuan, ed. *Tianjin jianzhi* (A short history of Tianjin). Tianjin: Tianjin renmin chubanshe, 1991.

Tianjin shizhi bianzuan chu, ed. *Tianjinshi gaiyao* (Essentials of Tianjin). Tianjin: Baicheng shuju, 1934.

Tianjin tebie shi weisheng gongshu weishengju, ed. *Tianjin tebie shi weisheng xingzheng yaolan* (Tianjin municipal public health administration highlights). Tianjin, 1940.

Tianjin tebie shi weisheng ju, ed. *Tianjin tebie shi weisheng yuekan* (Monthly journal of the Tianjin Municipal Health Bureau). Tianjin, 1929–31.

Tianjin tebieshi zhian weichi weiyuan hui, ed. *Fang yi bao gao* (Epidemic prevention report). Tianjin, 1938.

"Tianjin weisheng fangyi shiye de fazhan" (The development of epidemic prevention in Tianjin). In *Tianjin weisheng shiye sishinian* (Forty years of public health in Tianjin), ed. Tianjin weisheng shizhi bianxiu weiyuanui. Tianjin: Tianjin dikuangju ditiaodui yinshuachang, 1989.

Tianjin wenshi ziliao (Tianjin cultural and historical materials). Tianjin: Tianjin renmin chubanshe, 1986–93.

"Tianjin yiwu shiji" (A record of barbarian affairs in Tianjin). In *Di'erci yapian zhanzheng* (The second opium war, *DECYPZZ*) ed. Qi shihe. Vol. 2. Shanghai: Renmin chubanshe, 1978.

Tianjinshi zhengxie mishuchu, ed. *Tianjin badajia ji qi houyi* (Tianjin's eight great families and their descendants). Tianjin: Tianjinshi zhengxie, 1974.

Tianjin zizhiju wenjian luyao (Essential records of the Tianjin self-government bureau). Vols. 1–2. Tianjin, 1909.

Tianjin zongjiao zhi bianxiu weiyuanhui, ed., *Tianjin zongjiao ziliao xuan* (Historical materials on religion in Tianjin). Tianjin: Tianjin renmin chubanshe, 1986.

Tianjinshi jiaohui yiyuan qingkuang bao gao (Report on the missionary hospitals of Tianjin). Tianjin, 1950.

Tianjinshi dang'an guan, ed. *Tianjin shanghui dang'an huibian, 1903–1911* (Tianjin Chamber of Commerce archives). 2 vols. Tianjin: Tianjin renmin chubanshe, 1989.

Tianjinshi weisheng shizhi bianxiu weiyuan hui, ed. *Tianjin weisheng shiliao* (Historical materials on Tianjin public health). 10 vols. 1985–92.

Tianjinshi zhengfu. *Buzeng Tianjinshi tuixing zizhi gaikuang* (Supplementary report on carrying out self-government in Tianjin municipality). Tianjin, 1933.

———. *Tianjinshi zizhi diaocha* (Survey of self-government in Tianjin). Tianjin, 1934.

Tianjinshi zhengxie hui—wenshi ziliao yanjiu weiyuanhui, ed. *Lunxian shiqi de Tianjini* (Tianjin during the occupation period). Tianjin: Tianjin Jinghaixian yinshuachang, 1992.

———. *Tianjin jindai renwu lu* (Biographical dictionary of modern Tianjin). Tianjin: Tianjinshi difang shizhi bianxiu weiyuan hui zong bianji shi, 1987.

———. *Tianjin zujie* (The foreign settlements of Tianjin). Tianjin: Tianjin renmin chubanshe, 1986.

Tiegel, Ernst. *Eisei hanron* (Complete treatise on hygiene). Trans. Ôi Gendô. Tokyo: Hasunuma, [1880–81].

———. *Ifukuryô shikensetsu* (Report on comparative hygienic value of native and foreign clothing, including footwear). Trans. Katayama Kuniyoshi. Tokyo: Naimushô, Eiseikyoku, [1881].

Tomes, Nancy. *The Gospel of Germs: Men, Women, and the Microbe in American Life.* Cambridge, Mass.: Harvard University Press, 1998.

Tsao Yu. *Bright Skies.* Beijing: Foreign Language Press, 1960.

Tsin, Michael. *Nation, Governance, and Modernity in China: Canton, 1900–1927.* Stanford: Stanford University Press, 1999.

Tsuzuki, J. "Bericht uber meine epidemioligischen Beobachtungen und Forschundgen wahrend der Choleraepedemie im Nordchina im Jahre 1902" (Report on my epidemiological observations and researches during the cholera epidemic of 1902 in north China). In *Archiv für Schiffs und Tropen-Hygiene* (Archives for naval and tropical hygiene). Leipzig, 1904.

Tyrrell, Ian. *Woman's World/Woman's Empire: The Woman's Christian Temperance Union in International Perspective, 1800–1930.* Chapel Hill: University of North Carolina Press, 1991.

Unschuld, Paul. "Epistemological Issues and Changing Legitimation: Traditional Chinese Medicine in the Twentieth Century." In Charles Leslie and Allan Young, *Paths to Asian Medical Knowledge.* Berkeley: University of California Press, 1992.

———. *Medicine in China: Historical Artifacts and Images.* Munich and New York: Prestel, 2000.

———. *Medicine in China: A History of Ideas.* Berkeley and Los Angeles: University of California Press, 1985.

———. *Medicine in China: A History of Pharmaceutics.* Berkeley and Los Angeles: University of California Press, 1986.

Vaughan, Megan. *Curing Their Ills: Colonial Power and African Illness.* Cambridge: Cambridge University Press, 1991.

Vigarello, Georges. *Concepts of Cleanliness: Changing Attitudes in France Since the Middle Ages.* Trans. Jean Birrell. Cambridge: Cambridge University Press, 1988.

Virchow, Rudolf. *Collected Essays on Public Health and Epidemiology.* 2 vols. Ed. L. J. Rather. Canton, Mass.: Science History Publications, 1985.

Vogel, Morris J., and Charles E. Rosenberg, eds. *The Therapeutic Revolution: Essays in the Social History of American Medicine.* Philadelphia: University of Pennsylvania Press, 1979.

Vulliamy, C. E. *Crimea, The Campaign of 1854–56.* London: Jonathan Cape, 1939.

Wakeman, Frederic. "The Civil Society and Public Sphere Debate: Western Reflections on Chinese Political Culture." *Modern China* 19 (1993): 108–38.

———. *Policing Shanghai, 1927–1937.* Berkeley and Los Angeles: University of California Press, 1995.

———. *The Shanghai Badlands: Wartime Terrorism and Urban Crime, 1937–1941.* New York: Cambridge University Press, 1996.

Wang Guangren. *Zhongguo jindai kexue xianqu Xu Shou fu-zi yanjiu* (Pioneers of modern Chinese science: Xu Shou and son). Beijing: Qinghua daxue chubanshe, 1998.

Wang Huachang, ed. *Tianjin—yige chengshi de jueqi* (Tianjin—The rise of a city). Tianjin: Renmin chubanshe, 1990.

Wang Shixiong. *Huoluan lun* (Treatise on cholera). In *Qian zhai yi shu shi zhong* (Ten medical books from the subtle studio). 1838. Reprint, Taibei: Changjiang chubanshe, 1970.

Wang Shouxun. *Tianjin xian xin zhi* (A new gazetteer of Tianjin). Tianjin: n.p., 1938.

———. *Tianjin zhengsu yan'ge ji* (Records of the evolution of Tianjin's government and customs in Tianjin). Tianjin: n.p., 1938.

Wang, Shuo. *Please Don't Call Me Human (Qianwang bie ba wo dang ren).* Trans. Howard Goldblatt. New York: Hyperion, 2000.

Wang Xuehai. "Jiefang zhanzheng shiqi Guomindang de Tianjin chengfang" (Guomindang defenses of Tianjin during the war of liberation). *Tianjin lishi ziliao* 13 (1981): 1–16.

Wang Yangzong. "Gezhi huibian zhi Zhongguo bianjizhe zhi kao" (Investigations into the Chinese editor of the Gezhi huiban). *Wen xian* 63 (Jan. 1995): 237–43.

Warner, John Harley. *The Therapeutic Perspective: Medical Practice, Knowledge, and Identity in America, 1820–1885.* Cambridge, Mass.: Harvard University Press, 1986.

Watson, Burton. *The Complete Works of Chuang Tzu.* New York: Columbia University Press, 1968.

Watson, James. "Funeral Specialists in Cantonese Society: Pollution, Performance, and Social Hierarchy." In *Death Ritual in Late Imperial and Modern China*, ed. James Watson and Evelyn Rawski. Berkeley and Los Angeles: University of California Press, 1988.

Wear, Andrew. *Health and Healing in Early Modern England: Studies in Social and Intellectual History*. Brookfield, Vt.: Ashgate, 1998.

———. "The History of Personal Hygiene." In *Companion Encyclopedia of the History of Medicine*, vol. 2, ed. Roy Porter and W. F. Bynum. London: Routledge, 1993.

Weathersby, Katherine. "Deceiving the Deceivers: Moscow, Beijing, Pyongyang, and the Allegations of Bacteriological Weapons Use in Korea." *Cold War International History Project Bulletin*, 11 (winter 1998): 176–84.

Wei Dongbo. Tianjin difang zhi kaolue (A brief reference gazetteer of Tianjin). Changchun: Jilin sheng defang zhi bianzuan weiyuanhui, 1985.

Weisheng zazhi (Hygiene magazine; Tianjin), 1929–30.

Wells, David Ames. *Wells' Principles and Applications of Chemistry*. New York and Chicago: Ivison, Blakeman, Taylor, and Co., 1858.

White, Luise. *Speaking with Vampires: Rumor and History in Colonial Africa*. Berkeley: University of California Press, 2000.

Wile, Douglas. *Art of the Bedchamber: The Chinese Sexual Yoga Classics, Including Women's Solo Meditation Texts*. New York: SUNY Press, 1992.

Will, Pierre-Etienne. *Famine and Bureaucracy in Eighteenth-Century China*. Stanford: Stanford University Press, 1990.

Williams, Peter, and David Wallace. *Unit 731: The Japanese Army's Secret of Secrets*. London: Hodder and Stoughton, 1989.

Williams, Samuel Wells. *The Journal of S. Wells Williams, Secretary and Interpreter of the American Embassy to China during the Expedition to Tientsin and Peking in the Years 1858 and 1859*, edited by his son, Frederick Wells Williams. Shanghai: Kelly and Walsh, 1911.

Wohl, Anthony S. *Endangered Lives: Public Health in Victorian Britain*. London: J. M. Dent and Sons, 1983.

Wolseley, G. J. *Narrative of the War with China in 1860*. London: Longman, Green, Longman and Roberts, 1862.

Wright, David. "John Fryer and the Shanghai Polytechnic: Making Space for Science in Nineteenth-Century China." *British Journal of the History of Science*, 29 (1996): 1–16.

———. *Translating Science: The Transmission of Western Chemistry into Late Imperial China, 1840–1900*. Leiden and Boston: Brill, 2000.

Wu, Lien-teh, and K. C. Wong. *History of Chinese Medicine*. 1936. Reprint, Taibei: Southern Materials Center, 1985.

Wu Xianjian. *Tianjin kuailan* (Brief introduction to Tianjin). Shanghai: Shijie shuju, 1936.

Wu Yi-Li. "Transmitted Secrets: The Doctors of the Lower Yangzi Region and Popular Gynecology in Late Imperial China." Ph.D. diss., Yale University, 1998.

Xin Zhongguo yufang yixue lishi jingyan bian weiyuanhui, ed. *Xin Zhongguo yufang yixue lishi jingyan* (The historical experiences of preventive medicine in New China). Beijing: Renmin weisheng chubanshe, 1991.

Xiong Yuezhi. *Xi xue dong jian yu wan Qing she hui* (The dissemination of Western learning and late Qing society). Shanghai: Shanghai ren min chubanshe, 1994.

Xu Dachun. *The Forgotten Traditions of Ancient Chinese Medicine* (Yixue yuanliu lun). Trans. Paul Unschuld. N.p.: Paradigm Publications, 1990.

Xu Shiluan. *Jingxiang bishu* (Notes respectfully describing my home). 1932. Reprint, Tianjin fengtu congshu. Tianjin: Tianjin guji chubanshe, 1986.

———. *Yifang conghua* (Collected anecdotes on remedies). Tianjin: Tianjin xushi dieyuan, 1889.

Yamamoto Shun'ichi. *Nihon korera shi* (The history of cholera in Japan). Tokyo: Tokyo Daigaku Shuppankai, 1982.

Yan Renzeng. *Yan Xiu xiansheng nianpu* (Chronological biography of Mr. Yan Xiu). Jinan: Jilu shushe, 1990.

Yang Zhiyan. "Tianjinshi yiyuan shiliao jiyao" (Essential outline of historical materials on Tianjin's hospitals). *Tianjin wenshi congkan* 4 (1985): 175–91.

Yangcheng jiuke. *Jinmen jilue* (A brief record of Tianjin). 1898. Reprint, Tianjin: Tianjin guji chubanshe, 1986.

Yao Xiyun. "Tianjin Gulaodong Yaojia yishi." *Tianjin wenshi ziliao* (Tianjin historical materials, *TJWSZL*) 47 (1989): 204–42.

Yip, Ka-che. *Health and National Reconstruction in Nationalist China: The Development of Modern Health Services, 1928–1937.* Ann Arbor, Mich.: Association of Asian Studies, 1995.

Yishi bao (Social welfare; Tianjin), 1916–35.

Yoshizawa Seiichirô. *Tenshin no kindai* (Tianjin in the modern era). Nagoya: Nagoya University Press, 2002.

Young, Louise. *Japan's Total Empire: Manchuria and the Culture of Wartime Imperialism.* Berkeley: University of California Press, 1998.

Yuan Shikai zouzhe zhuanji (The palace memorials of Yuan Shikai). 8 vols. Taibei: National Palace Museum, 1970.

Zhang Chunze. "Chengshi yuanlin gaimao" (The general situation of the city's parks). In *Tianjin—yige chengshi de jueqi* (Tianjin—The rise of a city). Tianjin: Tianjin renmin chubanshe, 1990.

Zhang Qiong. "Demystifying Qi: The Politics of Cultural Translation and Interpretation in the Early Jesuit Mission to China." In *Tokens of Exchange: The Problem of Translation in Global Circulations,* ed. Lydia H. Liu. Durham, N.C.: Duke University Press, 1999.

Zhang Rongqing. "Fangyi gongzuo yu mianyi zhidu" (Epidemic prevention work and vaccination system). *Tianjin weisheng shiliao* (Historical materials on Tianjin's public health) 2 and 3 (1987): 47.

Zhang Shu Guang. *Mao's Military Romanticism: China and the Korean War, 1950–1953.* Lawrence: University of Kansas Press, 1995.

Zhang Tao. *Jinmen zaji* (Miscellaneous records of Tianjin). 1884. Reprint, Tianjin: Tianjin guji chubanshe, 1986.

Zhao Hongjun. *Jindai Zhongxiyi lunzhengshi* (History of the debates between Chinese and Western medicine). Anhui: Anhui Science and Technology Press, 1989.

Zheng Guanying. *Zheng Guanying ji* (The works of Zheng Guanying). Ed. Xia Dongyuan. Shanghai: Shanghai renmin chubanshe, 1982.

———. *Zhong wai weisheng yaozhi* (Chinese and foreign essentials of hygiene). 1890, 1895.

Zhibao (The Zhili gazzette [Tianjin]), 1894–1902.

Zhong gong Tianjinshi wei et al., eds. *Tianjin jieguan shilu* (Historical record of the taking over of Tianjin by the CCP). Beijing: Zhong gong dang shi chubanshe, 1991.

Zhongguo renmin zhengzhi xieshang huiyi Tianjin shi weiyuanhui. *Lun xian shi de Tianjin* (Tianjin during the Japanese occupation). Tianjin: n.p., 1992.

Zhongguo renmin zhengzhi xieshang huiyi Tianjin shi weiyuanhui, wen shi ziliao yanjiu weiyuan hui, ed.. *Jindai Tianjin renwu lu* (Biographical dictionary of modern Tianjin). Tianjin: Tianjinshi difang shizhi bianxiu weiyuan hui zong bianji shi, 1987.

Zhongyang dang'anguan, Zhongguo dier lishi dang'anguan, Jilinshen shehui kexueyuan, *Xijunzhan yu duqi zhan*. Beijing: Zhonghua shuju, 1989.

Zhouli jishuo. (Collected discussions on the rites of Zhou). *Electronic Si ku quan shu* (Complete collection of the Four Treasuries), *Wenyuange edition*. Hong Kong: Digital Heritage Publishing, 1999.

Zhu Chungu. *Douzhen dinglun* (Principles of smallpox). 1713. Reprint, Tianjin: Wang Xilun, 1898.

Zhu Qihua. *Tianjin quan shu* (Complete book of Tianjin). Tianjin: Tianjin renmin chubanshe, 1991.

Zhu Renxun, *Wenjian lu* (Recollections). Hand-copied manuscript, Tianjin: Tianjin Academy of Social Sciences, n.d.

Zhu Xi, *Lunyu jingyi.* (Essential meanings of the Analects of Confucius). *Electronic Si ku quan shu, Wenyuange edition*. Hong Kong: Digital Heritage Publishing, 1999.

Zimmerman, Jonathan. *Distilling Democracy: Alcohol Education in America's Public Schools, 1880–1925*. Lawrence: University of Kansas Press, 1999.

Zito, Angela, and Tani Barlow, eds. *Body, Subject, and Power in China*. Chicago: University of Chicago Press, 1994.

Index

acclimatization, 79–80, 116–17
alcohol, 34, 37, 44, 81, 98, 110, 112, 115–24, 148, 160, 161
Anderson, Warwick, 7, 9, 163, 173
Andrews, Bridie, 8, 253
Arnold, David, 7, 132
Arrow War, 73–74

bacteria, 8, 115, 150, 171, 173, 177–79, 181–82, 187–88, 205, 211, 225, 226, 230–36, 239, 245–49, 252–53, 266, 275, 281–83, 285, 287, 292, 294, 302, 304
bathrooms (*weisheng jian*), 1, 3, 190, 208, 224, 227, 231. *See also* sewers; toilets
Beiyang Army Medical Academy, 181–89, 190, 234, 274
Beiyang Epidemic Prevention Office (Beiyang *fangyi chu*), 188, 233
Beiyang Navy Medical Academy, 10, 161, 172
ben cao (materia medica), 31, 33–35, 94
blood, 7, 73, 80, 89, 90, 91, 92, 98, 114, 148, 152, 173, 226, 228–29, 250, 251, 255, 258, 259, 273. See also *xue*
Boxers, 165–167, 169, 170–171, 184, 185, 191, 263, 301
British Settlement, 83, 106, 132–34, 169, 187, 195–98, 200, 202–5, 211–13, 224, 262, 271, 292. *See also* Great Britain

Bureau of Health (*weisheng bu*), Tianjin: under Communists, 290–99; in Japanese Concession, 263–69; under Japanese occupation, 269–75; under Nationalists, 234–40; New Reforms period, 186–90, 205–7; under TPG, 172–80
burial practices, 70, 83–84, 174, 177, 180, 247. *See also* cemeteries
Buzhu wenyi lun, 59

Campaign to Suppress Counter-revolutionaries, 288
Cao Yu, 292
cemeteries, 56, 69, 70, 174, 177, 184. *See also* burial practices
cesspools, 86, 208, 239, 291, 296
Chadwick, Edwin, 76, 86, 100, 141
Changchun the Perfected One, 4–6
chemistry, 11, 90, 91, 104, 110–24, 148–50, 155, 161, 206, 304
Chinese Characteristics, 243
Chinese medicine, 96–98, 244–50, 253, 276–81, 304
Chinese Science Magazine (Gezhi huibian), 109
cholera, 95–100, 161–63, 179–83, 237, 245–49, 257, 271–73, 275–81, 283
Cold Damage School (Shanghan pai), 58, 59, 66, 73, 97, 246
Communists, 241, 283, 285–99
Confucius, 23, 25–26, 38

Text:	10/13 Aldus
Display:	Aldus
Compositor:	Integrated Composition Systems
Printer:	Thomson-Shore, Inc.